Public Health Ethics Analysis

Volume 3

Edited by

Michael J. Selgelid
Monash University, Melbourne, Australia

During the 21st Century, public health ethics has become one of the fastest growing subdisciplines of bioethics. This is the first book series dedicated to the topic of public health ethics. It aims to fill a gap in the existing literature by providing thoroughgoing, book-length treatment of the most important topics in public health ethics—which have otherwise, for the most part, only been partially and/or sporadically addressed in journal articles, book chapters, or sections of volumes concerned with public health ethics. Books in the series will include coverage of central topics in public health ethics from a plurality of disciplinary perspectives including: philosophy (e.g., both ethics and philosophy of science), political science, history, economics, sociology, anthropology, demographics, law, human rights, epidemiology, and other public health sciences. Blending analytically rigorous and empirically informed analyses, the series will address ethical issues associated with the concepts, goals, and methods of public health; individual (e.g., ordinary citizens' and public health workers') decision making and behaviour; and public policy. Inter alia, volumes in the series will be dedicated to topics including: health promotion; disease prevention; paternalism and coercive measures; infectious disease; chronic disease; obesity; smoking and tobacco control; genetics; the environment; public communication/trust; social determinants of health; human rights; and justice. A primary priority is to produce volumes on hitherto neglected topics such as ethical issues associated with public health research and surveillance; vaccination; tuberculosis; malaria; diarrheal disease; lower respiratory infections; drug resistance; chronic disease in developing countries; emergencies/disasters (including bioterrorism); and public health implications of climate change.

More information about this series at http://www.springer.com/series/10067

Drue H. Barrett • Leonard W. Ortmann
Angus Dawson • Carla Saenz • Andreas Reis
Gail Bolan
Editors

Public Health Ethics: Cases Spanning the Globe

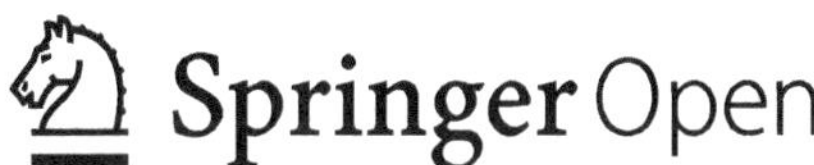

Editors
Drue H. Barrett
Office of Scientific Integrity, Office of the Associate Director for Science, Office of the Director
Centers for Disease Control and Prevention
Atlanta, GA, USA

Leonard W. Ortmann
Office of Scientific Integrity, Office of the Associate Director for Science, Office of the Director
Centers for Disease Control and Prevention
Atlanta, GA, USA

Angus Dawson
Center for Values, Ethics and the Law in Medicine, Sydney School of Public Health
The University of Sydney
Sydney, Australia

Carla Saenz
Regional Program on Bioethics
Office of Knowledge Management, Bioethics, and Research
Pan American Health Organization
Washington, DC, USA

Andreas Reis
Global Health Ethics
Department of Information, Evidence and Research
World Health Organization
Geneva, Switzerland

Gail Bolan
Division of STD Prevention
National Center for HIV/AIDS, Viral Hepatitis, STD and TB Prevention
Centers for Disease Control and Prevention
Atlanta, GA, USA

ISSN 2211-6680 ISSN 2211-6699 (electronic)
Public Health Ethics Analysis
ISBN 978-3-319-79538-6 ISBN 978-3-319-23847-0 (eBook)
DOI 10.1007/978-3-319-23847-0

Printed on acid-free paper

This Springer imprint is published by Springer Nature
The registered company is Springer International Publishing AG Switzerland

Disclaimer

The contents of this casebook represent the opinions, findings, and conclusions of the authors and do not necessarily reflect the official position, views, or policies of the editors, the editors' host institutions, or the authors' host institutions.

Preface

Public health ethics can be seen both as the application of principles and norms to guide the practice of public health and as a process for identifying, analyzing, and resolving ethical issues inherent in the practice of public health. Public health ethics helps us decide what we should do and why. Although the practice of public health has always considered ethical issues, the emergence of public health ethics as a discipline is relatively new. Although rooted in bioethics and clinical and research ethics, public health ethics has many characteristics that set it apart. The defining characteristics are its focus on achieving social goods for populations while respecting individual rights and recognizing the interdependence of people.

Currently there are few practical training resources for public health practitioners that consider ethical issues and dilemmas likely to arise in the practice of public health. In public health ethics training, we have found it advantageous to use cases to illustrate how ethical principles can be applied in practical ways to decision making. The use of cases encourages reflection and discussion of ethics, reinforces basic ethical concepts through application to concrete examples, highlights practical decision making, allows learners to consider different perspectives, and sensitizes learners to the complex, multidimensional context of issues in public health practice. The case-based approach (known as casuistry) contrasts with the theoretical approach to considering moral principles, rules, and theories. By describing scenarios, cases allow the learner to use ethical principles in the context of a realistic situation that sheds light on ethical challenges and illustrates how ethical principles can help in making practical decisions.

This casebook comprises a broad range of cases from around the globe to highlight the ethical challenges of public health. For those new to public health ethics, Section I introduces public health ethics. Chapter 1, "Public Health Ethics: Global Cases, Practice, and Context" by Ortmann and colleagues, summarizes basic concepts and describes how public health ethics differ from bioethics, clinical ethics, and research ethics. The chapter also includes an approach for conducting an ethical analysis in public health. In Chap. 2, "Essential Cases in the Development of Public Health Ethics," Lee, Spector-Bagdady, and Sakhuja highlight important events that shaped the practice of public health and explain how practitioners address and prevent ethical challenges.

Section II is organized into chapters that discuss the following public health topics:

- Resource allocation and priority setting
- Disease prevention and control
- Chronic disease prevention and health promotion
- Environmental and occupational public health
- Vulnerability and marginalized populations
- International collaboration for global public health
- Public health research

We have invited some of the leading writers and thinkers in public health ethics to provide an overview of the major ethical considerations associated with each topic. The topic overviews offer the authors' perspectives about applicable ethical theories, frameworks, and tools and draw attention to the cases that follow. The cases are meant to highlight the ethical issues in practice. Each represents the work of authors from around the globe who responded to a solicitation from the U.S. Centers for Disease Control and Prevention. We worked with the authors to ensure that each case included a concise articulation of a public health situation that raises ethical tensions, challenges, or concerns that require decisions or recommendations from public health officials or practitioners. The cases are presented in a standard format that includes a background, case description, discussion questions, and references. However, we also allowed for variation in the amount of detail provided in each section and the approach used to set up the case. Our goal was to include just enough contextual information to orient the reader who is not an expert in the case topic. We include the case setting, population, or intervention in question, legal or regulatory landscape, and questions to stimulate discussion on core ethical issues. Each case—although fictionalized—is as realistic as possible to reflect the ethical challenges that public health practitioners face daily. Sometimes the cases were based on actual or composite events. In these instances, the case details were modified to exclude identifying information that could be considered private, sensitive, or disputable by others involved in the case.

We deliberately did not attempt to provide a resolution or solution for the cases. Often in public health practice, there is no single correct answer. Instead, ethical analysis in public health is a process to identify the ethical dimensions of the options available and to arrive at a decision that is ethically justifiable, through deliberation and consideration of relevant facts, values, and contexts.

The cases and other writings in this book represent the opinions, findings, and conclusions of the authors and do not necessarily reflect the official position, views, or policies of the editors, the editors' host institutions, or the authors' host institutions. We decided which topic category to place the case in to best distribute the cases across chapters. However, you may note that some cases cross topic areas and could just as easily have been included in another chapter.

This casebook is written for public health practitioners, including frontline workers, field epidemiology trainers and trainees, and managers, planners, and decision makers with an interest in learning about how to integrate ethical analysis in their day-to-day public health practice. However, the casebook will also be useful to instructors in schools of public health and public health students as well as to academic ethicists who can use the book to teach public health ethics and distinguish it from clinical and research ethics.

Our hope is that the casebook will increase awareness and understanding of public health ethics and the value of ethical analysis in public health practice in all of its forms. This includes applied public health research; public health policy development, implementation, and evaluation; and public health decision making in national and international field settings and training programs. By emphasizing prospective practical decision making, rather than just presenting a theoretical academic discussion of ethical principles, we hope this casebook will serve as a useful tool to support instruction, debate, and dialogue about the nature of ethical challenges encountered in public health practice and how to resolve these challenges. We recommend discussing the cases in small groups and using the discussion questions, the ethical framework described in Chap. 1, and the information provided in the topic area overview sections as a starting place for exploring the ethical issues reflected in the cases. The ultimate goal of case-based learning is to develop skills in ethical analysis and decision making in daily public health practice. The ethical framework provides a convenient tool for putting our ideas into practice.

Atlanta, GA, USA — Drue H. Barrett, PhD
Atlanta, GA, USA — Leonard W. Ortmann, PhD
Sydney, Australia — Angus Dawson, PhD
Washington, DC, USA — Carla Saenz, PhD
Geneva, Switzerland — Andreas Reis, MD
Atlanta, GA, USA — Gail Bolan, MD

Contents

Section I Introduction to Public Health Ethics

1 **Public Health Ethics: Global Cases, Practice, and Context** 3
Leonard W. Ortmann, Drue H. Barrett, Carla Saenz, Ruth Gaare Bernheim, Angus Dawson, Jo A. Valentine, and Andreas Reis
1.1 Introduction 3
1.2 Public Health 5
1.3 Ethics 9
1.4 Public Health Ethics 19
1.5 Ethical Frameworks 27
1.6 A Three-Step Approach to Public Health Decision Making 28
References 33

2 **Essential Cases in the Development of Public Health Ethics** 37
Lisa M. Lee, Kayte Spector-Bagdady, and Maneesha Sakhuja
2.1 Introduction 37
2.2 Case Study: *Jacobson v. Massachusetts* 39
2.3 Case Study: U.S. Public Health Service Research on Sexually Transmitted Disease: Alabama and Guatemala 44
2.4 Case Study: *The New York City A1C Registry* 50
2.5 Conclusions and Implications 54
References 55

Section II Topics in Public Health Ethics

3 **Resource Allocation and Priority Setting** 61
Norman Daniels
3.1 Resource Allocation in Public Health 61
3.2 Collective Lessons from the Cases 62
3.3 Specific Ethical Issues in Resource Allocation 65

3.4 Decision-Making Process ... 69
References ... 70
3.5 Case 1: Priority Setting and Crisis of Public Hospitals in Colombia ... 71
References ... 74
3.6 Case 2: Intersection of Public Health and Mental Health: Meeting Family Needs ... 74
References ... 79
3.7 Case 3: Public-Private Partnerships: Role of Corporate Sponsorship in Public Health ... 80
References ... 83
3.8 Case 4: Black-White Infant Mortality: Disparities, Priorities, and Social Justice ... 84
References ... 86
3.9 Case 5: Priority Setting in Health Care: Ethical Issues ... 87
References ... 89
3.10 Case 6: Critical Care Triage in Pandemics ... 90
References ... 93

4 Disease Prevention and Control ... 95
Michael J. Selgelid
4.1 Introduction ... 95
4.2 Mandatory Treatment and Vaccination ... 95
4.3 Disease Screening and Surveillance ... 97
4.4 Stigma ... 98
4.5 Access to Care ... 99
4.6 Health Promotion Incentives ... 100
4.7 Emergency Response ... 101
4.8 Conclusion ... 102
References ... 103
4.9 Case 1: Mandatory Vaccination in Measles Outbreaks ... 103
References ... 107
4.10 Case 2: Public Health Approaches to Preventing Mother-to-Child HIV Transmission ... 108
References ... 111
4.11 Case 3: Newborn Bloodspot Screening: Personal Choice or Public Health Necessity? Storage and Ownership of Newborn Bloodspots ... 111
References ... 114
4.12 Case 4: Decoding Public Health Ethics and Inequity in India: A Conditional Cash Incentive Scheme—Janani Suraksha Yojana ... 116
References ... 119
4.13 Case 5: HIV Criminalization and STD Prevention and Control ... 120
References ... 124

4.14 Case 6: Ethics of Administering Anthrax Vaccine to Children 125
References ... 128
4.15 Case 7: Non-adherence to Treatment in Patients with Tuberculosis: A Challenge for Minimalist Ethics ... 129
References ... 132
4.16 Case 8: Mass Evacuation ... 132
References ... 135

5 Chronic Disease Prevention and Health Promotion ... 137
Harald Schmidt
5.1 Introduction ... 137
5.2 Individuals ... 140
5.3 Formal and Informal Health Workers ... 141
5.4 Governments (At Different Levels) ... 144
5.5 Corporate Entities ... 147
5.6 Case Studies ... 149
References ... 151
5.7 Case 1: Municipal Action on Food and Beverage Marketing to Youth ... 153
References ... 157
5.8 Case 2: Obesity Prevention in Children: Media Campaigns, Stigma, and Ethics ... 158
References ... 161
5.9 Case 3: Obesity Stigma in Vulnerable and Marginalized Groups ... 162
References ... 166
5.10 Case 4: Water Fluoridation: The Example of Greece ... 167
References ... 170
5.11 Case 5: The Prohibition of Smoking in Public Places in Bulgaria ... 172
References ... 175

6 Environmental and Occupational Public Health ... 177
Bruce Jennings
6.1 Environment and Workplace: Key Venues for Public Health ... 177
6.2 Population Benefits, Individual Rights, and Ethically Acceptable Risk ... 180
6.3 Systems and Power: The Ethical Importance of Ecological and Social Context ... 183
References ... 185
6.4 Case 1: Assessing Mining's Impact on Health Equity in Mongolia ... 186
References ... 190
6.5 Case 2: Exceptions to National MRSA Prevention Policy for a Medical Resident with Untreatable MRSA Colonization ... 191
References ... 194

6.6 Case 3: Safe Water Standards and Monitoring of a Well Construction Program 195
References 198
6.7 Case 4: Implementation of Global Public Health Programs and Threats to Personal Safety 199
References 201

7 Vulnerability and Marginalized Populations 203
Anthony Wrigley and Angus Dawson
7.1 Introduction 203
7.2 Different Approaches to the Concept of Vulnerability 204
7.3 Concerns Surrounding Approach (V2): Universal Condition 205
7.4 Concerns Surrounding Approach (V3): Specific Attributes, Contexts, or Groups 206
7.5 Concerns Surrounding Approach (V4): Overarching Concepts 207
7.6 Simplifying the Concept of Vulnerability (V5): The Moral-Marker Approach 208
References 210
7.7 Case 1: Reducing Sudden Infant Death Syndrome in a Culturally Diverse Society: The New Zealand Cot Death Study and National Cot Death Prevention Programme 211
References 215
7.8 Case 2: Medical Tourism and Surrogate Pregnancy: A Case of Ethical Incoherence 216
References 220
7.9 Case 3: Compulsory Treatment for Injection Drug Use after Incarceration 220
References 224
7.10 Case 4: Unanticipated Vulnerability: Marginalizing the Least Visible in Pandemic Planning 226
References 229
7.11 Case 5: Can Asylum Seeking Be Managed Ethically? 230
References 233
7.12 Case 6: Tuberculosis Screening, Testing, and Treatment among Asylum Seekers 235
References 239

8 International Collaboration for Global Public Health 241
Eric M. Meslin and Ibrahim Garba
8.1 Introduction 241
8.2 The Rise of Globalization and Global Health 242
8.3 Ethics Frameworks for Global Health 246
8.4 Summary 253
References 253
8.5 Case 1: The Ethics of HIV Testing Policies 256
References 259

8.6 Case 2: Just Allocation of Pre-exposure Prophylaxis Drugs in Sub-Saharan Africa ... 260
References ... 262
8.7 Case 3: Drug Trials in Developing Countries ... 263
References ... 265
8.8 Case 4: Ethical Issues in Responding to International Medication Stock-Outs ... 266
References ... 269
8.9 Case 5: Transmitting Cholera to Haiti ... 270
References ... 274
8.10 Case 6: Perilous Path to Middle East Peace: The Sanctions Dilemma ... 274
References ... 278
8.11 Case 7: Advancing Informed Consent and Ethical Standards in Multinational Health Research ... 279
References ... 283

9 Public Health Research ... 285
Drue H. Barrett, Leonard W. Ortmann, Natalie Brown, Barbara R. DeCausey, Carla Saenz, and Angus Dawson
9.1 Introduction ... 285
9.2 What Is Different About Public Health Research? ... 287
9.3 Ethical Considerations for Protecting the Public during Health Research ... 289
9.4 How Ethical Challenges Can Arise in Public Health Research: Lessons Learned from Cases ... 296
9.5 Conclusions ... 297
References ... 298
9.6 Case 1: To Reveal or Not to Reveal Potentially Harmful Findings: A Dilemma for Public Health Research ... 300
References ... 303
9.7 Case 2: Ethical Challenges in Impoverished Communities: Seeking Informed Consent in a Palestinian Refugee Camp in Lebanon ... 305
References ... 309
9.8 Case 3: Improving Review Quality and Efficiency of Research Ethics Committees to Enhance Public Health Practice in Africa ... 310
References ... 313
9.9 Case 4: Internet-Based HIV/AIDS Education and Prevention Programs in Vulnerable Populations: Black Men Who Have Sex with Men ... 314
References ... 317

Index ... 319

Contributors

Rima Afifi, PhD, MPH Department of Health Promotion and Community Health, Faculty of Health Sciences, American University of Beirut, Beirut, Lebanon

Waleed Al-Faisal, PhD Department of Family and Community Medicine, Faculty of Medicine, Damascus University, Damascus, Syrian Arab Republic

Primary Health Care, Dubai Health Authority, Dubai, United Arab Emirates

Silviya Aleksandrova-Yankulovska, MD, PhD, DSc Faculty of Public Health, Department of Public Health Sciences, Medical University of Pleven, Pleven, Bulgaria

Aikaterini A. Aspradaki, PhD, MA, DDS Joint Graduate Programme in Bioethics, University of Crete, Crete, Greece

Drue H. Barrett, PhD Office of Scientific Integrity, Office of the Associate Director for Science, Office of the Director, Centers for Disease Control and Prevention, Atlanta, GA, USA

Michael T. Bartenfeld, MA Children's Preparedness Unit, Disability and Health Branch, Division of Human Development and Disability, National Center on Birth Defects and Developmental Disabilities, Centers for Disease Control and Prevention, Atlanta, GA, USA

Carrie Bernard, MD MPH CCFP FCFP Department of Family and Community Medicine, University of Toronto, Toronto, ON, Canada

Department of Family Medicine McMaster University, Hamilton, ON, Canada

Ruth Gaare Bernheim, JD, MPH Department of Public Health Sciences, University of Virginia, Charlottesville, VA, USA

Divya Kanwar Bhati, BSc, MSc, MBA World Health Organization Collaborating Centre for District Health System Based on Primary Health Care, Indian Institute of Health Management Research University, Jaipur, Rajasthan, India

Dhrubajyoti Bhattacharya, JD, MPH, LLM Department of Population Health Sciences, School of Nursing and Health Professions, University of San Francisco, San Francisco, CA, USA

Erika Blacksher, PhD Department of Bioethics and Humanities, University of Washington, Seattle, WA, USA

Karin Johansson Blight, RGN, MSc, PhD The Policy Institute, Kings College London, London, UK

Gail Bolan, MD Division of STD Prevention, National Center for HIV/AIDS, Viral Hepatitis, STD and TB Prevention, Centers for Disease Control and Prevention, Atlanta, GA, USA

Renaud F. Boulanger, BA Biomedical Ethics Unit, McGill University, Montréal, QC, Canada

Andrew Boyd, MD Department of Medicine, Section of Hospital Medicine, Columbia University, New York, NY, USA

Natalie Brown, MPH Human Research Protections Office, Office of Scientific Integrity, Office of the Associate Director for Science, Office of the Director, Centers for Disease Control and Prevention, Atlanta, GA, USA

Cynthia H. Cassell, PhD Birth Defects Branch, Division of Birth Defects and Developmental Disabilities, National Center on Birth Defects and Developmental Disabilities, Centers for Disease Control and Prevention, Atlanta, GA, USA

Paul Christopher, MD Department of Psychiatry and Human Behavior, Warren Alpert Medical School, Brown University, Providence, RI, USA

Brian Cook, PhD Toronto Food Strategy, Toronto Public Health, Toronto, ON, Canada

Maite Cruz-Piqueras, BA Andalusian School of Public Health, Granada, Spain

Norman Daniels, PhD Department of Global Health and Population, Harvard T.H. Chan School of Public Health, Boston, MA, USA

Colleen Davison, MPH, PhD Clinical Research Centre and Department of Emergency Medicine, Kingston General Hospital, Kingston, ON, Canada

Department of Public Health Sciences, Queen's University, Kingston, ON, Canada

Angus Dawson, PhD Center for Values, Ethics and the Law in Medicine, Sydney School of Public Health, The University of Sydney, Sydney, Australia

Barbara R. DeCausey, MPH, MBA Clinical Research Branch, Division of Tuberculosis Elimination, National Center for HIV/AIDS, Viral Hepatitis, STD, and TB Prevention, Centers for Disease Control and Prevention, Atlanta, GA, USA

M. Gabriela Doberti, MD Hospital Padre Hurtado, Facultad de Medicina, Clínica Alemana–Universidad del Desarrollo, Santiago, Chile

Dora M. Dumont, PhD, MPH Division of Community, Family Health and Equity, Rhode Island Department of Health, Providence, RI, USA

Ewout Fanoy, MD Department of Infectious Disease Control, Municipal Health Service Utrecht, Zeist, The Netherlands

National Institute for Public Health and the Environment, Centre for Infectious Disease Control, Bilthoven, The Netherlands

Sherry Fontaine, PhD Department of Management, University of Wisconsin-La Crosse, La Crosse, WI, USA

Joseph B.R. Gaie, PhD Department of Theology and Religious Studies, University of Botswana, Gaborone, Botswana

Ibrahim Garba, MA, JD, LLM Indiana University Center for Bioethics, Indianapolis, IN, USA

Public Health Law Program, Office of State, Tribal, Local, and Territorial Support, Centers for Disease Control and Prevention, Atlanta, GA, USA

Rachel M. Glassford, BS School of Public Health and Health Services, George Washington University, Falls Church, VA, USA

Daniel S. Goldberg, JD, PhD Department of Bioethics and Interdisciplinary Studies, Brody School of Medicine, East Carolina University, Greenville, NC, USA

M. Inés Gómez, MD, Masters of Bioethics Centro de Bioética Facultad de Medicina, Clínica Alemana–Universidad del Desarrollo, Santiago, Chile

Susan D. Goold, MD, MHSA, MA Department of Internal Medicine and Department of Health Management and Policy, Center for Bioethics and Social Sciences in Medicine, University of Michigan, Ann Arbor, MI, USA

María del Pilar Guzmán Urrea, PhD Department of Community Medicine, El Bosque University, Bogotá, Colombia

Riripeti Haretuku, MEd Maori SIDS and Research, MauriOra Associates, Auckland, New Zealand

Alison Hayward, MD, MPH Department of Emergency Medicine, Yale School of Medicine, Yale University, New Haven, CT, USA

Uganda Village Project, Iganga, Uganda

Margaret Henning, MA, PhD International Health Systems Program, Harvard T. H. Chan School of Public Health, Boston, MA, USA

Health Science, Keene State College, Keene, NH, USA

Ildefonso Hernández-Aguado, MD, PhD Department of Public Health, History of Science and Gynecology, Universidad Miguel Hernández and CIBER de Epidemiología y Salud Pública, San Juan, Alicante, Spain

Sylvia Hoang, MPH Social and Epidemiological Research Department, Centre for Addiction and Mental Health, Toronto, ON, Canada

Matthew R. Hunt, PT, PhD School of Physical and Occupational Therapy, McGill University, Montréal, QC, Canada

Centre for Interdisciplinary Research on Rehabilitation, Montréal, QC, Canada

Hamid Hussain, MD, PhD Faculty of Medicine, University of Baghdad, Baghdad, Iraq

Dubai Residency Training Program and Public Health Consultant, Dubai Health Authority, Dubai, United Arab Emirates

Carel IJsselmuiden, MD, MPH Council on Health Research for Development, Geneva, Switzerland

School of Applied Human Sciences, South African Research Ethics Training Initiative, University of KwaZulu-Natal, Pietermaritzburg, South Africa

Craig Janes, PhD School of Public Health and Health Systems, University of Waterloo, Waterloo, ON, Canada

Bruce Jennings, MA Center for Biomedical Ethics and Society, Vanderbilt University, Nashville, TN, USA

Kipton E. Jensen, PhD Department of Philosophy and Religion, Morehouse College, Atlanta, GA, USA

Monique Jonas, PhD School of Population Health, Faculty of Medical and Health Sciences, The University of Auckland, Auckland, New Zealand

Amar Kanekar, PhD, MPH, MB, MCHES, CPH Department of Health, Human Performance and Sport Management, University of Arkansas at Little Rock, Little Rock, AR, USA

Mary Kasule, PhD Office of Research and Development, University of Botswana, Gaborone, Botswana

Carla Kessler, MA Ethics Institute, Utrecht University, Utrecht, The Netherlands

Sarah A. Kleinfeld, MD Department of Psychiatry, Medstar Georgetown University Hospital, Washington, DC, USA

Sarah Ann Kotchian, JD Education and Early Childhood Policy, Holland Children's Movement and the Holland Children's Institute, Omaha, NE, USA

Maria Kousis, PhD, MSc Center for Research and Studies in Humanities, Social Sciences and Pedagogics, University of Crete, Crete, Greece

André Krom, PhD Technology Assessment, Rathenau Institute, The Hague, The Netherlands

Juan Laguna-Sorinas, MD, MPH Department of Epidemiological Surveillance, Provincial Office of Health and Social Welfare of Granada

Department of Health and Social Welfare–Regional Government of Andalusia, Granada, Spain

Lory Laing, PhD School of Public Health, University of Alberta, Edmonton, AB, Canada

Drew E. Lee, MD, MA Department of Family Medicine, Advocate Lutheran General Hospital, Park Ridge, IL, USA

Lisa M. Lee, PhD, MA, MS Presidential Commission for the Study of Bioethical Issues, Washington, DC, USA

Justin List, MD, MAR, MSc Robert Wood Johnson/VA Clinical Scholars Program, University of Michigan, Ann Arbor, MI, USA

Oyunaa Lkhagvasuren, MD, MPH, MEd Leading Researchers, Ulaanbaatar, Mongolia

Lorna Luco, MD, Master of Bioethics Centro de Bioética, Facultad de Medicina, Clínica Alemana–Universidad del Desarrollo, Santiago, Chile

Blanca Lumbreras, PhD Department of Public Health, History of Science and Gynecology, Universidad Miguel Hernández and CIBER de Epidemiología y Salud Pública, San Juan, Alicante, Spain

Catherine L. Mah, MD, FRCPC, PhD Faculty of Medicine, Memorial University, St. John's, NL, Canada

Jihad Makhoul, DrPH, MPH Department of Health Promotion and Community Health, Faculty of Health Sciences, American University of Beirut, Beirut, Lebanon

Isabel Marin-Rodríguez, MD, MPH Provincial Office of Health and Social Welfare of Granada, Department of Health and Social Welfare–Regional Government of Andalusia, Granada, Spain

Christopher W. McDougall, MA Institute of Health Policy, Management and Evaluation, and Joint Centre for Bioethics, University of Toronto, Toronto, ON, Canada

Eric M. Meslin, PhD Indiana University Center for Bioethics, Indianapolis, IN, USA

Jennifer Milburn, MHA Newborn Screening Ontario, Children's Hospital of Eastern Ontario, Ottawa, ON, Canada

Joseph Millum, PhD Clinical Center Department of Bioethics and Fogarty International Center, National Institutes of Health, Bethesda, MD, USA

Raquel de Mock, MD Adult Health Program, Ministry of Health, University of Panama, Panama City, Panama

Boitumelo Mokgatla, BMedSc, MSc (Bioethics) Africa Office for Council on Health Research for Development, Gaborone, Botswana

Mapping African Research Ethics Review and Medicines Regulatory Capacity, Gaborone, Botswana

Indira Nair, MSc, PhD Department of Engineering and Public Policy, Carnegie Mellon University, Pittsburgh, PA, USA

Rima Nakkash, DrPH, MPH Department of Health Promotion and Community Health, Faculty of Health Sciences, American University of Beirut, Beirut, Lebanon

Stuart G. Nicholls, MSc, MRes, PhD School of Epidemiology, Public Health and Preventive Medicine, University of Ottawa, Ottawa, ON, Canada

Lloyd Novick, MD, MPH Brody School of Medicine, East Carolina University, Greenville, NC, USA

Leonard W. Ortmann, PhD Office of Scientific Integrity, Office of the Associate Director for Science, Office of the Director, Centers for Disease Control and Prevention, Atlanta, GA, USA

Georgina Peacock, MD, MPH, FAAP Division of Human Development and Disability, National Center on Birth Defects and Developmental Disabilities, Centers for Disease Control and Prevention, Atlanta, GA, USA

Anastas Philalithis, AKC, MBBS, PhD, MRCP, MS Department of Social Medicine, Faculty of Medicine, University of Crete, Crete, Greece

Daryl Pullman, MA, PhD Division of Community Health and Humanities, Faculty of Medicine, Memorial University, St. John's, NL, Canada

Andreas Reis, MD, MSc Global Health Ethics, Department of Information, Evidence and Research, World Health Organization, Geneva, Switzerland

Christy A. Rentmeester, PhD AMA Journal of Ethics, American Medical Association, Chicago, IL, USA

Josiah D. Rich, MD, MPH Department of Medicine, Warren Alpert Medical School, Brown University, Providence, RI, USA

Jorge Rodríguez, MD Sexual and Reproductive Health, Ministry of Health, Panama City, Panama

Panamanian Family Medicine Association, Panama City, Panama

Miguel Angel Royo-Bordonada, MD, MPH, PhD National School of Public Health, Madrid, Spain

Babette Rump, MD Department of Infectious Disease Control, Municipal Health Service Utrecht, Zeist, The Netherlands

Carla Saenz, PhD Regional Program on Bioethics, Office of Knowledge Management, Bioethics, and Research, Pan American Health Organization, Washington, DC, USA

Maneesha Sakhuja, MHS Presidential Commission for the Study of Bioethical Issues, Washington, DC, USA

Harald Schmidt, MA, PhD Department of Medical Ethics & Health Policy, Center for Health Incentives and Behavioral Economics, University of Pennsylvania, Philadelphia, PA, USA

Michael J. Selgelid, MA, PhD Centre for Human Bioethics, Monash University, Melbourne, Australia

Kasturi Sen, BA, Dip Soc Pol, PhD Global Public Health, Wolfson College (Common Room), University of Oxford, Oxford, UK

Pablo Simón-Lorda, MD, PhD Primary Health Care Centre Chauchina, UGC Santa Fe, Granada, Spain

Department of Health and Social Welfare–Regional Government of Andalusia, Granada, Spain

Maxwell J. Smith, MS Dalla Lana School of Public Health and the Joint Centre for Bioethics, University of Toronto, Toronto, ON, Canada

Jeremy Snyder, PhD Faculty of Health Sciences, Simon Fraser University, Burnaby, BC, Canada

Daniel M. Sosin, MD, MPH, FACP Office of Public Health Preparedness and Response, Centers for Disease Control and Prevention, Atlanta, GA, USA

Kayte Spector-Bagdady, JD, M Bioethics Presidential Commission for the Study of Bioethical Issues, Washington, DC, USA

Maribel Tamayo-Velázquez, PhD Andalusian School of Public Health, Granada, Spain

Emily Taylor, MA Dalla Lana School of Public Health, University of Toronto, Toronto, ON, Canada

Olinda Timms, DA, PGDMLE, PGDB Department of Health and Humanities, St. Johns Research Institute, Bangalore, Karnataka, India

Ioannis Tzoutzas, DDS, Dr. Odont., FIADR, FASM School of Dentistry, National and Kapodistrian University of Athens, Athens, Greece

Jo A. Valentine, MSW Division of STD Prevention, National Center for HIV/AIDS, Viral Hepatitis, STD, and TB Prevention, Centers for Disease Control and Prevention, Atlanta, GA, USA

Jim van Steenbergen, MD, PhD National Institute for Public Health and the Environment, Centre of Infectious Disease Control, Bilthoven, The Netherlands

Leiden University Medical Centre, Centre for Infectious Diseases, Leiden, The Netherlands

Claude Vergès, MD, EdD, MA (Bioethics, Law) Children's Hospital, University of Panama, Panama City, Panama

Marcel Verweij, PhD Department of Social Sciences, Communication, Philosophy and Technology: Centre for Integrated Development, Wageningen University, Wageningen, The Netherlands

A.M. Viens, PhD Centre for Health, Ethics and Law, Southampton Law School, University of Southampton, Southhampton, UK

Meghan Wagler, MPH Faculty of Health Sciences, Simon Fraser University, Burnaby, BC, Canada

Frank Wagner, MA, MHSc Department of Family and Community Medicine, Faculty of Medicine, University of Toronto, Toronto, ON, Canada

Toronto Central Community Care Access Centre and the University of Toronto Joint Centre for Bioethics Toronto, ON, Canada

Douglas Wassenaar, PhD South African Research Ethics Training Initiative, School of Applied Human Sciences, University of KwaZulu-Natal, Pietermaritzburg, South Africa

Marjan Wassenberg, MD, PhD Department of Medical Microbiology, Utrecht University Medical Centre, Utrecht, The Netherlands

Anthony Wrigley, PhD Centre for Professional Ethics, Keele University, Staffordshire, UK

Susan Zinner, MSJ, MHA, JD School of Public and Environmental Affairs, Indiana University Northwest, Gary, IN, USA

Section I
Introduction to Public Health Ethics

Chapter 1
Public Health Ethics: Global Cases, Practice, and Context

Leonard W. Ortmann, Drue H. Barrett, Carla Saenz, Ruth Gaare Bernheim, Angus Dawson, Jo A. Valentine, and Andreas Reis

1.1 Introduction

Introducing *public health ethics* poses two special challenges. First, it is a relatively new field that combines public health and practical ethics. Its unfamiliarity requires considerable explanation, yet its scope and emergent qualities make delineation difficult. Moreover, while the early development of public health ethics occurred in a Western context, its reach, like public health itself, has become global. A second challenge, then, is to articulate an approach specific enough to provide clear

The opinions, findings, and conclusions of the authors do not necessarily reflect the official position, views, or policies of the editors, the editors' host institutions, or the authors' host institutions.

L.W. Ortmann, PhD (✉) • D.H. Barrett, PhD
Office of Scientific Integrity, Office of the Associate Director for Science,
Office of the Director, Centers for Disease Control and Prevention, Atlanta, GA, USA
e-mail: lortmann@cdc.gov

C. Saenz, PhD
Regional Program on Bioethics, Office of Knowledge Management, Bioethics, and Research,
Pan American Health Organization, Washington, DC, USA

R.G. Bernheim, JD, MPH
Department of Public Health Sciences, University of Virginia, Charlottesville, VA, USA

A. Dawson, PhD
Center for Values, Ethics and the Law in Medicine, Sydney School of Public Health,
The University of Sydney, Sydney, Australia

J.A. Valentine, MSW
Division of STD Prevention, National Center for HIV/AIDS, Viral Hepatitis, STD, and TB Prevention, Centers for Disease Control and Prevention, Atlanta, GA, USA

A. Reis, MD, MSc
Global Health Ethics, Department of Information, Evidence and Research,
World Health Organization, Geneva, Switzerland

D.H. Barrett et al. (eds.), *Public Health Ethics: Cases Spanning the Globe*,
Public Health Ethics Analysis 3, DOI 10.1007/978-3-319-23847-0_1

guidance yet sufficiently flexible and encompassing to adapt to global contexts. Broadly speaking, public health ethics helps guide practical decisions affecting population or community health based on scientific evidence and in accordance with accepted values and standards of right and wrong. In these ways, public health ethics builds on its parent disciplines of public health and ethics. This dual inheritance plays out in the definition the U.S. Centers for Disease Control and Prevention (CDC) offers of public health ethics: "A systematic process to clarify, prioritize, and justify possible courses of public health action based on ethical principles, values and beliefs of stakeholders, and scientific and other information" (CDC 2011). Public health ethics shares with other fields of practical and professional ethics both the general theories of ethics and a common store of ethical principles, values, and beliefs. It differs from these other fields largely in the nature of challenges that public health officials typically encounter and in the ethical frameworks it employs to address these challenges. Frameworks provide methodical approaches or procedures that tailor general ethical theories, principles, values, and beliefs to the specific ethical challenges that arise in a particular field. Although no framework is definitive, many are useful, and some are especially effective in particular contexts. This chapter will conclude by setting forth a straightforward, stepwise ethics framework that provides a tool for analyzing the cases in this volume and, more importantly, one that public health practitioners have found useful in a range of contexts. For a public health practitioner, knowing how to employ an ethics framework to address a range of ethical challenges in public health—a know-how that depends on practice—is the ultimate take-home message.

We learn new things more readily when we can relate them to familiar things, and we understand complex things by breaking them into their components. Accordingly, throughout this introductory chapter, we will relate public health ethics to more familiar concepts and better-known related fields, while the immediately following section will explore the components of public health ethics that derive from its parent disciplines of public health and ethics. After describing public health's core activities, goals, and values, we will explain why ethical concepts like the right to health, social justice, and health equity directly follow as central concerns of public health. After defining ethics broadly in everyday terms, we will examine the complementary roles facts and values play in public health. This examination is important because the respective bases of the two parent disciplines differ considerably; public health science rests on the logic of scientific discovery, whereas ethics rests on the logic of right action and good decision making. We will then contrast the more familiar, everyday understanding of morality with the formal discipline of ethics as a prelude to considering three well-known ethical theories relevant to public health. Because both laws and ethical rules establish parameters for public health practice, their similarity and difference need to be clarified. This extended account, first of parent disciplines, then of kindred concepts, and finally of family resemblances between the related fields of clinical ethics, bioethics, and research ethics, will culminate in an effort to characterize what is distinctive about public health ethics.

1.2 Public Health

There are many definitions of public health. They often begin as descriptions of current practice but once established become prescriptions for subsequent practice. It is important, then, to consider definitions, because they shape not only public health practice, but also how we conceive of public health ethics (Dawson and Verweij 2007). The same logic applies to how we think about the individual concepts of health and the public. Defining health as the absence of disease or symptoms, for example, more readily fits allopathic medicine, which focuses on negating symptoms to treat disease. But it hardly fits public health's emphasis on preventive measures that address root causes rather than symptoms. Nor does it cover public health's promotion of health and well-being across a range of interventions. In this regard, the World Health Organization (WHO) offers a definition of health more suitable to public health: "A state of complete physical, mental, and social well-being and not merely the absence of disease or infirmity" (WHO 2006). But even this more holistic definition does not sufficiently clarify the meaning of "public" in public health. Dawson and Verweij (2007) identify two primary meanings of "public" in public health, each of which they break down into three senses. Public can mean population-wide and refer to (1) the epidemiologically measured health of a population or group, (2) the distribution of health in a population, or (3) the underlying social and environmental conditions impacting everyone's health. Public also can mean collectively accomplished and requiring (1) the concerted actions of many people and institutions whether governmental or nongovernmental; (2) the cooperation or involvement of the public, or (3) the public's joint participation to realize the health improvement.

In a practical field like public health, definition often takes the form of enumerating key activities, such as surveillance, sanitation, maintaining food and workplace safety, disease prevention and control, and promoting healthy behavior. The identification of the ten essential services of public health illustrates this enumerative approach (Fig. 1.1) (Public Health Functions Steering Committee 1994). These services fall under three overarching functions of assessment, policy development, and assurance that constitute an integrated cyclic process. The delivery of these services in local, regional, or national public health agencies accordingly defines public health practice. In this schema, research is a distinct practical service but also integral to all public health activities, providing insights and innovative solutions at every point. Public health ethics addresses the entire spectrum of ethical issues that arise in any area of public health practice but especially in those areas where no specific guidelines govern practice.

Such lists have the advantage of concretely specifying current activities but lack criteria that definitions normally provide for including or excluding additional activities as a field develops. In 1920, Charles Edward A. Winslow, an influential public health theorist and leader, pioneered a definition of public health that still informs many European and international public health institutions, including WHO (Marks et al. 2011).

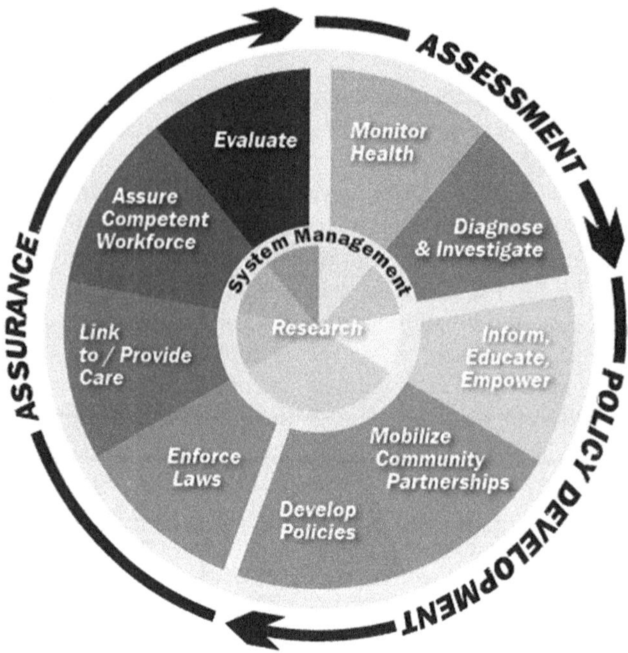

Fig. 1.1 Essential Public Health Services. (1) Monitor health status to identify community health problems. (2) Diagnose and investigate health problems and health hazards in the community. (3) Inform, educate, and empower people about health issues. (4) Mobilize community partnerships and action to identify and solve health problems. (5) Develop policies and plans that support individual and community health efforts. (6) Enforce laws and regulations that protect health and ensure safety. (7) Link people to needed personal health services and assure the provision of health care when otherwise unavailable. (8) Assure competent public and personal health care workforce. (9) Evaluate effectiveness, accessibility, and quality of personal and population-based health services. (10) Research for new insights and innovative solutions to health problems (From Public Health Functions Steering Committee 1994. *Essential Public Health Services*. Available at http://www.cdc.gov/nphpsp/essentialServices.html)

> Public health is the science and the art of preventing disease, prolonging life, and promoting physical health and efficiency through organized community efforts … and the development of the social machinery which will ensure to every individual in the community a standard of living adequate for the maintenance of health (Winslow 1920).

Even more succinctly, the U.S. Institute of Medicine (IOM) defines public health as "what we, as a society, do collectively to assure the conditions for people to be healthy" (IOM 1988).

These two definitions highlight the importance of collective action to address the health needs of populations. Public health's population focus distinguishes it from clinical medicine's focus on individual patients, though examples like vaccination indicate that the two fields can overlap. Epidemiologists statistically aggregate the health data of individuals to provide a picture of population health, but populations ultimately originate from *communities of individuals* who constitute social wholes.

Individuals in society stand in complex relations of interdependence, competition, and solidarity that can impact health in ways that transcend the individual. Thus, in addition to aggregating individual medical data, epidemiologists need to measure the impact of various social factors on health. To tackle the complex, often competing health needs of social groups, public health practitioners need to dialogue and partner with their communities. At a higher administrative level, public health officials need to manage intersectoral collaborations, navigate political processes, and formulate public health law. Four distinguishing features of public health practice—the pursuit of the collective good, a focus on prevention, the use of government or collective action, and an emphasis on an outcome-based (utilitarian) approach—generate most of the ethical challenges public health practitioners typically face (Faden and Shebaya 2010).

1.2.1 Core Values

People value many things such as friends and family, material goods and resources, knowledge, and art. Some things people value are ethical virtues like courage or honesty, whereas others are ethical principles like justice and equality. People generally value what they consider important, what matters to them, and what gives their lives meaning. Public health's primary goals and commitments reflect its core values, which are rooted in health, science, and the community (Public Health Leadership Society 2002). Everyone recognizes the value of health, but public health approaches health in relation to science and the community in its endeavor to prevent disease and injury, protect the public from harm, and promote health and well-being. But seeing how science and community represent values requires a word of explanation.

The commitment to science as a value stance often becomes apparent only in relation to people who distrust science or prioritize other value commitments such as economic interests or religion. Public health values science by endeavoring to base interventions and policies on the best available data and evidence-based practices. That endeavor entails a commitment to conduct surveillance and research, because only by understanding the social burden of disease and its underlying or structural causes can public health impact the health of the entire population. The qualifier "best available" is a reminder of the need to continuously improve practice and not rely on tradition or current practices. It also reminds us that during emergencies, time and resource constraints limit the ability to gather evidence.

Public health values community in two obvious senses. First, it recognizes that the success of most health interventions depends on a community's acceptance, cooperation, or participation. Second, it recognizes that to be successful, public health must respect the community's values and gain the trust of its members. Yet there is a third, deeper sense in which community represents a value. A community is, to emphasize again, neither a statistical abstraction nor a mere aggregate of individuals but rather a network of relationships and emotional bonds between people sharing a life in common organized through a political and moral order (Jennings 2007). The value that best reflects this fundamental, relational character of social life is *solidarity*. Solidarity can remain unspoken yet operative because it forms the basis of social life and collective action. Just as communities are not mere aggregates of individuals, neither are the agencies or organizations that make the collective decisions that affect the community. Personal interests, to be sure, can motivate individuals, but the felt recognition of a common plight, that we are all in it together, underlies the collective decisions society and public health must make to solve collective problems. To say that public health values community means that it values solidarity, even when solidarity remains unacknowledged as is often the case (Dawson and Jennings 2012).

1.2.2 Health Equity, Social Justice, and Social Determinants of Health

As the foregoing goals, definitions, core values, and commitments of public health clearly suggest, the right to health and health equity are central, not peripheral, to public health's mission. Chapter 8 on international collaboration will examine some practical challenges in addressing the right to health and social determinants of health, so the emphasis here will be on the rationale for achieving health equity as a matter of social justice.

Despite greater individual access to health care and advances in public health, high burdens of disease remain across much of the globe. Some differences in disease burden result from genetics and some from variable risks of exposure to infectious agents and other threats, but most of the differential burden arises from social, economic, and political conditions. These conditions include poverty, lack of education, and discrimination against particular social groups and often reflect historical injustices or long-standing systemic, structural deficiencies. Collectively, these conditions have come to be known as *social determinants of health* (Blane 1999). Greater access to individual health care can mitigate their effect, but an adequate response to them requires concerted public action to address their underlying causes.

Whether comparing countries or groups within countries, social stratification by social determinants correlates with differences in health status (Marmot 2007). These health differences have aroused widespread concern, but how one defines them significantly affects public health practice (Braveman 2006). In particular, distinguishing health disparity from health inequity is critical. As a comparative indicator of health status, health disparity is a neutral, epidemiologic term that need not imply an ethical obligation to remedy. Health disparities, however, can and frequently do reflect underlying inequities. WHO defines health inequities as health differences that are "socially produced; systematic in their distribution across the population; and unfair" (WHO 2007). Terms like "inequity" and "unfair" are ethical terms that imply an obligation to redress an injustice. Justice has a range of meanings that include giving people what they deserve or are owed and distributing goods and services fairly. Justice in a medical context often involves the individual's access to health services. In public health, discussions of health equity usually involve questions of how to distribute health benefits fairly or how to achieve better health outcomes among communities or groups that suffer health inequities. Attaining greater equity might involve the politically controversial strategy of disproportionally distributing resources within a population, by, for example, distributing more to those most in need. A less-controversial strategy is to improve health outcomes for all, even while devoting special efforts to those most in need. WHO defines health equity as "the absence of unfair and avoidable or remediable differences in health among population groups defined socially, economically, demographically, or geographically" (WHO 2007).

Achieving health equity is most urgent for groups who have experienced histories of marginalization and discrimination and who continue to experience higher rates of illness and premature deaths than members of the mainstream population. Especially for these groups, "social injustice is killing people on a grand scale" (WHO 2008). Realizing the goal of social justice with respect to health means achieving health equity. Doing so requires not only a fair distribution of health outcomes, it also means that "ideally everyone should have a fair opportunity to attain their full health potential" and that "no one should be disadvantaged from achieving this potential, if it can be avoided" (Whitehead 1992). For many, these goals imply that social justice obligates public health to improve any social condition that prevents people from maintaining a standard of life adequate to maintain health (Powers and Faden 2006). Although some believe that improving social conditions that affect health overextends public health's mandate, such a broad mandate is arguably consistent with both Winslow's and IOM's definitions of public health. Moreover, such a broad mandate has both nineteenth century precursors in the social medicine movement and more recent precedents in the "Health for All" strategy that emphasizes health promotion and the "Health in All Policies" strategy (Kickbusch 2003; Freiler et al. 2013). But a major milestone was reached with the 2008 report of the WHO Commission on Social Determinants of Health that sought to "marshal the evidence on what can be done to promote health equity, and to foster a global movement to achieve it" (WHO 2008). Although governments can guarantee human rights and essential services, establish policies that provide an equitable basis for health improvement, and gather and monitor data on health equity, achieving equity ultimately will depend on the cooperation of government and civil society (Blas et al. 2008).

1.3 Ethics

People strive to be "good," to do the "right" thing and to lead a "good life," but where do such basic, familiar moral values as good and right originate? Throughout history, religious people have explained these ideas as revelations of divine command.

Anthropologists, however, view morals as customs that govern social interactions, and because all cultures display such customs, interpret moral practices in terms of a survival function rooted in human nature. By contrast, many social and political thinkers emphasize that moral concepts result from social conventions or agreements that are subject to deliberation and change. Governments today often consult social scientists and health experts who empirically investigate what fosters or improves human life, health, and happiness. Where science informs law and policy, it helps define in a conventional sense what we mean by good and right. In particular, public health science helps establish what is considered good for the health of populations and communities. Further below we will examine three ethical theories prominent in public health ethics that offer contrasting perspectives on the nature and basis of morality. In the meantime, we will address three general questions that a public health practitioner first approaching the study of ethics might well ask: how does science relate to ethics, what is the difference between ethics and morality, and what sort of things count as principles or basic concepts in ethics?

1.3.1 Scientific Facts and Ethical Values

Public health practice increasingly requires appreciation of the complementary roles facts and values play in making and justifying decisions. Observation reveals facts, while scientific research controls and manipulates the experimental context to discover causation or correlation. Data on disease burden, research on intervention effectiveness, and estimates of the resultant health benefits for the population generally inform public health interventions. Health messaging can often inform the public about the scientific rationale underlying public health interventions. Nevertheless, in the mind of the public, scientific evidence does not always invalidate or outweigh other sources of evidence or appeals to emotions, interests, and values. While public health practitioners give more weight to community health and scientific evidence, they also need to consider how the public will respond to an intervention. Successfully implementing public health actions, then, will often entail weighing the public's attitudes, interests, and values in relation to public health's core values.

Two mundane features of public health practice often serve to conceal value assumptions: shared core values and standard practice. First, sharing values can render them invisible as assumptions, until they unexpectedly become contested. Unwelcome surprises occur when interventions that presuppose core values affect stakeholders who do not share those values, as when parents refuse to have children vaccinated based on media hearsay or individuals reject a highly effective program as governmental intrusion. Avoiding such surprises begins with becoming aware of one's own value presuppositions in relation to those of other stakeholders and community members. Second, routine use of evidence-based standards can conceal underlying value assumptions. If developed and tested to address a known health problem, as is common, an intervention's purpose and effectiveness is taken for granted. Standard interventions, then, generally require no more justification than noting their standard status or seeing that "the facts dictated" their use. "Dictating" facts are indicators that trigger use of a standard intervention (e.g., meeting the criteria of a case definition or documenting exposure to a dangerous level of a contaminant). Such "dictating facts," more properly speaking, only *indicate* the appropriate intervention but cannot literally *dictate* that anything be done. What in the end dictate actions are the values, goals, and obligations that the standard intervention presupposes and that practitioners tacitly ratify each time they apply the standard. In other words, values, goals, and obligations, even when tacit, form a necessary bridge between knowledge and action.

Though standard practices tacitly incorporate ethical principles, they seldom raise ethical challenges. Challenges more typically arise in unusual or extreme situations where standards are not yet in place, are changing, or are competing. These situations include emergency operations, foreign cultural settings, emergent fields with innovative interventions, or periods of severe budget constraints that force prioritization of programs. In such challenging situations where no value consensus exists or where evidence does not point to a single course of action, public health ethics provides a process to determine and justify a course of action. That justification can incorporate a number of factors: evidence base for the intervention, cost effectiveness, analysis of relevant ethical rules and stakeholder values, a creative design of options or alternatives that embody these values, and a fair and transparent decision-making process that incorporates stakeholder contributions.

Recognizing one's own value assumptions in relation to those of the public will be critical for implementing new interventions wherever success depends on public acceptance. The public will not embrace interventions that embody or presuppose values that clash with community values or whose relative importance is low compared to other community values. Members of the public generally are more committed to their political views, ethical and religious values, and an intervention's impact on them personally than to scientific evidence or community impact. Public health practitioners need to recognize that no matter how compelling to them, community impact and scientific rationale seldom resonate as deeply with the public. Consequently, in communicating, public health practitioners need to supplement scientific messaging with dialogue, an appeal to common values, or enlistment of spokespersons who share the value orientation of the relevant stakeholders or community. Regarding some controversial matters, ultimate success in implementing an intervention may require building a social consensus (Ortmann and Iskander 2013).

In certain situations, untangling factual claims based on science from value judgments is critical for success. For example, suppose independent investigators have scientifically verified the level of worker exposure to a toxic chemical used in industry. Determining what level of exposure would be safe, however, remains a value judgment that depends on the degree of concern that people have about safety. Placing a higher value on safety might result in stricter controls that decrease risk for workers, but the financial costs of decreasing risks could cut industry profits or jobs, even as health costs fall. Stakeholders representing industry, workers, or public health practitioners might have different positions regarding a safe level of exposure.

To make a good decision about a safe exposure level, the value of safety might have to be discussed and weighed in relation to business, employment, and health considerations. However, these varying positions regarding safety need not imply disregard for safety or disagreement on the underlying facts. Rather, they illustrate that conflicting value judgments can coexist despite a consensus on both the underlying facts and the importance of a particular value such as safety.

Directly addressing the value conflicts in such situations through ethical deliberation makes more sense than calling into question the underlying facts and can lead to better, fairer, and more transparent decisions. It is also important to recognize that doubting the science often represents an underlying value dispute masquerading as a scientific dispute (Brunk et al. 1991). Sowing doubt on scientific assessments merely as a tactic to oppose an evidence-based policy or recommendation undermines science. This doubt can exert pressure to test and retest results, raising the bar for scientific validity ever higher (Michaels 2008). The solution is not to litigate, as it were, the science, but to recognize that communicating risk is a social process that goes beyond science messaging and must take cultural attitudes, perceptions, and symbolic meanings into account (Krimsky and Plough 1988). Where profound value disagreements prevail, public health legitimately prioritizes its core values but cannot speak for everyone. Stakeholder views require a fair hearing, whether through media research, stakeholder analysis, or direct solicitation of input from individuals, focus groups, or public meetings. By design, a fair, transparent ethical decision-making procedure can help determine what value tradeoffs are feasible and what values may be nonnegotiable. Such a deliberative procedure can help to gain public acceptance and become part of the justification for a course of action.

To those accustomed to rigorous research methods and evidence-based standards of practice, navigating the world of ethical values and rules can be perplexing. Values, as the term itself implies, manifest valences, that is, variable degrees of commitment or estimations of importance along a continuum. Individuals rank values differently, change their rankings, and will alter their relative ranking of values in different contexts. The range of options for ethical rules are far more limited, namely, to obey or not obey. Nevertheless, the ethical rules governing particular situations also vary from country to country or even from jurisdiction to jurisdiction within a country. Despite this variability in values and ethical rules, reducing ethical judgment to mere opinion or to a consensus of opinion relative only to personal or cultural preferences would be a mistake. Ethical values and rules enjoy the approval of history, custom, law, and religious tradition, but they also find anchor biologically, psychologically, and socially in human life. Value judgments and ethical determinations, then, are not relative as much as correlative; that is, they correlate and resonate with these deeper roots of human life that we share. If humans indeed share a set of fundamental values, then ethical conflicts primarily reflect differences in prioritizing values in a particular context, rather than a fundamental disagreement about values. This point of view provides grounds for optimism about the possibility of finding a deeper basis for understanding and mutual respect, if not agreement, when ethical tensions surface.

1.3.2 Ethics and Morality

Although many use the terms ethics and morality interchangeably, we will distinguish the formal discipline of ethics from the common morality that guides everyday actions and behavior. Morality refers to a society's shared, stable beliefs about what is good and bad, right and wrong. Through upbringing and socialization, each generation passes this common morality to the next. Common morality envelopes the individual like an ecosphere of shared customs, rules, and values. For most circumstances, people habitually rely on this common morality to guide their conduct, and it serves them well, just as standard practice generally serves professional practitioners well. Still, common morality can fall short where its rules conflict, where it inadequately illuminates novel moral problems, or where intense disagreement prevails among rival stakeholders. In such instances, the formal discipline of ethics offers a deliberate, systematic way of addressing troubling moral issues, conflicts, and dilemmas. Ethics can assist in:

- Recognizing ethical issues and distinguishing them from factual issues;
- Providing a vocabulary to systematically discuss ethics;
- Identifying appropriate ethical principles to guide action in a particular context;
- Using these principles to analyze actions in regard to their ethical acceptability;
- Understanding the competing moral claims and values of stakeholders;
- Designing alternative courses of action that incorporate these claims and values;
- Evaluating which alternative best fits a given context, all things considered
- Establishing a procedurally just, transparent process for decision making; and
- Justifying decisions regarding recommendations, policies, or interventions.

1.3.3 Ethical Principles

Principles are general categories, rules, or guidelines that form the basis of a discipline. In ethics, there are various kinds of principles and many examples of each kind. The kinds include basic ethical categories (e.g., virtues, values, or rights), ethical commands or rules of conduct (e.g., not stealing, not harming, or treating others with respect), and guidelines for weighing outcomes (e.g., achieving the greatest good for the greatest number, distributing burdens and benefits fairly, or properly proportioning benefit to harm). Ethical principles like justice or respect for autonomy are simultaneously values, ideals, and the basis for deriving rules of conduct. Such rules serve as ethical standards to evaluate past and pending actions, programs, and policy recommendations. When addressing complex or controversial issues or issues involving numerous stakeholders, many different principles can come into play. But because ethical decision making depends on context (e.g., on local circumstances, community stakeholders, and decision makers), no formula can determine the most relevant ethical principles. Nevertheless, most ethicists and practitioners working in a field would agree that certain principles, theories, or frameworks provide more helpful guidance for that field. Given the need for flexibility, some prefer to speak not of ethical principles but of "general moral considerations" that can provide guidance in public health practice (Childress et al. 2002). At any rate, a complex ethical challenge involving stakeholders with competing moral claims frequently demands consideration of a variety of ethical principles and theories to address the situation and justify a proposed intervention. For these reasons, it will be useful both to examine below several ethical theories used in public health ethics and to provide at the end of the chapter a framework that is generally applicable to ethical issues that arise in public health.

1.3.4 Ethical Theories

As used here, an ethical framework refers to a tool or approach for practically addressing ethical challenges that often includes a stepwise procedure. An ethical framework may rely heavily on just one ethical theory, but frameworks generally take a pragmatic approach that procedurally allows for using a variety of theories or principles as the issue or context demands. Whereas an ethical framework has a practical orientation, an ethical theory also addresses more fundamental questions, so-called "metaethical" questions. Does morality originate in divine command, human nature, or human convention? Is it essentially a habit, intuition, form of reasoning, or a quality or purpose of an action? An ethical theory will offer a distinct, coherent understanding of the source and nature of morality that will shape how one reasons about moral issues and determine which principles are most important. Two persons employing the same theory, however, will not necessarily reach the same conclusion about an ethical issue; much will depend on which aspects of the issue they deem most important and on how they weigh different factors. Nevertheless, because a particular ethical theory tends to favor certain principles or types of principles, using the same theoretical approach will lead to similar lines of reasoning and selection of principles.

The diversity of ethical theories does not imply their mutual opposition so much as points to the extensive range of the moral landscape and the need to illuminate its various contours. A helpful way of illuminating this landscape is to distinguish theories depending on whether they focus on the actor, the action, or the results of action. To illustrate this particular way of carving up the moral landscape, Table 1.1 describes some well-known ethical theories.

Aristotle's virtue ethics is an ethical theory that focuses on the moral character of the actor or agent (Bartlett and Collins 2011). Classic virtues are dispositions or stable patterns of behavior that lie between extremes of vice; courage, for example, lies between the extremes of cowardice and foolhardiness in taking risks. Habit and practice are necessary to develop virtues whose possession we equate with good character and that equip a person to be effective in society or an organization. Because good character translates into virtuous action that others aspire to emulate,

Table 1.1 Ethical theories

Theory	Agent-centered	Deontology	Utilitarianism
Focus	Agent	Action	Result of action
Key figure	Aristotle	Immanuel Kant	John Stuart Mill
Main concept	*Virtues*: Acquired habits, skills, or dispositions that make people effective in social or professional settings	*Duties*: Ethical rules or commands that constrain one's action or define obligations owed to others	*Results*: Good or bad outcomes of actions and policies or their beneficial or harmful effects on individuals and society
Examples	Honesty, courage, modesty, trustworthiness, transparency, reliability, and perseverance	Ethical and religious commandments, obligations to seek justice or respect persons and their rights	Burdens, risks, harms, or costs versus the benefits, advantages, or savings resulting from interventions or policies
Ethical action	Doing what a virtuous person would do in a given situation	Fulfilling an obligation or duty owed to oneself or society	Maximizing the net balance of benefits over harms
Uses	Assessing skills and capacities needed for success in a community, organization, or profession	Establishing compliance rules and regulations, and setting standards for evaluating actions and behavior	Conducting population-level cost-benefit, risk-benefit, or cost-effectiveness analyses

we tacitly invoke virtue ethics whenever we ask how an outstanding public figure or health leader would handle a situation. In a modern professional context, virtues also include the skills the profession has identified that lead to success in that profession and which professional education and training instill in practitioners. Once established, virtues readily become the standards of obligation and accountability to evaluate professional performance and function similarly to the rules and principles of duty discussed below. Holding public health institutions accountable for the professional competence of their employees illustrates virtue ethics (Public Health leadership Society 2002). More recently, the capabilities approach has exploited the potential of virtue ethics to guide decisions about policy or interventions in a way that goes beyond matters of professional training and responsibilities. This approach takes a broader developmental view of human agency and capacity building. It conceives health as a fundamental capability necessary for individuals to succeed in society, one on which many further capabilities depend (Sen 2009; Ruger 2010).

An ethical theory that focuses on action or, more properly, the rules governing action, is deontology. The word deontology comes from the ancient Greek word, *deontos*, which means duty. Because duties oblige us to obey rules that govern actions or conduct, they bind or constrain the will ahead of action. In judging whether an action is right or wrong, deontology ignores consideration of harmful or beneficial consequences and relies on these rules of duty to serve as the standard of judgment. People usually have rules of duty or obligation in mind when they speak of ethical standards or worry that standards are breaking down. Examples of these rules include religious commandments to honor parents, not lie, or not steal and rules of social interaction such as treating people fairly, doing them no harm, or respecting their rights. Rights often are said to stand in reciprocal relation to duties. Thus, the right to free speech presupposes a duty to respect the right of others to speak or the public health obligation to ensure conditions for maintaining health presupposes a right to health.

Deontology as a theory owes most to Immanuel Kant's view of the "good will" and his closely linked account of autonomy. A person of morally good will does the right thing for its own sake, which means acting purely for the sake of duty. Duties are moral rules or laws that bind the will and limit the scope of action. For Kant, basing decision for one's action solely on duty without regard to the potential good or bad consequences of the action is the only legitimate basis for moral action. Kant even goes so far as to say that "a free will and a will under moral laws are one and the same" (Gregor et al. 2012).

Kant conceives duty as the quintessential expression of autonomy, which may come as a surprise to those who equate autonomy with rational free choice or even just following one's preferences without interference. However, the meaning of autonomy for Kant derives from its literal meaning in Greek, *autos* (self) and *nomos* (law); namely, self-legislating. Autonomy enacts from within the moral rules and principles that bind the will and guide action. However, not every self-originating impulse should be obeyed; only actions conceivable as universal laws morally bind the will. Morally laying down the law for oneself entails legislating for everyone, but universally legislating does not mean asserting one's will over others. Nor does it mean that the ethical content of a moral law or duty is valid eternally and everywhere. Rather, it refers to the "categorical imperative" an unconditional requirement for an action to be moral. To qualify as a duty, a rule that commands action must apply to every rational person. Stealing, for example, could never qualify as a duty, because a situation where everyone steals from everyone else would undercut the one-sided advantage of stealing that the thief hopes to exploit. Although self-directed, autonomous action is necessarily other-regarding.

Kant maintains that the categorical imperative can be expressed in two other ways equivalent to universality, namely, "respect for humanity" and a "kingdom of ends" (Gregor et al. 2012). In each, this other-regarding dimension of autonomy is evident. Respecting humanity means never treating persons as mere means or objects but always treating them as ends, that is, regarding them as fellow autonomous agents. Autonomously agreeing on actions, interventions, or policies requires that decision makers mutually consider and understand their reasons for action and be willing to abide by the rules derived from these reasons as laws they collectively impose upon themselves (O'Neill 2002).

The idea of a fellowship of mutual consideration comes out most clearly in Kant's concept of a kingdom of ends. This concept is really the ideal of a systematic union or commonwealth of autonomous individuals making laws that apply to everyone. This ideal presupposes that ethical deliberation places respect for others as ends, as autonomous agents, above self-interest. The core idea is that we only consider actions that could gain acceptance by a community in which all see themselves as sovereigns who lay down universal laws binding on themselves and others.

The hope is that the body of law governing society progressively embodies this ideal. Such mutual regard in laying down the moral laws that will bind one's actions differs significantly from insistence on noninterference with individual free choice, let alone with personal preferences. Conversely, the aspiration behind Kant's view of autonomy harmonizes well with the public health obligation to address collective problems through collective action.

For utilitarianism, judging the rightness of an action depends on an estimation of its subsequent practical outcome or result rather than on its conformity to principles of duty. Utilitarianism considers ethically best that course of action that will result in the greatest net benefits over harms. A utilitarian approach underlies cost-benefit analyses that weigh an intervention's costs (risks, harms, burdens, or disadvantages) against its benefits (advantages, utility, improvements, cost savings). In addition to its focus on consequences, utilitarianism is egalitarian, communitarian, and scientific in outlook. It is egalitarian in considering everyone's benefit and equally weighting each person's good, as opposed to privileging certain people. It is communitarian in attempting to increase benefits to society rather than individuals, seeking the "greatest good for the greatest number." It endeavors to be scientific by quantifying harms and benefits, accounting for probability, and calculating net benefit. Calculating net benefits over harms is less problematic when relevant factors employ a common scale of measurement, for example, weighing the financial costs of treating a disease with the cost savings from preventing that disease. Comparing different outcomes (e.g., financial costs versus quality-adjusted life years) sometimes involves difficult judgments about the relative value of each outcome. Because the utilitarian approach seeks to determine and promote the collective good based on aggregate measures, it readily lends itself to justifying public health interventions.

1.3.5 Law Versus Ethics

Laws share certain deontological features with ethical principles of action (and with religious commandments). They all define one's obligations or duties and typically take the form of rules or commands regarding what one should or should not do. They can lay down positive requirements to fulfill but more commonly establish parameters that prohibit certain actions or constrain liberty in some way. Laws do not differ from ethical rules primarily based on content, because an ethical rule can become a law without changing the rule's content. For Kant, at least, the crucial difference between ethics and law concerns one's reason for obeying; namely, whether one acts purely voluntarily out of a sense of duty or merely in external conformity with duty, either to appear to be moral or out of fear of penalty or punishment. Laws are rules enforced by penalty or punishment, which many people might otherwise break. Society can tolerate the flouting of some rules, but disobedience of more important rules can disrupt society or create danger. For these reasons, society establishes and enforces laws regarding socially important matters, not leaving their compliance up to individual prerogative. An ethical rule's enactment as law, therefore, implies agreement by society or the law's enactors on the importance of strictly regulating the behavior the law governs. Law can be a blunt instrument that effectively compels compliance, which suffices to satisfy the reasons for its enactment, even if it cannot coax voluntary obedience from an inward sense of duty.

In theory, deontologically evaluating a past or proposed action is a straightforward binary determination of compliance or noncompliance with a legal or ethical rule. In practice, however, defining a rule's scope or determining exactly which actions fall under it can prove difficult. Moreover, when different rules apply, determining which should take precedence often becomes problematic, especially when they conflict. Lying to protect a relative, for example, can put the duty to speak truthfully into conflict with familial obligations. Determining which rule takes precedence can involve reasoning clearly from ethical principles, weighing the underlying values embodied in the law, or considering the practical impact of the intervention in context. Because laws demand compliance, they are more rigid. Additional legal stipulations can prioritize or specify how to apply laws in certain situations, but doing so increases their complexity. Ethical guidelines operate more flexibly than rigid, compulsory laws and more readily accommodate compromise. With ethical guidelines, decision makers can consider and rank the underlying values the ethical rules serve to promote. Doing so allows for trade-offs between competing ethical considerations and for deciding which values it makes sense to prioritize in the given context. Conversely, law's comparative rigidity can be a virtue where only stricter oversight and enforcement will ensure compliance and establish order.

Across cultures, legal, ethical, and religious rules prohibiting basic offenses such as lying, theft and murder show considerable overlap. However, cultures vary in exactly which rules are matters of individual choice and which are matters of legal enforcement and punishment. This variability also applies to the status of rules and standards governing research on human subjects. Even within a country, significant variability can prevail in whether human subjects' research rules and standards are legal regulations or ethical guidelines (U.S. Department of Health and Human Services 2015). Some see the lack of legal regulation as a breach in protections, but others prefer guidelines, arguing that regulations tie reviewer hands, making it more difficult to make trade-offs or nuanced judgments based on moral discernment of the particulars of each case (Verweij and Dawson 2009). Because each approach offers advantages and disadvantages, political culture and local context must ultimately decide whether human subjects' research rules exist as enforceable regulations or ethical guidelines.

Regardless of whether it takes the form of guidelines or law, research ethics will govern only a fraction of the ethical issues that the field of public health must address. In many areas of public health practice, there are no specific ethical guidelines or regulations. To address ethical challenges in these areas or to address emergent challenges, the ethical practice of public health therefore requires the ability to use general ethical frameworks. Such frameworks can employ checklists of questions and stepwise procedures. However, because novel challenges continually emerge and changing contexts introduce nuances no set of rules can anticipate, public health professionals ultimately need to practice ethical decision making over time in order to cultivate moral judgment and discernment.

By laying down and enforcing what may, must, or cannot be done, legal rules function as boundaries of acceptable behavior. Ethics, science, budgets or politics, each in its own way, also can restrict the scope of action. Public health practitioners and officials therefore first need to conduct a feasibility analysis to determine the relevant limits on possible interventions or policies. Determining these limits seldom will restrict the scope of action to a single possible course. Given multiple possibilities, most people will aspire to the best course of action beyond the legal floor of minimally acceptable behavior yet within the other relevant limits. As a result, the ethical challenges public health practitioners face seldom involve stark choices between right or wrong, good or evil. A good feasibility analysis will have ruled out any unethical or illegal options or alternative courses of action in advance. Rather, the tough choices more frequently involve selecting the best alternative from among competing goods, each of which to a greater or lesser degree realizes the public health goal and embodies relevant stakeholder values.

Whereas determining and complying with the various limits on action is largely an analytic process, designing alternatives is a synthetic, creative process. Alternatives should all realize the public health goal and incorporate the perspectives and values of subject matter experts and relevant stakeholders. Deciding upon the best alternative must take into account how it will realize the public health goal in a particular context and with respect to the stakeholders. For example, advocating contraceptives to reduce unwanted teen pregnancy might seem to promise success based on efficacy studies, but ethical controversy could render such a program less than optimal in some contexts. Political culture or social norms can confer partisan advantage or disadvantage to some alternatives, while other alternatives may enjoy an advantage because of the experience and expertise of a health department. Whatever alternative practitioners finally choose, their choice will presuppose a prioritizing of values. The foregoing account highlights why public health practitioners need to see ethics as something more than a compliance matter. It transcends compliance because public health ethics also involves practical decision making, which should include stakeholder analysis, the incorporation of stakeholder values in the design of alternatives, and a fair, transparent deliberative process to evaluate alternatives.

1.4 Public Health Ethics

Compared with more established fields of practical ethics such as clinical ethics, research ethics, and bioethics, the field of public health ethics is relatively new. Consequently, many public health practitioners may be better acquainted with these more established fields than with public health ethics. In particular, practitioners may already be acquainted with the four principles these fields rely on for ethical evaluation: beneficence, nonmaleficence, respect for persons (autonomy), and justice (U.S. Department of Health, Education, and Welfare 1979; Beauchamp and Childress 2012). Being applicable to health and research, these four principles also are relevant to public health, but having arisen to address issues in other fields, they need to be adapted to a public health context. Even then, they still fall short in addressing the ethical challenges that arise in public health. Examining these related ethics fields and showing how the four principles fit into a public health context can serve by way of contrast to indicate what is distinctive about public health ethics.

1.4.1 Research Ethics, Clinical Ethics, and Bioethics: Principlism and the Four Principles

Research ethics entails the wider notion of scientific integrity but is best known and most developed in relation to medical research involving human subjects. The development of human subjects' research ethics guidelines can neither be divorced from breaches of ethical conduct in human subjects' research nor wholly reduced to a reaction to these events. But beginning with the *Nuremberg Code* (1947), balancing risks and benefits to research subjects and getting their informed consent have been cornerstones of international research ethics guidelines. Far more influential than the *Nuremberg Code*, the *Declaration of Helsinki* from the World Medical Association (WMA) is a fundamental document in international human subjects' research ethics guidelines. Its initial 1964 version included provisions for proxy consent for those with diminished autonomy. Its 1975 revision called for review of research by an independent committee, now known as an ethics review committee (WMA 1964, 1975, 2013). The use of such committees began spreading under the aegis of WHO and then in response to the HIV/AIDS pandemic, as the number of large-scale vaccine and drug trials grew in developing countries. In the United States, research regulations set forth in the Common Rule govern ethics review committees as well as all human subjects' research that receives U.S. government funding (U.S. Department of Health and Human Services 2009). In the United States, a standing ethics review committee generally functions within a specific governmental or university institution and therefore is referred to as an institutional review board (IRB). Beginning in 1982, the Council for International Organizations of Medical Sciences (CIOMS), in collaboration with WHO, proposed international ethical guidelines for biomedical research involving human subjects (CIOMS 2002).

Our discussion of these documents has only highlighted key provisions of what is required to ensure the safety of human subjects. CIOMS's most recent research guidelines (2002), for example, contain more than 60 pages of text, explanation, and commentary. But ensuring ethical conduct and scientific integrity in research requires more than the oversight function of ethical review committees. It also requires extensive training not only in research ethics but also in a number of related areas. Training and guidelines should cover, among other things, mentoring of junior researchers, authorship and publications policy, conflicts of interest that arise in partnerships and collaborative science, and data acquisition, management, sharing and ownership. Ethics training can help develop moral judgment. The hope is that training and application will enable practitioners to reason about new, difficult, or ambiguous cases in morally discerning ways.

Clinical ethics address the ethical issues that arise in clinical practice. Until the advent of bioethics, medical professionalism emphasized the health care provider's obligation to prioritize the patient's welfare, the health care provider's professional judgment about what would most benefit the patient, and the importance of establishing patient trust. The traditional model of clinical ethics was frankly paternalistic. Under the influence of bioethics, many health care providers began embracing a more patient-centered model of care that emphasized patient autonomy and informed consent. This patient-centered model conceives care as a contract between patient and provider. The emphasis on contracts strikes some as an inappropriate consumerist model that undervalues professional judgment and undermines patient trust in the medical profession. Tensions between these two models have led to a compromise that reasserts the importance of medical professionalism and clinical judgment, while acknowledging the importance of respecting patient autonomy (ABIM Foundation et al. 2002).

Bioethics has a range of meanings, the first of which applies to ethical issues brought about by advances in biomedicine and biotechnology. Ethical issues that arise from using life-sustaining technologies in end-of-life and beginning-of-life care epitomize this sense of bioethics. But bioethics also arose in response to medical paternalism and to the abuse of human subjects in medical research. Bioethics has championed informed consent, patient autonomy in doctor-patient relationships and the safety of human subjects in research. However, many bioethicists think the focus on clinical ethics and on personal autonomy unduly restricts bioethics' purview. They advocate a more holistic, social justice approach in bioethics, which has been referred to as "population-based bioethics" or "integrative bioethics" (Sodeke 2012). It can be argued that this expansion of bioethics beyond clinical ethics into population issues moves bioethics into the arena of public health ethics (Callahan and Jennings 2002).

Principlism came into being in a 1979 document called the *Belmont Report* (U.S. Department of Health, Education, and Welfare 1979). The report was the work of the U.S. National Commission for the Protection of Human Subjects of Biomedical and Behavioral Research, which convened in 1974 partly in response to the exposé of the U.S. Public Health Service Tuskegee Syphilis Study. The *Belmont Report* became the basis for revising 45 CFR 46, the so-called Common Rule, part of the legally binding U.S. Code of Federal Regulations, governing the protection of human subjects (U.S. Department of Health and Human Services 2009). The *Belmont Report* clearly explained the underlying ethical principles that informed existing regulations and provided an ethical framework for thinking about subsequent regulations. Principlism has remained the predominant ethical framework in biomedical ethics (Beauchamp and Childress 2012). Its explanatory groundwork accounts for much of its success, but its relevance to medicine and research, the prestige that attaches to these fields, and its compatibility with liberal individualism also have played a role.

Beneficence (doing good) and *nonmaleficence* (doing no harm) date back to the Hippocratic Oath as medical principles. Collapsing them both into beneficence, as the *Belmont Report* does, underscores the practical consideration that biomedical decisions generally aim to optimize net benefit over harm, rather than to maximize only benefits or minimize only harms or risks. However, these principles are distinct, not mere opposites. Not doing harm has a certain priority (first, do no harm), because not benefitting someone seems a less serious offense than doing that person harm. That priority partly reflects the human tendency more readily to forgive overlooked benefits (errors of omission) than deliberate actions resulting in harm (errors of commission).

Justice has several meanings that include due process and fair deliberative procedure, properly assessing what people are owed or due, and equitable distribution of burdens and benefits. According to philosophic tradition, justice has always functioned dually, applying to individuals but more importantly serving as an overarching principle for adjudicating competing claims in relation to the group or to other members of society. The phrase, "social justice," then, is redundant but in political contexts marked by individualism serves as a reminder of justice's social dimension. In fact, this phrase came into vogue in public health circles to counter the ideology of "market justice," which views the equal access of individuals to the free market as a valid, reliable, and preferred means for sorting out issues of economic and social justice (Beauchamp 1976). The notion of health equity, which compares different groups, primarily refers to this social dimension of justice, although denial of access to health care, a contributing factor to health inequity, violates what the individual is owed.

Respect for persons emphasizes that individuals, as agents in charge of their own lives and bodies, have the right to make decisions and choices free from undue interference. Respect for persons forms the basis of informed consent, namely, the right of patients and human research subjects to be informed of, and to assent to, medical or research procedures they might undergo, especially procedures that pose potential harm or risk. Conducting research on human subjects or performing medical procedures on patients without their prior knowledge or consent in most cases violates their personal autonomy. However, health professionals have a special (i.e., paternal) obligation to look out for the welfare of people with diminished decisional capacity—such as those in a coma or the very young—and to protect them from harm.

These four principles were originally conceived as *prima facie* principles, that is, each expressed a self-evident though not absolutely binding obligation and none had an inherent priority over another. However, in many Western countries and in the United States in particular, respect for persons has dominated discussion in bioethics, clinical ethics, and research ethics where it often takes precedence as a moral consideration over the other principles. This ascendancy most likely reflects the high value that these countries place on liberty and freedom. At any rate, in public discourse generally and in public debate about public health interventions, respect for persons often amounts to an insistence on noninterference with individual free choice or with personal preferences. Although Kant's other-regarding idea of moral autonomy, harmonizes well with collective decision making, the insistence on non-interference with personal choice often creates impediments to the implementation of public health interventions. In part for this reason, the social justice movement has had to challenge the emphasis on respect for persons in order to promote the public good and health equity.

1.4.2 Contrast between Clinical Ethics and Public Health Ethics

Table 1.2 contrasts the individual focus of clinical ethics with the community/population focus of public health ethics. Because public health and clinical practice can overlap, the items in the respective columns represent tendencies along a continuum rather than stark opposites. Where separate agencies carry out public health services and medical care, these contrasts may be more pronounced. The overlap between public health and clinical practice makes it even more important to highlight their differences to bring out distinctive features of public health ethics.

The table makes clear that the Belmont principles of beneficence (seeking benefits), nonmaleficence (avoiding harm), respect for persons, and justice remain important in public health, but must be extended to accommodate the broader scope

Table 1.2 Comparison of areas of focus/tendency in clinical ethics and public health ethics

Clinical ethics focus/tendency	Public health ethics focus/tendency
Treatment of disease and injury	Prevention of disease and injury
Medical interventions by clinical professionals	Range of interventions by various professionals
Individual benefit seeking and harm avoidance based on health care provider's fiduciary relation to a patient	Social, community, or population benefit seeking and harm avoidance based on collective action
Respect for individual patients	Relational autonomy of interdependent citizens
Professional duty to place the interests of the patient over that of provider	Duty to the community to address health concerns that individuals cannot solve and that require collective action
Authority based on the prestige and trustworthiness of the physician and the medical profession as a whole	Authority based on law, which is a principal tool of public health policy for creating health regulations
Informed consent sought from an individual patient for specific medical interventions	Community consent and building a social consensus through ongoing dialogue and collaboration with the public
Justice concerns largely limited to treating patients equally and ensuring universal access to health care	Central concern with social justice regarding health and achieving health equity

of public health interventions. This broader scope entails many types of professionals, interventions and policies that display a political and social dimension, and a wider range of activities such as community engagement, intersectoral collaboration, collective decision making, and governmental administration. As a result, prevailing political philosophies and culture will necessarily shape the way public health functions. The crucial point is that differences of scale that produce a higher order of complexity also produce qualitative differences that introduce different patterns of causation. Among other things, this means that social factors do not merely represent aggregated individual factors and so cannot always be addressed in the same way as individual factors.

1.4.3 Individual Versus Relational Autonomy

For understanding what is qualitatively distinct about public health, the contrast between respect for individual persons and the relational autonomy of community members is key. Respect for persons upholds an individual's right to make *independent* decisions free from undue pressure, but relational autonomy emphasizes that individual actions occur in the context of other people whom these actions will affect. The potential harmful impact of individual action on the welfare of others sets a limit to individual action. Relational autonomy draws attention, then, to the *interdependence* of people living in communities and to the solidarity that arises from the emotional bonds that shared lives create. Anthropology teaches that people always find themselves in a network of social relations, while evolutionary biology has shown how profoundly people are built from the physiological ground up as sociopolitical beings. Because it presupposes the social context of language and reasoning ability, individual autonomy also depends developmentally on relational autonomy. That is, people only become autonomous through relations and interactions with others. As African humanism (ubuntu philosophy) epitomizes it, *umuntu ngumuntu ngabantu*, "a person is a person through other persons" (Louw 2008). Familial and communal deliberate processes are foundational for the development of individual autonomy and provide an even deeper basis for collective decisions than the type of solidarity that comes to the fore in crises or in the face of common predicaments. Kant would reject any suggestion that developmental context, emotional bonds or feelings of solidarity underpin moral autonomy. Nevertheless, moral autonomy and relational autonomy both display an inner-directed, but other-oriented feature that readily aligns with collective decision making.

These points about the foundational character of social relatedness, solidarity, interdependence, and communal decision making do not readily align with certain features of social contract theory, on whose principles liberal democracy is based. Whereas virtually every other political tradition conceives the sociopolitical realm as a natural feature of human life, social contract theory posits humankind's original state, the state of nature, as one of solitary individualism. In this view, society or at least civil society come into existence voluntarily through a contract that creates government through the consent of the governed (Riley 1982). Although never seriously advanced as a scientific account of society's origins, social contract theory nevertheless has exerted a powerful influence as a political founding myth. As such, it has made personal liberty, free choice, and consent of the governed presumptive values of societies whose governing political philosophy rests on social contract theory. By "presumptive," we mean that the value, norm, or claim is assumed to be valid or have priority, so that the onus is on the person who objects to the presumption to justify a different value, norm, or claim.

1.4.4 Personal Autonomy as a Presumptive Value of Liberal Democracy

Personal autonomy in a clinical and research context generally means respect for the patient's right to receive an explanation of a medical procedure or research intervention, to be informed of any potential benefits or harms, and to freely choose whether to accept the procedure or participate in the research. More generally and in other contexts, personal autonomy has come to mean an insistence on liberty, free choice, and noninterference with personal preferences. Personal autonomy in this more general sense owes more to John Stuart Mill's nineteenth-century views on liberty than to Kant's eighteenth-century idea of autonomy (O'Neil 2002; Dawson 2011). An important aspect of Mill's view of liberty is the "harm principle," which holds that "the only purpose for which power can be rightfully exercised over any member of a civilized community, against his will, is to prevent harm to others" (Mill 1989). What people choose to do regarding themselves is no business of government. Interfering with this private sphere of self-determination constitutes governmental paternalism. This interference diminishes the sphere of liberty that affords individuals the chance to direct their own lives and develop their talents and character to the highest degree. A chief advantage of democratic society, one that benefits the entire society, is the creative social dynamism that emerges from the synergism between individuals who are developing their talents and abilities.

Arguably, the primary aim of the harm principle is to promote the kind of individual self-development that benefits society rather than to champion every exercise of free choice. At any rate, some have sought to distinguish this edifying version of personal autonomy from an all-encompassing version that demands undue deference to any and all personal choices and preferences merely because they are personal (O'Neill 2002; Dawson 2011; Powers et al. 2012). Presuming, or insisting on, the validity of personal autonomy makes more sense in the delimited context of medicine and biomedical research on human subjects where an individual's body is the focus of activity. It makes less sense in the far wider sphere of public health activity where social interactions and the interdependence of people come into play. Absolutizing personal autonomy in the sphere of public health would give effective veto power over every collective decision aimed at the public good to any individual who felt constrained by that decision. A more moderate version might distinguish levels of importance of personal choices and exercises of liberty. A collective decision concerning the public good could override some personal choices and limit liberty, even when they did not involve direct harm to others. Such decisions, when made in the context of a fair, transparent process of ethical deliberation involving stakeholders, are more likely to get buy-in from a community and less likely to be labeled paternalistic.

Because public health considers the relation between individuals and the collective good, it necessarily has a political dimension. How a country's political culture balances this relation will drive and constrain public health practice and so shape the nature of the ethical frameworks that are appropriate to a country's politics (Hyder et al. 2008). In the brief history of public health ethics, the most important ethics frameworks have emerged in the political context of liberal democracy. Many of these frameworks reflect the tensions between public health's obligation to act collectively for the common good and the presumptive value of personal autonomy. The principle of least infringement and Kass's *code of restraint* illustrate the effort to mediate such tensions (Kass 2001). The code of restraint strives to balance autonomy claims against the obligation to safeguard community health by determining what intervention most effectively protects health while minimally infringing on liberty. In a liberal political context that recognizes Mill's harm principle, this strategy justifies the trumping of personal autonomy as long as imminent harm threatens the populace, for example, in a deadly outbreak of contagious disease. But where the threat of harm to others is indirect or not immediate, as with the obesity epidemic, the harm principle less readily justifies a liberty-limiting intervention such as banning or taxing certain foods. Utilitarian approaches that weigh the health advantages of intervention and the disadvantages of obesity clearly support obesity intervention, but limiting interventions to those that do not restrict personal choices also have limited effectiveness. In Chap. 6, Jennings considers the relative merits of these approaches in his overview of the ethical issues in environmental and occupational public health. His discussion raises the question of the extent to which an ethical framework should adapt itself to the presumptive values of the political context or should reflect the nature of the practical field under investigation. To some extent, it must do both.

The three-step framework offered in the next section is designed to guide decision makers, through questions, to assess the ethical dimensions of a case, including which moral considerations (e.g., population utility or liberty) may have more weight than others, given the issue or context. This contextual approach provides the flexibility and starting point for deliberation to accommodate the issues globally and to uncover the varying perspectives of stakeholders with potentially different presumptive moral norms (e.g., solidarity versus individual rights).

1.5 Ethical Frameworks

What at first glance demarcates public health ethics from related fields of health ethics are the ethical problems that public health professionals typically encounter in their practice and the ethical frameworks used in practice to address these problems. Regarding these ethical problems, this casebook offers a representative, but not exhaustive, sample. Regarding ethical frameworks, this chapter has suggested two competing criteria for choosing. On the one hand, ethical frameworks should be grounded in their topics. Dawson (2011) expresses the point succinctly by arguing that public health should be the foundation of public health ethics. Accordingly, we have presented a view of public health ethics that builds on the definitions of public, health, and public health, and on the goals of public health practice. But we have also defined ethics and indicated how public health ethics draws on numerous ethical theories and can provide a moral guide grounded in the norms of benefiting others, preventing harms, and providing utility. We have pointed out its distinguishing principles based on the facts of community and interdependence. Lastly, we have situated public health ethics within the process of ethical decision making about which options are the most justifiable means to achieve public health goals in a particular context. In the end, grounding public health ethics in public health may require public health leaders to have the courage to advocate public health values and goals, even when that position is unpopular. Such a stance may be justified, for example, where the feasibility of a much-needed public health intervention requires a long-range strategy to change social norms or build social consensus.

On the other hand, precisely because public health itself is practical, pragmatic, and community oriented, an ethical framework designed for it must accommodate itself to a country's presumptive values and political culture. This consideration illustrates that the feasibility of public health interventions usually depends on their alignment with the political culture, while their success usually implies public acceptance. Many established frameworks, like that of Kass, seem designed with a liberal political context in mind that gives presumptive weight to individual liberty, which may limit the range of interventions that can be justified. Newer approaches to ethical analysis in public health place more emphasis on social values like equity and solidarity, although these newer approaches often are difficult to put into practice (Lee 2012). In addition, while newer approaches may offer clear reasons to justify a broader range of interventions, the reasons may be less persuasive if they do not consider the presumptive values in context. For example, in Chap. 3, Daniels discusses the ethical conflicts that arise during pandemics between the standard goal of improving population health and emergency contexts that demand allocating scarce resources in a way that treats people fairly. He asks, if in the pandemic context we believe that saving the most lives trumps giving priority to those who are sickest, can we justify revising the usual priority given to the sickest in health care?

Arguably, what would be most useful is not a set of frameworks designed for specific presumptive values, but, rather, a framework that can accommodate any presumptive values and consider them in relation to values rooted in public health or in context. The three-step framework that follows is a straightforward tool to help practitioners analyze the ethical tensions in a particular context. It addresses Daniels' tough question directly by considering health care's presumptive prioritization of the sickest in relation to the public health value of saving the most lives in a pandemic.

1.6 A Three-Step Approach to Public Health Decision Making

We offer the following framework, drawn from public health practice and described by Bernheim et al. (2007), as an example of an analytic tool that can guide decision makers through reasoning and deliberation. It is not meant to introduce a rigid application of ethical principles, nor does it presume that any one moral norm has greater weight that trumps other norms. Instead, the questions are designed to help decision makers clarify whether a particular moral norm (e.g., solidarity or liberty or equity) is weightier than others in context, and if so, then strong reasons must be offered to override the presumptive moral norm. For example, during an epidemic, equity may carry presumptive weight and trump other moral norms in some contexts. Ethicists at the Joint Centre for Bioethics offered the following insight from the SARS experience:

> In the case of an epidemic, it is important to control the spread of the disease, but as much attention should be paid to the rights of the noninfected patients who need urgent medical care. There may be as many people who died from other illnesses and could not get into hospital as there were who died from SARS. Equity is required in the amount of attention given to a wide array of people, including patients with and without SARS. Accountability for making reasonable decisions, transparency and fairness are expected …. (Singer et al. 2003)

The questions clarify the relevant factors, such as stakeholder claims, alternative actions, and possible justifications for deciding on one course of action.

1.6.1 An Approach to Ethical Analysis and Justification in Context

Step I: Analyze the Ethical Dimensions of the Public Health Issue and Context

- What are the risks, harms, or concerns?
- What are the appropriate public health goals in this context?
- What is the scope and legitimacy of legal authority, and which laws and regulations apply?
- What are the moral norms and claims of stakeholders, and how strong are they?

- Are precedent legal or ethical cases relevant for identifying the presumptive moral norms?
- Which features of the social-cultural-historical context apply?
- Do professional codes of ethics provide guidance?

Step II: Formulate Alternative Courses of Action and Evaluate their Ethical Dimensions

- What are the short- and long-term options, given the assessment of the public health issue and context in Step I?
- What are the ethical dimensions and tensions of each option?
  - Utility: Does the public health action produce the best balance of benefits over harms and other costs?
  - Equity and Justice: Is health equity advanced? Are the benefits and burdens distributed fairly (distributive justice)? Is there appropriate public participation, including the participation of affected parties (procedural justice)?
  - Respect for Individual and Community Interests: Does the public health action respect self-determination and human rights, as well as civic roles and community values (e.g., trustworthiness, solidarity) (Dawson and Jennings 2012)?
- Other Moral Considerations in Public Health: Are there other moral considerations in public health that are important to consider? (For example, reciprocity, solidarity, protecting privacy and confidentiality; keeping promises and commitments; or disclosing information and speaking honestly, sometimes grouped as transparency.)

Step III: Provide Justification for a Particular Public Health Decision

- Effectiveness: Is the public health action likely to be effective?
- Proportionality: Will the probable benefits of the action outweigh the infringed moral considerations?
- Necessity: Is the action necessary (i.e., will overriding a conflicting ethical norm achieve an important public health goal)?
- Least Infringement: Is the public health action the least restrictive means available?
- Public Justification: Can decision makers offer public justification in the political and cultural context that stakeholders, the public, and those most affected find acceptable?

Consider the following scenario described by Melnick (2015a). A family adopted several children from a developing country with a high tuberculosis (TB) prevalence, including multidrug-resistant TB (MDR-TB). Screening on arrival revealed that the children were infected with TB but did not have active disease and were not contagious. The family has strong religious beliefs about medical care and refused treatment, immunizations, and other preventive care. The children were homeschooled, but they did attend community activities. Soon after arrival one of the teenage children developed TB symptoms, and after several months the family consulted a pediatrician who diagnosed active pulmonary TB. Cultures revealed that the child had MDR-TB. Directly observed treatment (DOT) is part of the standard of care for active TB in the United States, and the local health department nurse visited the family to provide DOT. The parents objected to the home visit, stating that DOT was an invasion of their privacy and parental rights. The health department has the statutory authority to require in-person DOT and even impose isolation of the case and removal from the family to protect the public's health. What should health officials do? Drawing on questions in Step I, health officials might first clarify the harms and risks and the goals of public health action. The public health goals are to prevent TB transmission and ensure the child receives appropriate care. Requiring DOT creates risks for the child such as side effects from treatment and social and behavioral harms associated with isolation and loss of privacy during visits, and potential community harm, by driving cases underground. Who are the stakeholders, and what are their moral claims?

> There are several stakeholders: the child, the child's family (including parents but also several siblings), and the public, which expects the health department to protect the community from TB. Regarding moral claims, the child has some expectations of freedom of movement, and privacy; the family has similar expectations regarding privacy, respect for parental rights, and the freedom to administer medications to their child at a convenient time and place. However, these claims are not absolute, and competing moral claims can outweigh them. The child has a moral claim that could compete with her parent's claim, specifically, that receiving DOT will reduce the risk of inappropriate treatment and relapse compared to having her parents administer the medications. In addition, the public has a moral claim based on two expectations: (*1*) that the health department will protect the community from TB, and (*2*) that people contagious for TB and other infectious diseases will protect others by behaving in an appropriate manner, including staying home when contagious and cooperating with treatment recommendations. This is especially concerning in this case because the immigration health officials had discussed the risks with the parents, warning them to seek treatment as soon as the child developed symptoms, yet the parents waited several months before taking the child to a pediatrician (Melnick 2015a, 175).

Consider another short scenario that illustrates the value of exploring options under Step II. A new policy is being considered that would require parental consent for newborn screening. Parental consent currently is not required, although newborn testing is not conducted if there are parental objections. The health department has been asked to take a position on the pending policy. What position should the health department take? What are the options?

Options include mandatory screening without consent, routine screening with advance notification (Opt In), routine screening without advance notification (Opt Out) (i.e., screening and testing done unless the parents object), voluntary screening (i.e., screening requires full consent and might also include a pre- and post-counseling session with each new mother). Some arguments that might be offered against requiring parental consent focus on the fact that (1) the benefits of screening are obvious and substantial, relative to potential harms; (2) parents have few good reasons to justify parental refusal and place their child at risk for harm; (3) obtaining consent from each parent is difficult, costly, and an unwarranted expenditure of time and money; and (4) the history of newborn screening has become acceptable and routine. Some arguments that may be raised for requiring parental consent include (1) parental consent is necessary because refusal of newborn screening is reasonable given the increasing list of diseases included in the battery of newborn tests and the low probability of many of these diseases; (2) newborn screening can have adverse consequences such as psychological harms associated with false positive tests; (3) long-term parental caretaking is enhanced when parents are included in all clinical decisions about their children; and (4) the process of obtaining consent need not be time-consuming or burdensome but rather can help enhance the health professional-patient relationship (CDC 2012). Which arguments are stronger, and which of the options are the most ethically justifiable? The answer may depend on the social and political context in which the issue is considered, and which ethical values carry weight in that context. Whether there were presumptive values in place would be explored through the questions in Step I, which examines previous cases, the applicable laws and policies, and stakeholder claims in context. So, for example, in a society that has a strong moral norm or presumption for solidarity, there could be a presumption for continuing population newborn screening without parental consent. On the other hand, for a society that has a liberal political context that has a presumption for individual liberty, there may be a presumption for an option that seeks more explicit consent from parents. In either context, the presumptive moral norms are not determinative but are rebuttable, so the arguments or reasons to override those norms must be stronger.

Consider a third case from public health practice in which a person (the index case) infected with primary syphilis and HIV refuses to provide contact information for his wife, insisting that he and his wife had not had sexual relations for several years. Contact tracing and partner notification have been important tools historically for public health officials, although these interventions can involve thorny ethical tensions, requiring health officials to justify their decisions. In this type of situation, health officers will consider several options, starting with those that infringe least on the index case's choices. For example, they might first provide to the index case additional information and assurance about confidentiality while allowing him to notify his wife voluntarily, either alone or with the help of public health workers. If this proves unsuccessful, other interventions might be considered, such as incentives, the threat of restrictions such as isolation, or attempts to notify the wife without his knowledge or consent. Each of these options would be determined in context, using the questions in Step III. Questions considered may include (1) Would the options likely accomplish the goal of warning and testing the wife without risking greater harm or possible adverse outcomes for the wife (e.g., domestic violence, loss of income, or loss of housing)? (2) Is there significant concern about a risk of harm to others, such as family members or children, so that the burdens and benefits of the action would not be distributed fairly? (3) Is the option the least restrictive of the important moral claims of the stakeholders? (4) Is it necessary now to override conflicting claims to achieve the public health goal? Answering the questions in Step III helps decision makers consider whether actions are justifiable. As one health officer explains, "Public health officials should justify their decisions with deliberations that build not only community support and trust, but also build support and trust from the individuals and families directly affected" (Melnick 2015b).

As the scenarios illustrate, public health is a social and political undertaking. Thus, making difficult choices in public health implicates important social, cultural, and political norms embedded in a particular context and community of stakeholders (Childress and Bernheim 2008). Regardless of whether decision makers work in a government public health agency, community nonprofit, nongovernmental organization (NGO) from another country, or a global organization, decision makers must rigorously assess the public health issue *in context*, to minimally be able to act "in ways that preserve the moral foundations of social collaboration" at the core of collective health activity (Calabresi and Bobbitt 1978).

The context specifically includes attention to stakeholders and relationships among public health stakeholders and community members, including the common understanding of their roles, obligations, and collaborations. Especially in global public health, it is important to note that even the decision makers are stakeholders, in some sense, and often, when they are health professionals, they have their own social-cultural norms and their own professional codes that can provide guidance. Appeals to the codes of particular professions, however, do not provide a sufficient justification for a public health decision, since justifications should be grounded in a society's widely shared ethical values and norms.

Engaging stakeholders and addressing claims, especially those of the people most affected by a public health issue, in ethical analysis, is especially important and can sometimes support and strengthen the collaboration and cohesion needed for public acceptance of a decision. The ways to engage and reason with stakeholders in an ethical analysis will vary in different settings and communities, depending on community values, cohesion, and expectations, and can range from establishing an ethics board for deliberation, to gathering information from focus groups or social media, to including stakeholder representatives on the decision-making team. Stakeholder norms and claims are a critical feature for an ethical analysis in order to achieve a primary goal in public health—the development and maintenance of relationships of trust, defined in a report from IOM as "the belief that those with whom one interacts will take one's interests into account, even in situations in which one is not in a position to recognize, evaluate, or thwart a potentially negative course of action by those trusted" (IOM 1996).

Ethical analysis is a dynamic process and, particularly for the practice of public health, is best accomplished through group deliberations that involve understanding others' perspectives and thinking independently and imaginatively. Public health professionals often have to decide how best to realize numerous important societal norms and values when pursuing public health goals. Ethical tensions do occur in public health and at times require overriding an important principle, value, or moral consideration to undertake a justifiable public health action. However, a structured ethical analysis can often lead to imaginative alternatives that transcend or minimize ethical tensions and to decisions that most or many stakeholders find acceptable.

References

ABIM Foundation, ACP–ASIM Foundation, and European Federation of Internal Medicine. 2002. Medical professionalism in the new millennium: A physician charter. *Annals of Internal Medicine* 136: 243–246.

Bartlett, R., and S. Collins. 2011. *Aristotle's Nicomachean ethics*. Chicago/London: University of Chicago Press.

Beauchamp, D.E. 1976. Public health as social justice. *Inquiry* 13(1): 3–14.

Beauchamp, T.L., and J.F. Childress. 2012. *Principles of biomedical ethics*, 7th ed. New York: Oxford University Press.

Bernheim, R.G., P. Nieburg, and R.J. Bonnie. 2007. Ethics and the practice of public health. In *Law in public health practice*, 2nd ed, ed. R.A. Goodman, 110–135. New York: Oxford University Press.

Blane, D. 1999. The life course, the social gradient, and health. *Social Determinants of Health* 2: 54–77.

Blas, E., L. Gilson, M.P. Kelly, et al. 2008. Addressing social determinants of health inequities: What can the state and civil society do? *Lancet* 372(9650): 1684–1689.

Braveman, P. 2006. Health disparities and health equity: Concepts and measurement. *Annual Review of Public Health* 27: 167–194.

Brunk, C.E., L. Haworth, and B. Lee. 1991. *Value assumption in risk assessment: A case study of the alachlor controversy*. Waterloo: Wilfrid Laurier University Press.

Calabresi, G., and P. Bobbitt. 1978. *Tragic choices*. New York: Norton.

Callahan, D., and B. Jennings. 2002. Ethics and public health: Forging a strong relationship. *American Journal of Public Health* 92(2): 169–176.

Centers for Disease Control and Prevention (CDC). 2011. *Advancing excellence & integrity of CDC science. Public health ethics*. http://www.cdc.gov/od/science/integrity/phethics/. Accessed 14 Feb 2014.

Centers for Disease Control and Prevention. 2012. Unit 2: Ethics and the law. In *Public Health Law 101: A foundational case for public health practices*. Public Health Law Program, Centers for Disease Control and Prevention. http://www.cdc.gov/phlp/publications/phl_101.html. Accessed 24 June 2015.

Childress, J.F., and R.G. Bernheim. 2008. Public health ethics: Public justification and public trust. *Bundesgesundheitsblatt, Gesundheitsforschung, Gesundheitsschutz* 51(2): 158–163. doi:10.1007/s00103-008-0444-6.

Childress, J.R., R.R. Faden, R.D. Gaare, et al. 2002. Public health ethics: Mapping the terrain. *Journal of Law, Medicine & Ethics* 30(2). 170–178.

Council for International Organizations of Medical Sciences (CIOMS). 2002. *International ethical guidelines for biomedical research involving human subjects*. Geneva: Council for International Organizations of Medical Sciences. http://www.cioms.ch/publications/layout_guide2002.pdf. Accessed 14 Feb 2014.

Dawson, A. 2011. Resetting the parameters: Public health as the foundation for public health ethics. In *Public health ethics: Key concepts and issues in policy and practice*, ed. A. Dawson, 1–19. Cambridge: Cambridge University Press.

Dawson, A., and B. Jennings. 2012. The place of solidarity in public health ethics. *Public Health Reviews* 34: 65–79.

Dawson, A., and M. Verweij. 2007. The meaning of "public" in public health. In *Ethics, prevention, and public health*, ed. A. Dawson and M. Verweij, 13–29. Oxford: Clarendon Press.

Faden, R., and S., Shebaya. 2010. Public health ethics. In *Stanford encyclopedia of philosophy*, ed. E. N. Zalta. http://plato.stanford.edu/archives/sum2010/entries/publichealth-ethics/. Accessed 14 Feb 2014.

Freiler, A., C. Muntaner, K. Shankardass, et al. 2013. Glossary for the implementation of Health in All Policies (HiAP). *Journal of Epidemiology and Community Health* 67: 1068–1072. doi:10.1136/jech-2013-202731.

Gregor, M., J. Timmermann, and C.M. Korsgaard (eds.). 2012. *Kant: Groundwork of the metaphysics of morals*. New York: Cambridge University Press.

Hyder, A., M. Merritt, J. Ali, N. Tran, K. Subramaniam, and T. Akhtar. 2008. Integrating ethics, health policy and health systems in low- and middle-income countries: Case studies from Malaysia and Pakistan. *Bulletin of the World Health Organization* 86(8): 606–610.

Institute of Medicine (IOM). 1988. *The future of public health*. Washington, DC: National Academy Press.

Institute of Medicine. 1996. *Healthy communities: New partnerships for the future of public health*. Washington, DC: National Academy Press.

Jennings, B. 2007. Public health and civic republicanism. In *Ethics, prevention, and public health*, ed. A. Dawson and M. Verweij, 30–58. Oxford: Oxford University Press.

Kass, N. 2001. An ethics framework for public health. *American Journal of Public Health* 91(11): 1776–1782.

Kickbusch, I. 2003. The contribution of the World Health Organization to a new public health and health promotion. *American Journal of Public Health* 93(3): 383–388.

Krimsky, S., and A. Plough. 1988. *Environmental hazards: Communicating risks as a social process*. Dover: Auburn House.

Lee, L.M. 2012. Public health ethics theory: Review and path to convergence. *Journal of Law Medicine & Ethics* 40(1): 85–98.

Louw, D.J. 2008. The African concept of ubuntu and restorative justice. In *Handbook of restorative justice: A global perspective*, ed. D. Sullivan and L. Tifft, 161–171. New York: Routledge.

Marks, L., D.J. Hunter, and R. Alderslade. 2011. *Strengthening public health capacity and services in Europe: A concept paper*. Geneva: World Health Organization. http://www.euro.who.int/__data/assets/pdf_file/0007/152683/e95877.pdf. Accessed 10 Dec 2013.

Marmot, M. 2007. Achieving health equity: From root causes to fair outcomes. *Lancet* 370: 1153–1163.

Melnick, A.L. 2015a. Chapter 8, Containing Communicable Diseases: Personal Control Measures. In Essentials of public health ethics, ed. R.G. Bernheim, J.F. Childress, R.J. Bonnie, and A.L. Melnick, Burlington: Jones & Bartlett Learning.

Melnick, A.L. 2015b. Chapter 6, Case finding: Screening, testing, and contact tracing. In Essentials of public health ethics, ed. R.G. Bernheim, J.F. Childress, R.J. Bonnie, and A.L. Melnick, Burlington: Jones & Bartlett Learning.

Michaels, D. 2008. *Doubt is their product: How industry's assault on science threatens your health*. New York: Oxford University Press.

Mill, J.S. 1989. In *On liberty and other writings*, ed. S. Collini. Cambridge: Cambridge University Press.

Nuremberg Code. 1947. *Trials of war criminals before the Nuremberg Military Tribunals under Control Council Law No. 10*, vol. 2, 181–182. Washington, DC: U.S. Government Printing Office, 1949. http://www.hhs.gov/ohrp/archive/nurcode.html. Accessed 3 June 2014.

O'Neill, O. 2002. *Autonomy and trust in bioethics (Gifford lecture)*. Cambridge: Cambridge University Press.

Ortmann, L., and J. Iskander. 2013. The role of public health ethics in vaccine decision making: Insights from the Centers for Disease Control and Prevention. In *Vaccinophobia and vaccine controversies of the 21st century*, ed. A. Chatterjee, 291–305. New York: Springer.

Powers, M., and R. Faden. 2006. *Social justice: The moral foundations of public health and health policy*. New York: Oxford University Press.

Powers, M., R. Faden, and Y. Saghai. 2012. Liberty, mill and the framework of public health ethics. *Public Health Ethics* 5(1): 6–15.

Public Health Functions Steering Committee. 1994. *Essential public health services*. http://www.health.gov/phfunctions/public.htm. Accessed 2 Jan 2014.

Public Health Leadership Society. 2002. *Principles of the ethical practice of public health*. http://phls.org/CMSuploads/Principles-of-the-Ethical-Practice-of-PH-Version-2.2-68496.pdf. Accessed 1 Feb 2013.

Riley, P. 1982. *Will and political legitimacy: A critical exposition of social contract theory in Hobbes, Lock, Rousseau, Kant, and Hegel*. Cambridge, MA: Harvard University Press.

Ruger, J. 2010. *Health and social justice*. New York: Oxford University Press.

Sen, A. 2009. *The idea of justice*. London: Allen Lane.

Singer, P.A., S.R. Benatar, M. Bernstein, et al. 2003. Ethics and SARS: Lessons from Toronto. *British Medical Journal* 327(7427): 1342–1344.

Sodeke, S. 2012. Tuskegee University experience challenges conventional wisdom: Is integrative bioethics practice the new ethics for the public's health? *Journal of Health Care for the Poor and Underserved* 23(4): 15–33. doi:10.1353/hpu.2012.0169.

U.S. Department of Health and Human Services. 2009. *Code of Federal Regulations, Title 45, Part 46, Protection of Human Subjects*. http://www.hhs.gov/ohrp/humansubjects/guidance/45cfr46.html. Accessed 3 June 2014.

U.S. Department of Health and Human Services. 2015. *International Compilation of Human Research Standards*. Office for Human Research Protections. http://www.hhs.gov/ohrp/international/intlcompilation/2015internationalcompilation.doc.doc. Accessed 23 June 2015.

U.S. Department of Health, Education, and Welfare. 1979. *The Belmont report: Ethical principles and guidelines for the protection of human subjects of research*, Publication No. (OS) 78-0012. Washington, DC: U.S. Government Printing Office.

Verweij, M., and A. Dawson. 2009. Public health ethics: A research agenda. *Public Health Ethics* 2(1): 1–6.

Whitehead, M. 1992. The concepts and principles of equity and health. *International Journal of Health Services* 22(3): 429–445.

Winslow, C.-E.A. 1920. The untilled fields of public health. *Science* 51(1306): 23–33.

World Health Organization (WHO). 2006. *Constitution of the World Health Organization–Basic documents*, 45th ed., suppl. www.who.int/governance/eb/who_constitution_en.pdf. Accessed 29 Apr 2014.

World Health Organization (WHO). 2007. *A conceptual framework for action on the social determinants of health (Discussion paper draft)*. Geneva: Commission on Social Determinants of Health, World Health Organization. http://www.who.int/social_determinants/resources/csdh_framework_action_05_07.pdf. Accessed 4 Mar 2014.

World Health Organization (WHO). 2008. *Closing the gap in a generation: Health equity through action on the social determinants of health*, Final Report of the Commission on Social Determinants of Health. Geneva: Commission on Social Determinants of Health, World Health Organization. http://whqlibdoc.who.int/publications/2008/9789241563703_eng.pdf. Accessed 4 Mar 2014.

World Medical Association (WMA). 1964, 1975, 2013. *WMA Declaration of Helsinki—Ethical principles for medical research involving human subjects*. http://www.wma.net/en/30publications/10policies/b3/. Accessed 4 Mar 2014.

Chapter 2
Essential Cases in the Development of Public Health Ethics

Lisa M. Lee, Kayte Spector-Bagdady, and Maneesha Sakhuja

2.1 Introduction

While "public health" has been defined as what society does to "assure the conditions for people to be healthy" (Institute of Medicine 2003, xi), public health *ethics* is a "systematic process to clarify, prioritize, and justify possible courses of public health action based on ethical principles, values and beliefs of stakeholders, and scientific and other information" (Schools of Public Health Application Service 2013). Despite several important characteristics that distinguish public health from clinical medicine, at its start public health ethics borrowed heavily from clinical ethics and research ethics (see Chap. 1). In the 1980s, with the onset of the AIDS epidemic and unprecedented advances in biomedicine, the inability of clinical ethics to accommodate the ethical challenges in public health from existing frameworks led pioneering ethicists to reframe and adapt clinical ethics from an individual and autonomy focused approach to one that better reflected the tension between individual rights and the health of a group or population (Bayer et al. 1986; Beauchamp 1988; Kass 2001; Childress et al. 2002; Upshur 2002). Others called for public health ethics to emphasize relational ethics and political philosophy (Jennings 2007). More recently, some authors have suggested outlining foundational values from which operating principles for public health ethics can be articulated only after careful consideration of the goals and purpose of public health. This approach would require us to establish a clear definition of the moral endeavor of public

---

The opinions, findings, and conclusions of the authors do not necessarily reflect the official position, views, or policies of the editors, the editors' host institutions, or the authors' host institutions.

L.M. Lee, PhD, MA, MS (✉) • K. Spector-Bagdady, JD, M Bioethics
M. Sakhuja, MHS
Presidential Commission for the Study of Bioethical Issues, Washington, DC, USA
e-mail: lisa.lee@bioethics.gov

D.H. Barrett et al. (eds.), *Public Health Ethics: Cases Spanning the Globe*,
Public Health Ethics Analysis 3, DOI 10.1007/978-3-319-23847-0_2

health as a field (Lee 2012) and construct an ethical framework stemming from the nature of it (Dawson 2011).

A versatile framework for public health ethics must accommodate public health in practice and research. In public health practice, an ethics framework must guide decisions about activities like infectious disease control, primary prevention, and environmental health, as well as newer expectations of public health such as chronic disease control and preparedness. In public health research, biomedical and behavioral research ethics provide a great deal of guidance—but research that focuses on population-based outcomes and community concerns reveals additional ethical considerations.

A fundamental tension in public health is one between individual- and population-based interests. Various political traditions place different value on each, and these values can fluctuate within the same political structure over time. When authorities intervene to affect population health, they must find an equilibrium between individual and population interests in all political contexts, whether authoritarian, socialist, or liberal individualist. To consider individual interests as well as population interests, regardless of the philosophical tradition within which these interests are valued, is a challenge for a public health ethics framework. The cases we present in this chapter illustrate how this equilibrium between individual and population interests has been established in the context of dynamic political and historical influences.

One way of approaching public health ethics deliberation is through the method of casuistry, defined as "the interpretation of moral issues, using procedures of reasoning based on paradigms and analogies, leading to the formulation of expert opinion about the existence and stringency of particular moral obligations, framed in terms of rules or maxims that are general but not universal or invariable, since they hold good with certainty only in the typical conditions of the agent and the circumstances of action" (Jonsen and Toulmin 1988, 297). Consideration of case studies and the use of casuistic methods of resolution of morally similar cases through interpretation of ethical principles have played important roles in the development of public health ethics—particularly before public health ethics was viewed as distinct from clinical ethics. Individual case studies enable discussions about which ethical norms we should adopt for the practice of public health and how public health professionals should deliberate to resolve ethical problems in practice (Centers for Disease Control and Prevention [CDC] 2012). In this chapter, we review several seminal cases that shaped the ethics of public health research and practice over the past century to provide the foundation of current public health ethics and lay the groundwork for a casebook to enable casuist analysis.

Our first case example is *Jacobson v Massachusetts*, set in the beginning of the twentieth century. *Jacobson* is a foundational U.S. public health legal case that supports states' rights to create and enforce laws and regulations that limit individual autonomy to protect the public's health and stop the spread of communicable disease. Our second case study, from the mid-1900s, looks at two ethically troubling U.S. Public Health Service (PHS) protocols for studying sexually transmitted diseases (STDs) in the U.S. state of Alabama and Guatemala. These experiments, like most research protocols, were not intended to benefit the subjects; rather their intent was the broader benefit of the public's health. They show however, that researchers, despite the apparent motivation to advance public health, can breach public health research ethics and harm research subjects. The final case, a contemporary example of the New York City A1C Registry to monitor and address the diabetes epidemic in the city, demonstrates how addressing the ethical dimensions of public health interventions can facilitate their implementation. This case moves our focus from public health interventions targeting communicable diseases to those supporting secondary prevention of noncommunicable diseases. It focuses on the ethical dimensions that can arise when technological advances in communication might affect individual privacy. Unlike the consistent movement forward with which casuistry has moved clinical ethics, (Jonsen 1991), the outcomes in the cases we describe here shaped, and sometimes jolted, the nascent field of public health ethics.

These three case studies, occurring within the same political structure over the span of a century, illustrate the tension between individual autonomy and protection of public health in very different ways. The first case depicts a situation where the balance tipped in favor of protection of the public's health in the context of infectious diseases. The second case demonstrates unconscionable exploitation of vulnerable research subjects for the benefit of other communities. Finally, the third case presents a situation in which solutions to public health problems based on technological advances and access to data can strike a balance with individual health privacy concerns. Each case illustrates the quest for equilibrium between individual and population interests.

2.2 Case Study: *Jacobson v. Massachusetts*

The earliest activities associated with modern public health are sanitation and infectious disease control. From the first public health surveillance system in colonial America that required tavern keepers in Rhode Island to report contagious disease, to John Snow removing the Broad Street pump handle in London to end the 1854 cholera epidemic, control of communicable diseases has been firmly in the jurisdiction of public health (Thacker 2010). Discovery of the physiological mechanisms of vaccines in the eighteenth century gave us new tools to control infectious diseases but also raised critical questions about how to carry out—effectively and ethically—policies and plans that support individual and community health.

2.2.1 *Background*

By the turn of the twentieth century, public health campaigns—including improved hygiene, sanitation, and access to safer food and water—had already extended the average life expectancy in the United States (CDC 1999). But infectious diseases were still the leading cause of mortality, with tuberculosis, pneumonia, and diarrheal disease accounting for 30 % of U.S. citizen deaths (Cohen 2000). Evolving support for the government's involvement in protecting public health led to the establishment of hygienic laboratories in 1887 (Kass 1986). These laboratories continue today to provide essential services such as diagnostics, public health surveillance, research, and vaccine development.

Edward Jenner, who discovered that a vaccine for smallpox could be created using cowpox lesions, sent his vaccine from England to Benjamin Waterhouse at Harvard University in 1800 (Riedel 2005). After successfully vaccinating the members of his household, Waterhouse began selling the vaccine in Boston, Massachusetts (Kass 1986). Not all physicians vaccinated as meticulously as Waterhouse however, and in one unfortunate incident, adulterated smallpox vaccine caused an epidemic in the Boston area (Kass 1986).

As interest in and concern about the vaccine grew, the Board of Health of Boston decided to perform one of the first controlled clinical trials in U.S. history, which eventually demonstrated effectiveness of the vaccine (Kass 1986). A century later, Massachusetts had established vaccination campaigns, but smallpox persisted: One hundred cases were reported in Massachusetts in 1900 with 2314 cases by 1902 (Parmet et al. 2005). The Board of Health had originally promoted a voluntary vaccination scheme until January 1902 when two children, one in Boston, died of post-vaccination complications within a month of each other (Willrich 2011). After voluntary efforts stalled, the Board ordered mandatory vaccination in February, but did not enforce the order. After an outbreak sent another 50 adults and children to the hospital and caused seven deaths, the Board voted that the regulations needed to be enforced (Willrich 2011).

Local public health officials employed creative ways to follow enforcement orders, "many of which were scientifically sound but not all of which were apt to inspire public trust" (Parmet et al. 2005, 653). The Boston Herald, for example, reported in March 1902 that public health doctors and guards forcibly vaccinated "Italians, negroes and other employees" (Parmet et al. 2005, 653). Despite the success of the smallpox vaccine in curtailing disease, anti-vaccinationists described compulsory vaccination as "the greatest crime of the age" and as "more important than the slavery question, because it is debilitating the whole human race" (Washington Post 1905; Gostin 2008, 122). Pro-vaccinationists were as polarizing, describing the debate as "a conflict between intelligence and ignorance, civilization and barbarism" (New York Times 1885; Gostin 2008, 122).

2.2.2 Case Description

It was in this context that the U.S. Supreme Court heard *Jacobson v. Massachusetts*, which despite, and perhaps because of, the vastly different ways it has been interpreted and applied since then, is arguably the most important legal public health case ever decided in the United States (Gostin 2005). Under the doctrine of "police power," it had already been established in the late 1800s that states had the authority to enforce "sanitary laws, laws for the protection of life, liberty, health or property within its limits [and] laws to prevent persons and animals suffering under contagious or infectious diseases …" within their own boundaries (R. R. Co. v. Husen 1877, 465, 472). In 1885, the Supreme Court confirmed that this included ensuring conditions essential to the "safety, health, peace, good order and morals of the community" as "even liberty itself… is only freedom from restraint under conditions essential to the equal enjoyment of the same right by others" (Crowley v. Christensen 1890, 86, 89).

In 1902, in response to the increase in smallpox cases discussed above, the Cambridge, Massachusetts Board of Health issued an order, which became law, requiring citizens be vaccinated against smallpox or pay a $5 fine (the equivalent of about $135 in 2015) (Massachusetts Revised Laws 1902; Commonwealth v. Henning Jacobson 1903; Mariner et al. 2005). Henning Jacobson, a Cambridge minister, refused both the vaccination *and* to pay the fine. He argued he had previously received the smallpox vaccination in Sweden as a child and had experienced "great and extreme suffering, for a long period" as a result and that one of his sons had experienced adverse events from vaccination as well (Commonwealth v. Henning Jacobson 1903, 246). Jacobson argued that the law was thus "hostile to the inherent right of every freeman to care for his own body and health in such way as to him seems best …." (Jacobson v. Massachusetts 1905, 26). The case went to trial.

At trial, Jacobson argued that his history of adverse reaction to the smallpox vaccine should grant him an exception from the law. However, the law did not actually provide for such exceptions for adults (as it did for children). Jacobson was found guilty of "the crime of refusing vaccination" (Willrich 2011, 285). He appealed to the superior court, where the judge again ruled that Jacobson's medical history was "immaterial" to his legal violation. The judge also refused Jacobson's plea to tell the jury that the law was a violation of the constitutions of Massachusetts and the United States because it offered no such exception. The court again found Jacobson guilty (Willrich 2011).

Jacobson fared no better in the Massachusetts Supreme Court. It too rejected Jacobson's evidence of his prior adverse experience with the vaccination as well as his son's as "matters depending upon his personal opinion, which could not be taken as correct, or given effect, merely because he made it a ground of refusal to comply with the requirement" (Commonwealth v. Henning Jacobson 1903, 246). Moreover, it pointed out that even if Jacobson *could* prove that he would suffer adverse effects from the vaccine, the statute did not offer an exception for such a case. In response to Jacobson's argument that this deficiency rendered the statute unconstitutional, the court responded that the "theoretical possibility of an injury in an individual case as a result of its enforcement does not show that as a whole it is unreasonable. The application of a good law to an exceptional case may work hardship" (Commonwealth v. Henning Jacobson 1903, 247). However, the Massachusetts court held that if citizens refused to be vaccinated it was not within the power of public health authorities to vaccinate them by force (as the Boston Herald had reported occurring) (Commonwealth v. Henning Jacobson 1903; Parmet et al. 2005).

When the *Jacobson* case finally made its way to the U.S. Supreme Court, the Court found that the vaccination statute was generally a reasonable protection of the public health while maintaining individual liberty. The Supreme Court did conclude that to subject someone to vaccination who was unfit because of a health condition "would be cruel and inhuman in the last degree;" it stipulated that "we are not inclined to hold that the statute establishes the absolute rule that an adult must be vaccinated if it be apparent or can be shown with reasonable certainty that he is not at the time a fit subject of vaccination or that vaccination, by reason of his then condition, would seriously impair his health or probably cause his death" (Jacobson v. Massachusetts 1905, 38–39). However, the Court found that Jacobson was "in perfect health and a fit subject of vaccination" and that he simply "refused to obey the statute and the regulation adopted in execution of its provisions for the protection of the public health and the public safety, confessedly endangered by the presence of a dangerous disease" (Jacobson v. Massachusetts 1905, 39). The Court ordered Jacobson to submit to vaccination or pay the fine (Jacobson v. Massachusetts 1905). Three years after his legal fight began, Jacobson paid the $5 penalty (Willrich 2011).

2.2.3 Discussion

Legal cases since 1890 had allowed states to require citizens be vaccinated, but around the turn of the century, limits to that right began appearing that included a "present danger" standard requiring a real and immediate threat and adherence to the harm avoidance principle protecting citizens from undue burden as much as possible (Willrich 2011). *Jacobson* has endured as a fundamental philosophical foundation of the reconciliation of individual interests with those of the public's health in a political system emphasizing liberal individualism.

Despite the limitations of the facts in *Jacobson*, it has been interpreted in many ways to support numerous public health activities over the past century. Notably, the Supreme Court did not require that otherwise healthy citizens submit to vaccination, only that it was constitutional to require citizens to be vaccinated *or* pay a fine. Also, while the Court found that a lack of a health exception to the vaccination mandate would be unconstitutional, it did not grant Jacobson this exception for himself.

However, as with so many examples in the lexicon of medical ethics, one of the most important practical effects of historical cases is how they have been interpreted and applied to future circumstances. Part of *Jacobson's* legacy has been the Court's "community oriented philosophy" based in social-contract (or compact) theory (Gostin 2005, 578): "a fundamental principle of the social compact [is] that the whole people covenants with each citizen, and each citizen with the whole people, that all shall be governed by certain laws for 'the common good ....'" (Jacobson v. Massachusetts 1905, 26). While the Court recognized individual liberty interests protected by the Constitution, it found that these interests did not impart an absolute right of freedom from restraint because "on any other basis organized society could not exist with safety to its members" (Jacobson v. Massachusetts 1905, 26). It noted that no citizen could enjoy full liberty in a society that recognized "the right of each individual person to use his own [liberty] … regardless of the injury that may be done to others" (Jacobson v. Massachusetts 1905, 26).

The Court also found that reasonable regulations to protect the public health and safety were among these constitutional limits on liberty (Jacobson v. Massachusetts 1905). Despite the fact that Jacobson found mandatory vaccination distressing and objectionable, it was the responsibility of the city board of health to "not permit the interests of the many to be subordinated to the wishes or convenience of the few" (Jacobson v. Massachusetts 1905, 29). As discussed above, the Court found that exceptions were needed for citizens with established concerns for their health—but did not apply this exception in Jacobson's case.

The social contract implied in this case also needed to be reconciled with limits on government and constitutional protections of individual liberty. While the Court had already established a standard of fair application of public health interventions (e.g., not targeting a specific race-based group) (Jew Ho v. Williamson 1900; Gostin 2008), *Jacobson* built on several cases to further explain standards of constitutional protections (i.e., there must be a public health threat to the community, and the state or board of health must design the public health intervention to combat that threat). The Court found that the intervention must be proportionately tailored to that threat creating a "reasonable balance … between the public good and the degree of personal invasion" and should not harm citizens in and of itself (Gostin 2008, 126–127).

While it is hard to reconcile some of the facts of *Jacobson* with its lofty constitutional deliberation, it is the Court's desire to reconcile individual interests with those of the public health in a society that values liberal individualism that has become its enduring legacy. Many court decisions following *Jacobson* reaffirmed states' use of police power for the public health (Gostin 2005), and in 1922 the Supreme Court agreed that states could require vaccinations for children who attend school (Zucht v. King 1922). *Jacobson* was an important step in the lengthy public health battle against smallpox, culminating in its eradication in 1977 (Cohen 2000).

The legal and ethical boundaries between the individual and public health remain mobile in public health law and policy despite the *Jacobson* decision. Notwithstanding its rejection of forced vaccination, coercion—as opposed to the modern emphasis on education—continued as a public health tactic, employed frequently and often directed toward vulnerable citizens (e.g., quarantined sex workers during World War I) (Colgrove and Bayer 2005). And despite the liberty protections it carved out, the Court itself struggled with upholding both individual rights and constitutional liberties. In 1927, citing *Jacobson*, the Court upheld a forced-sterilization law in Virginia of "mental defectives." The *Buck v. Bell* decision reasoned that "[i]t is better for all the world, if instead of waiting to execute degenerate offspring for crime, or to let them starve for their imbecility, society can prevent those who are manifestly unfit from continuing their kind. The principle that sustains compulsory vaccination is broad enough to cover cutting the fallopian tubes" (Buck v. Bell 1927, 207).

In more communitarian-leaning societies, *Jacobson's* value serves less as a map for navigating public good in an individualist context, and more as an illustration of how individual and community interests can be balanced within the political and social structure. Even within the United States, however, *Jacobson* has been interpreted over the decades to be a foundation for diverse legal opinions supporting remarkable expansions of federal power—including warrantless entry into homes in time-sensitive circumstances of compelling need and a defense of the federal government's right to detain U.S. citizens without due process as "enemy combatants" (in a dissenting opinion) (Willrich 2011). Many of these cases, and certainly *Buck v. Bell* serve as a stark reminder that federal powers ostensibly in the public interest cannot be used solely to maximize perceived public benefit—they must be tempered by justice and fairness to both communities and individuals (Lombardo 2008). But as the legal community continued to struggle with what the implications and contours of what *Jacobson* should be in the United States, officials continued to press on in what was then an unregulated field—that of public health research.

2.3 Case Study: U.S. Public Health Service Research on Sexually Transmitted Disease: Alabama and Guatemala

Since the 1940s, contemporary research ethics has developed rapidly through a desire to protect human participants in research. Internationally, the Nuremberg Trials for Nazi war criminals, including the trial of Nazi physicians who conducted torturous medical experiments on subjects, resulted in the *Nuremberg Code* (1947), a compilation of guidelines for conducting research with human participants. In 1964, the World Medical Association's (WMA) *Declaration of Helsinki* further refined ethical guidance for research with humans, and in particular the participation of vulnerable populations (WMA 1964).

The next case study focuses on two separate mid-century U.S. PHS experiments on sexually transmitted diseases in the U.S. state of Alabama and Guatemala. While one of the ten essential public health services is to "conduct research to attain new insights and innovative solutions to health problems" (CDC 2013b; Harrell et al. 1994, 29), these experiments demonstrate how an imbalance of population and individual interests—coupled with disregard for respect for persons—can lead to tragic results.

2.3.1 *Background*

In the early 1900s, STDs—and syphilis in particular—were major concerns for public health. Conservative estimates suggested that syphilis affected 10–15 % of the U.S. population (Jabbour 2000) with symptoms ranging from sores to paralysis, blindness, and death (CDC 2013a). One leading expert at the time described syphilis as a plague "which, in these times of public enlightenment, is still shrouded in obscurity, entrenched behind a barrier of silence, and armed, by our own ignorance and false shame, with a thousand times its actual power to destroy…" (Stokes 1920, 7). In 1905, German scientists isolated the microbe that caused syphilis, and in 1910 other scientists proposed salvarsan (a preparation of arsenic) as the cure (Jones 1993). Salvarsan treatment involved a painful set of injections over a long period and ultimately turned out to be highly toxic (Jones 1993).

In 1912, the U.S. government established PHS to join other federal public health efforts to improve administration and distribution of public health aid to the states, to oversee interstate infectious diseases and sanitation, and to conduct public health research (Jones 1993). In 1918, PHS established a Division of Venereal Disease to organize and support state prophylactic and treatment work (Jones 1993). World War I had highlighted the harmful effect of STDs on the U.S. armed forces, but after interest in the disease from a wartime perspective abated, public health workers focused on syphilis as a poverty-linked disease—and a disease that reportedly affected African Americans in particular. Some physicians even argued that syphilis was a "quintessential black disease" and African Americans a "notoriously syphilis-soaked race" (Jones 1993, 24, 27).

Funding for and interest in preventing and treating STDs waned during peacetime, though they remained a public health problem. With World War II on the horizon, the director of the PHS Venereal Disease Research Laboratory argued that "[t]he prevention of the primary invasion of the male by the syphilis spirochete, as a means of minimizing the loss of effectiveness which is incident to established disease, still constitutes one of the most pressing problems of military medicine" (Mahoney 1936, 78–79). When the United States became involved in World War II, public health officials once again became concerned about STD rates in American troops and predicted "approximately 350,000 fresh infections with gonorrhea [in the armed forces], [which] will account for 7,000,000 lost man days per year, the equivalent of putting out of action for a full year the entire strength of two full armored divisions or of ten aircraft carriers" (Presidential Commission for the Study of Bioethical Issues [PCSBI] 2011, 12). The cost of treating the anticipated infections was $34 million (about $465 million in 2015, adjusted for inflation) (PCSBI 2011, 12).

2.3.2 Case Description

In search of a more effective treatment for syphilis, U.S. PHS researchers in the 1930s had turned to African-American communities for public health research in part because of the perception of high rates of infection, as discussed above. PHS surveyed six southern counties and found the highest syphilis rates among black men in Macon County, Alabama, where the city of Tuskegee serves as the county seat. Created in part by a confluence of economic, social, and clinical factors—including the Great Depression, lack of public and private funds for continuation of development projects, pervasive racism in American medicine, and failed attempts in the pre-penicillin era to treat syphilis with heavy metals—public health researchers decided to conduct a study to observe the "natural progression" of untreated syphilis (Brandt 1978; U.S. Department of Health, Education, and Welfare [HEW] 1973).

The Tuskegee syphilis study or, more accurately, the *U.S. Public Health Service Study of Untreated Syphilis in the Male Negro, Macon County, Alabama*, was an observational study of 399 men with syphilis, and 201 men without, conducted from 1932 through 1972. After 40 years, it finally ended when a PHS STD investigator, Peter Buxton, went to the press with allegations of gross ethical violations, including a lack of informed consent for participation, deception, withholding treatment, as well as racism and lack of scientific soundness (Jones 1993; Brandt 1978).

During this study, public health researchers posed as physicians and told the men, who were already infected with syphilis, that they were going to *treat* them for "bad blood" (which, in common vernacular referred to a range of chronic conditions of unknown origin that could have included anything from syphilis to anemia). In reality, the researchers were not treating the subjects for any of these diseases. While during the salvarsan-era, nontreatment would not necessarily have made a large difference *clinically*, once the Venereal Disease Research Laboratory established that penicillin was a safe, effective, and inexpensive cure for syphilis in 1943, the profound clinical detriment of being a study participant became clear. After 1943, the researchers actively kept subjects from receiving penicillin for other ailments so as not to interfere with their ability to analyze the primary outcome of interest, which was the natural progression of untreated syphilis (CDC 2013c).

Throughout the study, the public health researchers practiced active deceit resulting in 399 infected men being kept from penicillin treatment until their death or 1972 when the study was stopped. The Assistant Secretary for Health and Scientific Affairs, under the then U.S. Department of Health, Education, and Welfare, chartered an advisory panel to investigate the circumstances surrounding the study. The panel later issued the Final Report of the Tuskegee Study Ad Hoc Advisory Panel in April 1973 (HEW 1973).

Meanwhile, the experience of soldiers during World War II had confirmed the need for improved diagnosis and treatment of STDs. After the war, these efforts were revitalized by animal studies that demonstrated the effectiveness of a new post-exposure prophylaxis called "orvus-mapharsen." PHS was interested in whether this solution would be effective in humans, and it was believed that establishing efficacy in humans required controlled intentional exposure in humans—preferably via the "natural method" of sexual intercourse. Because, in part, commercial sex work was legal in the prison in Guatemala City, Guatemala, the researchers planned to conduct prophylaxis experiments there. The plan was to intentionally expose prisoners to STDs through sexual intercourse with commercial sex workers carrying infection (PCSBI 2011).

As a result, from 1946 through 1948, the U.S. government funded, via a federal grant from the National Institutes of Health and approved by the highest echelons of

PHS (including Surgeon General Thomas Parran), STD, serological, and inoculation experiments in Guatemala (Spector-Bagdady and Lombardo 2013). The researchers, led on the ground by a senior surgeon in the PHS, John C. Cutler, soon discovered that they could not reliably infect prison subjects with STDs through sexual intercourse with commercial sex workers; the researchers were thus unable to compare the effectiveness of the prophylaxis regimen they were testing. In an effort to increase infection rates, researchers expanded to other vulnerable populations, such as soldiers and psychiatric patients, and engaged in more invasive methods of intentional exposure, such as abrasion of genitals and manually applying syphilitic emulsion—despite objections of their PHS supervisors that the latter methods of inoculation were scientifically unsound (PCSBI 2011).

By the end of these experiments, considered by some at the time to be "ethically impossible" in design (Kaempffert 1947), public health researchers intentionally exposed approximately 1300 Guatemalan prisoners, soldiers, commercial sex workers, and psychiatric patients to syphilis, gonorrhea, and/or chancroid without informed consent. The researchers documented some form of treatment for only half of the subjects they exposed to infection (PCSBI 2011).

The Guatemala STD experiments ended in 1948 when the researchers decided not to apply for a continuation of funding due to concerns about reporting project activities to the approving study section and the new surgeon general in the United States (PCSBI 2011). The Guatemala STD experiments remained undiscovered for nearly 65 years until Cutler's papers, uncovered in 2003, were brought to the attention of the U.S. government and presented at a professional meeting in 2010 (PCSBI 2011; Reverby 2011). Upon learning of the experiments, President Barack Obama requested that his Presidential Commission for the Study of Bioethical Issues (Bioethics Commission) conduct a historical review and ethical analysis of the studies in Guatemala. The Bioethics Commission concluded its analyses and reported its results to President Obama in September 2011 (PCSBI 2011).

2.3.3 *Discussion*

The U.S. PHS Study of Untreated Syphilis in the Negro Male unmasked a range of important ethical issues that fit into three fields of bioethics we now call professional ethics, public health ethics, and research ethics. Through the lens of professional ethics, the untreated syphilis study calls into question what it means to be an ethical scientist, an ethical physician, and an ethical government steward of public trust. Through the public health ethics lens, it raises issues of imposing the risk of harm to individuals to benefit the community, appropriate engagement with the affected community, and justice and fairness.

Far and away, however, the untreated syphilis study in Tuskegee had the most substantial impact on research ethics. It was not the first study to egregiously disrespect personal autonomy and grossly exploit vulnerable populations. Indeed, by 1966, Henry Beecher had outlined 22 such studies in clinical research, some involving children, mentally and physically compromised patients, and incarcerated individuals (Beecher 1966). Nor was it the first instance of African Americans being mistreated by the medical establishment (Gamble 1997), but it was the first unethical study of this magnitude scandalously exposed by the mainstream media involving and funded by the U.S. federal government. While the original intent of the untreated syphilis study in Tuskegee was to contribute to the greater and seemingly more urgent social good, it has been remembered for withholding treatment from a socially and politically vulnerable group by actively deceiving them.

Comprehensive scholarship has examined the legacy of the untreated syphilis study. Its impact is as deep as it is broad in the bioethics community and the social culture of the United States. This case study examines only the policy outcomes that resulted from the ethical review and analysis of the untreated syphilis study, which is but a small slice of its legacy, yet one that has profoundly shaped the way clinical and public health research is conducted in the United States.

The Tuskegee Study Ad Hoc Advisory Panel (Advisory Panel) submitted its final report to then Assistant Secretary for Health, Charles C. Edwards, in April 1973 (HEW 1973). The Advisory Panel found that the study was ethically unjustified in 1932 due to the lack of evidence that any consent was obtained from participants, breaking "… one fundamental ethical rule…that a person should not be subjected to avoidable risk of death or physical harm unless he freely and intelligently consents" (HEW 1973, 7). Also, the lack of a study protocol or plan left the study's scientific soundness highly suspect, especially in light of the "disproportionately meager" scientific data it produced (HEW 1973, 8).

Besides the lack of informed consent, other important ethical violations noted by the Advisory Panel included researchers lying and withholding penicillin even after it was established to be effective as a treatment for syphilis. The insults to basic dignity and respect for persons forced on the men in the study convinced the Advisory Panel to recommend a permanent body to regulate all federally supported research involving human participants. This permanent body was to formulate policies for establishing institutional review boards (IRBs), compensating research participants who suffer research-related injury, and reviewing protocols at local institutions before beginning research studies. It also called for creating local subject advisory groups to monitor consent procedures (HEW 1973). While the U.S. Department of Health, Education, and Welfare (now the U.S. Department of Health and Human Services) had guidelines for research grants and contracts, the Advisory Panel recommended "… that serious consideration should be given to developing, through Congressional action, rules and procedures which apply to the entire human research enterprise without reference to the source of funding" (HEW 1973, 37).

The Advisory Panel report paved the way for creation of the first congressionally formed national bioethics committee: the National Commission for the Protection of Human Subjects of Biomedical and Behavioral Research (National Commission). As a direct consequence of the ethical investigation into the untreated syphilis study, and acknowledgment that this was not an isolated incident, the National Commission began work in 1974 developing national guidelines for research involving human participants.

The National Commission's most cited work, the *Belmont Report*, outlined three ethical principles for research still in use today: respect for persons, beneficence, and justice (National Commission for the Protection of Human Subjects of Biomedical and Behavioral Research 1979). It also provided guidance on informed consent, special rules for vulnerable populations, and requirements for review of protocols by IRBs. These recommendations, later codified into federal regulations that govern federally funded research with human participants, continue to influence human research today—helping ensure the respectful and ethical treatment of participants in biomedical and public health research (U.S. Department of Health and Human Services 2009).

A more subtle, but enduring impact of the National Commission's efforts specific to public health research was its focus on engaging the community in which research is to be conducted. Although only anecdotally reported, a lack of trust in government, health care, and research is widely believed to be a lasting consequence of the untreated syphilis study (Gamble 1993; Swanson and Ward 1995). Empirical data suggest, however, that the untreated syphilis study itself did not deter participation (Katz et al. 2008), but rather a lack of trust stemming from a larger social legacy of racism and fears of exploitation originating in the era of slavery in the United States (Gamble 1993). In recent times, these fears resurfaced at the onset of the AIDS epidemic in the 1980s in the form of suspicion of intentional infection and genocide (Jones 1993). This mistrust resulted in the distribution of misinformation and difficulties in delivering education and care for those at high risk for HIV (Thomas and Quinn 1991). Since then, methods and best practices for community engagement have been developed and published both in the United States (Barnett 2012; U.S. Department of Health and Human Services 2011) and internationally (World Health Organization [WHO] 2012; UNAIDS 2011).

When analyzing the effect of the Guatemala STD experiments on public health ethics, it is important to note that while the experiments took place in the 1940s, they were critically investigated only recently—65 years after their occurrence. Despite the stark contrast of today's regulated research context with research conducted in the 1940s, scholars continue to examine the original research documents, and our ability to learn from past errors continues. That the U.S. government, at least, had learned lessons from the Tuskegee study is evident by the swiftness of its response to the discovery of the Guatemala STD experiments. While it took 25 years for a U.S. president to apologize to the Tuskegee syphilis study participants, families, and community (The White House 1997), President Barack Obama called President Alvaro Colom of Guatemala to apologize for the STD research immediately following the announcement of its discovery to the public in 2010.

The PHS research studies in Tuskegee and Guatemala demonstrate the serious consequences that can result when the relative interests of the individual and the population are inappropriately reconciled. Indeed, these abuses of individual research subjects have created an enduring legacy of cautionary tales that, together with an orientation toward liberal individualism, have provided a lasting and powerful check on public health authority in the United States. Major policy changes were put into practice after the discovery of the syphilis studies in Alabama.

These policies were intended to protect research participants from being treated as mere means to an end, to bring back into equilibrium the individual and population interests that public health must reconcile. Still, public health interventions continue to face resistance to actions perceived to limit individual choice—making substantive engagement of the relevant community even more critical for turn-of-the-century public health campaigns. The case that follows describing the New York City A1C Registry highlights how, even after all of the regulatory and ethical work accomplished over the past four decades, innovative approaches to public health advances interpreted to curtail some individual liberty can still inspire debate about the optimal role of government in promoting public health.

2.4 Case Study: *The New York City A1C Registry*

Public health increasingly has focused on secondary prevention, or the prevention of disability from disease. As the burden of disease in the United States has shifted from communicable diseases like smallpox and STDs to noncommunicable diseases, public health professionals face new ethical challenges related to monitoring chronic conditions and inspiring individuals to improve their health. The following case illustrates how new technologies affect public health interventions and can limit the precedent set by *Jacobson* when health risks are neither communicable nor imminent. Such cases call for a recalibration of population and individual interests when considering dramatically different health and social settings.

2.4.1 Background

Although infectious diseases accounted for more than 80 % of deaths in the United States in the 1900s (Steinbrook 2006), in 2011, WHO estimated that *noncommunicable* diseases were responsible for 66 % of deaths worldwide (WHO 2013). These changes in the causes of morbidity and mortality are typical of an "epidemiologic transition," a population health phenomenon that occurs when populations carry out public health measures such as sanitation and immunization, which decrease death rates from infectious diseases, increase life expectancy, and simultaneously begin to increase risk for noncommunicable conditions (McKeown 2009).

Of noncommunicable disease deaths worldwide in 2008, deaths from diabetes alone accounted for 1.3 million (WHO 2011). In the United States, 8.3 % of the population (about 25.8 million people) had diabetes in 2011 (CDC 2011). Because of the significant impact that noncommunicable diseases, such as diabetes, have on health systems, WHO has promoted lifestyle modifications and other public health interventions (WHO 2011).

Several interventions, such as providing advice about physical activity and a healthy diet to people with impaired glucose tolerance, have lowered rates of diabetes (Dornhorst and Merrin 1994; Ramachandran et al. 2006). Research also has shown that controlling blood sugar levels (measured by A1C levels), blood pressure, and LDL cholesterol can reduce the risk of long-term complications and death among people with diabetes (Chamany et al. 2009). Some evidence suggests improvements from educating patients in diabetes management, but more evidence is needed (Chamany et al. 2009).

Although there are effective ways of controlling risk factors for complications once diabetes is diagnosed, management of these risk factors across the United States has been deemed inadequate (Chamany et al. 2009). In New York City the percentage of adults who reported having diabetes more than doubled from 3.7 % in 1994 to 9.2 % in 2004 (Chamany et al. 2009). A 2005 report of the New York City Department of Health and Mental Hygiene (NCY DOHMH) showed that diabetes prevalence was higher among non-white residents (NCY DOHMH 2007; NCY DOHMH 2006a). In 2004, NCY DOHMH found that diabetes was the fourth leading cause of death in the city's population (NCY DOHMH 2004), and a survey of New York City adults in 2004 showed that fewer than 10 % of those with diabetes were able to manage blood sugar, blood pressure, and cholesterol satisfactorily according to city public health standards (Chamany et al. 2009). In New York City, 37 % of diabetes patients on state and federally funded Medicaid had an A1C level (reflecting average blood sugar) greater than 9 %—which suggests poor glycemic control (Barnes et al. 2007). WHO has found that policies that promote management of these risk factors have potential to reduce spending for individuals and the public (WHO 2011).

2.4.2 Case Description

In December 2005, the NCY DOHMH submitted a proposal to the New York City Board of Health that would require laboratories with electronic reporting capabilities to submit A1C test results for New York City residents to the NCY DOHMH (NCY DOHMH 2005a). After a period for public comment, the New York City Board of Health approved this proposal, creating the first U.S. program requiring public health reporting of A1C results. Supported by evidence from the success of other disease control programs (such as programs targeting lead poisoning and tuberculosis), this program established a public health surveillance system to track diabetes in the population and to support those who could benefit from diabetes control (Chamany et al. 2009).

The mandate required applicable laboratories to submit A1C test results to the NCY DOHMH within 24 h of completion. Data to be reported included date of the test; name of the testing facility; name and address of the ordering facility or provider; and name, address, and date of birth of the individual tested (Chamany et al. 2009). The NCY DOHMH proposed to use the reported A1C results to generate a registry to monitor glycemic control in the New York City population and to provide mechanisms to support patients and physicians in controlling diabetes

(NCY DOHMH 2005a). The data in the registry were analyzed by various factors including age, location, and type of health care facility to determine distinctions in testing patterns, health care usage, and glycemic control. However, race and ethnicity data were not reported and therefore not included in the longitudinal analysis (Chamany et al. 2009).

After the A1C test results reached the NCY DOHMH, if the average blood sugar level exceeded a predetermined threshold, the patient and provider were notified. Providers were mailed a roster of their patients ordered from highest to lowest A1C level, listing the patients' two most recent test results calling special attention to A1C levels greater than 9 % (NCY DOHMH 2006b). Patients at least 18 years of age with an A1C level greater than 9 % or who were overdue for testing also received a letter informing them of their test results, advising them on how to control their A1C level, and specifically recommending a follow-up appointment with their provider. The letter was printed in English and Spanish (NCY DOHMH 2005a).

The goals of the provider and patient notification program were to increase providers' knowledge about glycemic control in their patient population, facilitate providers in assisting and guiding patients at high risk for complications, and inform and aid patients at high risk for devastating sequelae (NCY DOHMH 2012). While patients had the option to opt-out of the provider and patient notification program, laboratories were still required to report their data to the registry (NCY DOHMH 2005b). Reported data were held confidentially and were unavailable to insurers, licensure organization, or employers (NCY DOHMH 2005c). In 2009, 3 years after initiation of the program, 4.2 million A1C test results for almost 1.8 million individuals were registered with the NCY DOHMH (Chamany et al. 2009).

2.4.3 Discussion

The mandated reporting of A1C results in New York City and the interventions that followed stimulated discussion about the role of government in preventing noncommunicable diseases. Mandated communicable disease reporting is a longstanding and widely accepted essential public health practice, but the modern technology available to collect, analyze, and respond to health data today is unprecedented. While there are clear population interests in controlling the sequelae of diabetes—preventing limb amputations and reducing care disparities, for example—there are also individual interests such as privacy and self-determination at stake. Current public health ethics frameworks must consider the tension between individual and population interests in conjunction with the social, epidemiologic, technologic, and economic context of the case.

Proponents of the A1C Registry argued that outreach for noncommunicable disease is an integral part of public health practice and indeed is an obligation of public health agencies, especially for a disease deemed epidemic (WHO 2011). They argued that the A1C Registry allowed practitioners to identify patients in greatest need of follow-up or referral—often patients with fewest resources—and develop disease management strategies (Chamany et al. 2009). One of the program's goals in mailing test results to patients was to enable them to better manage their own diabetes (e.g., only 10 % of people with diabetes know their own A1C level) (Berger and Silver 2008).

Others criticized some of New York City Mayor Michael Bloomberg's public health policies and interventions as creating a "nanny state" (characterized by being overly controlling of the lives of its citizens) (Magnusson 2014). Some patients believed that the A1C Registry represented an unwarranted invasion of privacy (Barnes et al. 2007), and some providers considered it an intrusion in the provider–patient relationship (Goldman et al. 2008). Many who argued against public health interventions such as the A1C Registry view choices about food and health—even when damaging—as choices that should enjoy a high degree of autonomy uninfluenced by government (although they generally are silent about the influence of food and beverage industry advertising). A public health entity with fiscal and moral interests in the well-being of its citizenry should also work to ensure that individuals have accurate and actionable information with which to make their health decisions (Thaler and Sunstein 2008).

Unlike the early 1900s when *Jacobson* was decided, or the 1940s when the U.S. PHS STD research was conducted in Alabama and Guatemala, we now have several public health ethics frameworks that help us approach ethical issues more systematically (Kass 2001; Childress et al. 2002; Baum et al. 2007; Bernheim et al. 2007). These frameworks reflect attempts to reconcile individual and population interests outlined by the *Jacobson* Court. For example, the A1C Registry case raised issues relating to principles of least infringement, social justice, health equity, and evidence of benefit.

When applying these ethical precepts to the A1C Registry case, the principle of least infringement requires that public health pursue the least intrusive course of action that still achieves the public health goals. The A1C Registry attempted to accommodate this principle by allowing people to opt out, which prevented NCY DOHMH from contacting patients and their clinicians, but did not relieve the laboratory from submitting reports to the registry. While the opt-out mechanism gives individuals some control over how their data are used, it can still allow a public health entity to seek to improve constituents' well-being with minimal infringement.

Policy makers must also explain the aims of the program and whether benefits and burdens are expected to be distributed equitably throughout the population. In the A1C Registry case, these foundational values of social justice and health equity in large part motivated the reporting system. In New York City, substantial differences in morbidity and mortality by race/ethnicity and neighborhood income level were evident. NCY DOHMH use of the data to identify and then reduce these differences promoted public health goals. One challenge in addressing such disparities is to ensure efforts do not inadvertently increase disparities or cause other social harms, including stigma or loss of social capital.

Finally, policy makers have a duty to ensure public health programs are effective, including empirically evaluating programs to provide evidence of this effectiveness. In developing the A1C Registry, policy makers compiled evidence from effective public health programs to help explain the need and potential effectiveness of this program. As the NCY DOHMH evaluates the program and collects evidence of the A1C Registry's effect on diabetes in the city, it might alter policies and procedures. Empirical data on the effectiveness of the registry are pending, and those results will certainly play an important role in assessing the program's scientific and ethical rationale. As this brief analysis demonstrates, contemporary frameworks to guide ethical public health decision making offer additional nuance to the foundational tension between individual and population interests.

The case of the A1C Registry draws attention to important implications of the *Jacobson* precedent and the continued influence of major historic breaches of public health ethics. The current agreed-upon equilibrium in the United States emphasizes individualism, even as similar noncommunicable disease public health campaigns continue to be established (e.g., attempting to control the addition of trans fats to foods and the size of sugar-sweetened beverages) (Gostin 2013). These contemporary cases in the United States are being established and deliberated in a climate of changing health care policy and in the absence of an agreed-upon framework for public health ethics. The challenges they elucidate, however, are likely to have an important impact on the future role of public health in health care.

2.5 Conclusions and Implications

The cases discussed here demonstrate how providing essential public health services requires ethical principles and analysis as varied as the goals they hope to achieve. Clinical and research ethics play a role, but are not sufficient for the consideration of competing public health values. More substantial limits on liberty and privacy can be justified as public health ethics aims to alleviate the "collective hazard," as opposed to individual risk, for both motivation and validation of interventions (Bayer and Fairchild 2004). However, as the cases in Alabama and Guatemala underscore, limitations on power are as important as justifications.

In different ways, the cases outlined here shaped public health practices and ethical expectations in the United States. However, as our world grows more connected and our work increasingly crosses jurisdictional boundaries, it is clear that there are common values that motivate public health ethics even in vastly different political, social, and economic contexts. The global setting in which many public health professionals work requires attention to such contextual factors.

Many of the cases outlined in the chapters that follow uncover additional ethical considerations affecting daily public health practice wherever that practice occurs. Whether it is social duty or political feasibility of the negative right to noninterference, case studies can clarify ethical dimensions, help us examine alternatives for approaching decisions, and remind us that ethical decision making in public health is not an optional endeavor in *any* case. These case studies underscore the need to identify decision-making frameworks that lead to careful consideration of individual and public interests, as a disregard for one or the other is perilous to both.

References

Barnes, C.G., F.L. Brancati, and T.L. Gary. 2007. Mandatory reporting of noncommunicable diseases: The example of the New York City A1C Registry (NYCAR). *American Medical Association Journal of Ethics* 9(12): 827–831.

Barnett, K. 2012. *Best practices for community health needs assessment and implementation strategy development: A review of scientific methods, current practices, and future potential. Report of proceedings from a public forum and interviews of experts*. Oakland: The Public Health Institute.

Baum, N.M., S.E. Gollust, S.D. Goold, and P.D. Jacobson. 2007. Looking ahead: Addressing ethical challenges in public health practice. *Journal of Law, Medicine, & Ethics* 35(4): 657–667.

Bayer, R., and A.L. Fairchild. 2004. The genesis of public health ethics. *Bioethics* 18(6): 473–492.

Bayer, R., C. Levine, and S.M. Wolf. 1986. HIV antibody screening: An ethical framework for evaluating proposed programs. *Journal of the American Medical Association* 256: 1768–1774.

Beauchamp, D.E. 1988. *The health of the republic: Epidemics, medicine and moralism as challenges to democracy*. Philadelphia: Temple University Press.

Beecher, H.K. 1966. Ethics and clinical research. *New England Journal of Medicine* 274(24): 1354–1360.

Berger, D.K., and L.D. Silver. 2008. *Improving diabetes care for all New Yorkers*. http://www.nyc.gov/html/doh/downloads/pdf/diabetes/diabetes-presentation-a1c-registry.pdf. Accessed 8 June 2015.

Bernheim, R.G., P. Nieburg, and R.J. Bonnie. 2007. Ethics and the practice of public health. In *Law in public health practice*, 2nd ed, ed. R.A. Goodman, 110–135. New York: Oxford University Press.

Brandt, A.M. 1978. Racism and research: The case of the Tuskegee syphilis study. *Hastings Center Report* 8(6): 21–29.

Buck v. Bell, 274 U.S. 200, 207 (1927).

Centers for Disease Control and Prevention (CDC). 1999. *Achievements in public health, 1900–1999: Control of infectious diseases*. http://www.cdc.gov/mmwr/preview/mmwrhtml/mm4829a1.htm. Accessed 9 June 2015.

Centers for Disease Control and Prevention. 2011. *National diabetes fact sheet 2011*. http://www.cdc.gov/diabetes/pubs/pdf/ndfs_2011.pdf. Accessed 9 June 2015.

Centers for Disease Control and Prevention. 2012. *Good decision making in real time: Practical public health ethics for local health officials, student guide*. Atlanta: Centers for Disease Control and Prevention. http://www.cdc.gov/od/science/integrity/phethics/trainingmaterials.htm. Accessed 12 June 2015.

Centers for Disease Control and Prevention. 2013a. *Syphilis: CDC fact sheet*. http://www.cdc.gov/std/syphilis/STDFact-Syphilis.htm. Accessed 9 June 2015.

Centers for Disease Control and Prevention. 2013b. *The public health system and the 10 essential public health services*. http://www.cdc.gov/nphpsp/essentialservices.html. Accessed 9 June 2015.

Centers for Disease Control and Prevention. 2013c. *U.S. Public Health Service syphilis study at Tuskegee. The Tuskegee timeline*. http://www.cdc.gov/tuskegee/timeline.htm. Accessed 9 June 2015.

Chamany, S., L.D. Silver, M.T. Bassett, et al. 2009. Tracking diabetes: New York City's A1C Registry. *Milbank Quarterly* 87(3): 547–570.

Childress, J.R., R.R. Faden, R.D. Gaare, et al. 2002. Public health ethics: Mapping the terrain. *Journal of Law, Medicine & Ethics* 30(2): 170–178.

Cohen, M.L. 2000. Changing patterns of infectious disease. *Nature* 406(6797): 762–767.

Colgrove, J., and R. Bayer. 2005. Manifold restraints: Liberty, public health, and the legacy of Jacobson v Massachusetts. *American Journal of Public Health* 95(4): 572–573.

Commonwealth v. Henning Jacobson, 183 Mass. 242 (1903).

Crowley v. Christensen, 137 U.S. 86, 89 (1890).

Dawson, A. 2011. Resetting the parameters: Public health as the foundation for public health ethics. In *Public health ethics: Key concepts and issues in policy and practice*, ed. A. Dawson. New York: Cambridge University Press.

Dornhorst, A., and P.K. Merrin. 1994. Primary, secondary and tertiary prevention of non-insulin-dependent diabetes. *Postgraduate Medical Journal* 70(826): 529–535.

Gamble, V.N. 1993. A legacy of distrust: African Americans and medical research. *American Journal of Preventive Medicine* 9(suppl 6): 35–38.

Gamble, V.N. 1997. Under the shadow of Tuskegee: African Americans and health care. *American Journal of Public Health* 87(11): 1773–1778.

Goldman, J., S. Kinnear, J. Chung, and D.J. Rothman. 2008. New York City's initiatives on diabetes and HIV/AIDS: Implications for patient care, public health, and medical professionalism. *American Journal of Public Health* 98(5): 807–813.

Gostin, L.O. 2005. Jacobson v Massachusetts at 100 years: Police power and civil liberties in tension. *American Journal of Public Health* 95(4): 576–581.

Gostin, L.O. 2008. *Public health law: Power, duty, restraint*, 2nd ed. Berkeley: University of California Press.

Gostin, L.O. 2013. Bloomberg's health legacy: Urban innovator or meddling nanny. *Hastings Center Report* 43(5): 19–25.

Harrell, J.A., E.L. Baker, and The Essential Services Working Group. 1994. The essential services of public health. *Leadership in Public Health* 3(3): 27–30.

Institute of Medicine. 2003. *The future of the public's health in the 21st century*, 2nd ed. Washington, DC: National Academies Press.

Jabbour, N. 2000. Syphilis from 1880 to 1920: A public health nightmare and the first challenge to medical ethics. *Essays in History* 42. http://www.uri.edu/artsci/com/swift/HPR319UDD/Syphilis.html#n3. Accessed 9 June 2015.

Jacobson v. Massachusetts, 197 U.S. 11 (1905).

Jennings, B. 2007. Public health and civic republicanism: Toward an alternative framework for public health ethics. In *Ethics, prevention, and public health*, ed. A. Dawson and M. Verweij. New York: Oxford University Press.

Jew Ho v. Williamson, 103 Cal. 10 (1900).

Jones, J.H. 1993. *Bad blood: The Tuskegee syphilis experiment*. New York: Free Press.

Jonsen, A. 1991. Casuistry as methodology in clinical ethics. *Theoretical Medicine* 12: 295–307.

Jonsen, A.R., and S. Toulmin. 1988. *The abuse of casuistry: A history of moral reasoning*. Berkeley: University of California Press.

Kaempffert, W. 1947. Notes on science: Syphilis preventive. *New York Times*, April 27.

Kass, E.H. 1986. A brief perspective on the early history of American infectious disease epidemiology. *Yale Journal of Biology and Medicine* 60(4): 341–348.

Kass, N.E. 2001. An ethical framework for public health. *American Journal of Public Health* 91: 1776–1782.

Katz, R.V., B.L. Green, N.R. Kressin, et al. 2008. The legacy of the Tuskegee Syphilis Study: Assessing its impact on willingness to participate in biomedical studies. *Journal of Health Care for the Poor and Underserved* 19(4): 1168–1180.

Lee, L.M. 2012. Public health ethics theory: Review and path to convergence. *Journal of Law, Medicine & Ethics* 40: 85–98.

Lombardo, P.A. 2008. *Three generations, no imbeciles: Eugenics, the Supreme Court, and Buck v. Bell*. Baltimore: Johns Hopkins University Press.

Magnusson, R. 2014. Bloomberg, Hitchens, and the libertarian critique. *Hastings Center Report* 44(1): 3–4.

Mahoney, J.F. 1936. An experimental resurvey of the basic factors concerned in prophylaxis in syphilis. *Military Surgeon* 351: 78–79.

Mariner, W.K., G.J. Annas, and L.H. Glantz. 2005. Jacobson v Massachusetts: It's not your great-great-grandfather's public health law. *American Journal of Public Health* 95(4): 582.

Massachusetts Revised Laws c. 75, §137. 1902.

McKeown, R.E. 2009. The epidemiologic transition: Changing patterns of mortality and population dynamics. *American Journal of Lifestyle Medicine* 3(suppl 1): 19–26.

National Commission for the Protection of Human Subjects of Biomedical and Behavioral Research. 1979. *The Belmont report: Ethical principles and guidelines for the protection of human subjects of research*. http://www.hhs.gov/ohrp/humansubjects/guidance/belmont.html. Accessed 8 June 2015.

New York City Department of Health and Mental Hygiene (NCY DOHMH). 2004. *Press release: Diabetes is now the fourth leading cause of death in New York City*. http://www.nyc.gov/html/doh/html/press_archive04/pr164-1222.shtml. Accessed 8 June 2015.

New York City Department of Health and Mental Hygiene. 2005a. *Notice of adoption to amend article 13 of the New York City health code*. http://www.nyc.gov/html/doh/downloads/pdf/public/notice-adoption-a1c.pdf. Accessed 8 June 2015.

New York City Department of Health and Mental Hygiene. 2005b. *New York City A1C Registry: "Do Not Contact" request*. http://www.nyc.gov/html/doh/downloads/pdf/diabetes/diabetes-a1coptout-form.pdf. Accessed 8 June 2015.

New York City Department of Health and Mental Hygiene. 2005c. *Diabetes prevention and control*. http://www.nyc.gov/html/doh/html/diabetes/diabetes-nycar.shtml. Accessed 10 Feb 2014.

New York City Department of Health and Mental Hygiene. 2006a. *Summary of vital statistics 2005: The city of New York*. http://www.nyc.gov/html/doh/down- loads/pdf/vs/2005sum.pdf. Accessed 10 Feb 2014.

New York City Department of Health and Mental Hygiene. 2006b. *A1C Registry. Frequently asked questions*. http://www.nyc.gov/html/doh/downloads/pdf/csi/diabeteskit-hcp-a1c-faq.pdf. Accessed 10 Feb 2014.

New York City Department of Health and Mental Hygiene. 2007. *More than 100,000 New Yorkers face complications due to seriously out-of-control diabetes*. http://www.nyc.gov/html/doh/html/pr2007/pr002-07.shtml. Accessed 10 Feb 2014.

New York City Department of Health and Mental Hygiene. 2012. *The New York City A1C Registry: Supporting providers & patients in diabetes care*. http://www.nyc.gov/html/doh/downloads/pdf/diabetes/diabetes-a1c-reg-serv.pdf. Accessed 8 June 2015.

New York Times. 1885. Editorial. 26 September.

Nuremberg Code. 1947. Trials of War Criminals before the Nuremberg Military Tribunals under Control Council Law No. 10, vol. 2, 181–182. Washington, DC: U.S. Government Printing Office, 1949. http://www.hhs.gov/ohrp/archive/nurcode.html. Accessed 8 June 2015.

Parmet, W.E., R.A. Goodman, and A. Farber. 2005. Individual rights versus the public's health—100 years after Jacobson v. Massachusetts. *New England Journal of Medicine* 352(7): 652–654.

Presidential Commission for the Study of Bioethical Issues (PCSBI). 2011. "*Ethically Impossible*": *STD research in Guatemala from 1946 to 1948*. Washington, DC: PCSBI.

R. R. Co. v. Husen, 95 U.S. 465, 472 (U.S. 1877).

Ramachandran, A., C. Snehalatha, S. Mary, et al. 2006. The Indian Diabetes Prevention Programme shows that lifestyle modification and metformin prevent type 2 diabetes in Asian Indian subjects with impaired glucose tolerance (IDPP-1). *Diabetologia* 49: 289–297.

Reverby, S.M. 2011. "Normal Exposure" and inoculation syphilis: A PHS "Tuskegee" doctor in Guatemala, 1946–48. *Journal of Policy History* 23(2): 6–28.

Riedel, S. 2005. Edward Jenner and the history of smallpox and vaccination. *Baylor University Medical Center Proceedings* 18(1): 21–25.

Schools of Public Health Application Service. 2013. *Glossary–program areas*. http://www.sophas.org/glossaryofterms.cfm. Accessed 8 June 2015.

Spector-Bagdady, K., and P.A. Lombardo. 2013. "Something of an adventure": Postwar NIH research ethos and the Guatemala STD experiments. *Journal of Law, Medicine & Ethics* 41(3): 697–710.

Steinbrook, R. 2006. Facing the diabetes epidemic—Mandatory reporting of glycosylated hemoglobin values in New York City. *New England Journal of Medicine* 345(6): 545–548.

Stokes, J.H. 1920. *The third great plague: A discussion of syphilis for everyday people*. Philadelphia: W. B. Saunders Company.

Swanson, G.M., and A.J. Ward. 1995. Recruiting minorities into clinical trials: Toward a participant-friendly system. *Journal of the National Cancer Institute* 87(23): 1747–1759.

Thacker, S.B. 2010. Historical development. In *Principles and practice of public health surveillance*, 3rd ed, ed. L.M. Lee et al. New York: Oxford University Press.

Thaler, R.H., and C.R. Sunstein. 2008. *Nudge: Improving decisions about health, wealth, and happiness*. New Haven: Yale University Press.

The White House. 1997. *Remarks by the president in apology for the study done in Tuskegee* (May 16). http://clinton4.nara.gov/New/Remarks/Fri/19970516-898.html. Accessed 8 June 2015.

Thomas, S.B., and S.C. Quinn. 1991. The Tuskegee Syphilis Study, 1932–1972: Implications for HIV education and AIDS risk education programs in the black community. *American Journal of Public Health* 81(11): 1498–1505.

U.S. Department of Health and Human Services. 2009. *Public Welfare Code of Federal Regulations. Protection of Human Subjects. 45 CFR. Part 46*. http://www.hhs.gov/ohrp/policy/ohrpregulations.pdf. Accessed 12 June 2015.

U.S. Department of Health and Human Services. 2011. *Guidance for integrating culturally diverse communities into planning for and responding to emergencies: A toolkit*. http://www.hhs.gov/ocr/civilrights/resources/specialtopics/emergencypre/omh_diversitytoolkit.pdf. Accessed 8 June 2015.

U.S. Department of Health, Education, and Welfare (HEW). 1973. *Final report of the Tuskegee syphilis study Ad hoc advisory panel (Advisory panel)*. Washington, DC: U.S. Department of Health, Education, and Welfare. http://biotech.law.lsu.edu/cphl/history/reports/tuskegee/tuskegee.htm. Accessed 8 June 2015.

UNAIDS. 2011. *Good participatory practice: Guidelines for biomedical HIV prevention trials*. http://www.unaids.org/sites/default/files/media_asset/JC1853_GPP_Guidelines_2011_en_0.pdf. Accessed 9 June 2015.

Upshur, R.E.G. 2002. Principles for the justification of public health intervention. *Canadian Journal of Public Health* 93: 101–103.

Washington Post. 1905. Vaccination a crime: Porter Cope, of Philadelphia, claims it is the only cause of smallpox. 29 July. F7.

Willrich, M. 2011. *Pox: An American history*. New York: Penguin Press.

World Health Organization (WHO). 2011. *Global status report on noncommunicable disease 2010*. http://www.who.int/nmh/publications/ncd_report_full_en.pdf. Accessed 8 June 2015.

World Health Organization (WHO). 2012. *Engage-TB: Integrating community-based tuberculosis activities into the work of nongovernmental and other society organizations: Operational guidance*. http://apps.who.int/iris/bitstream/10665/75997/1/9789241504508_eng.pdf. Accessed 8 June 2015.

World Health Organization (WHO). 2013. *The top 10 causes of death*. http://www.who.int/mediacentre/factsheets/fs310/en/index2.html. Accessed 8 June 2015.

World Medical Association (WMA). 1964. *WMA Declaration of Helsinki–ethical principles for medical research involving human subjects*. http://www.wma.net/en/30publications/10policies/b3/. Accessed 8 June 2015.

Zucht v. King, 260 U.S. 174 (1922).

Section II
Topics in Public Health Ethics

Chapter 3
Resource Allocation and Priority Setting

Norman Daniels

3.1 Resource Allocation in Public Health

There has been much discussion of resource allocation in medical systems, in the United States and elsewhere. In large part, the discussion is driven by rising costs and the resulting budget pressures felt by publicly funded systems and by both public and private components of mixed health systems. In some publicly funded systems, resource allocation is a pressing issue because resources expended on one disease or person cannot be spent on another disease or person. Some of the same concern arises in mixed medical systems with multiple funding sources.

Although much has been written on resource allocation issues in medicine, there has been less discussion about how resource allocation affects public health. Federal, state, and local public health budgets in the United States constrain investments in health at those levels. In this regard, they are more like some foreign medical systems than the more fragmented and mixed public-private medical system of the United States. In the context of budget cuts domestically and in many countries responding to an economic downturn, how to invest (and allocate) public health resources is a pressing issue.

Most investments in public health aim to reduce population health risks, but some risks are greater than others, and resource allocation decisions must respond to risks. Sometimes resource allocation decisions focus on the immediate payoff of reducing risks from a specific disease, whereas other resource allocation decisions affect the infrastructure needed to respond to health risks over time. In addition, resource allocation decisions may determine who faces risks—the distribution of

The opinions, findings, and conclusions of the author do not necessarily reflect the official position, views, or policies of the editors, the editors' host institutions, or the author's host institution.

N. Daniels, PhD (✉)
Department of Global Health and Population, Harvard T.H. Chan School of Public Health, Boston, MA, USA
e-mail: ndaniels@hsph.harvard.edu

D.H. Barrett et al. (eds.), *Public Health Ethics: Cases Spanning the Globe*, Public Health Ethics Analysis 3, DOI 10.1007/978-3-319-23847-0_3

risks matters, not just the aggregate impact. Resource allocation in public health thus focuses on deciding *what* risks to reduce—which depends in part on their seriousness as population factors and who faces them—and *how* to reduce risks.

The cases in this chapter that discuss resource allocation force us to contemplate decisions about priorities in public health as opposed to the more frequently discussed medical issues about health care priorities. Later we suggest that making decisions about these issues should be part of a deliberative process that emphasizes transparency, stakeholder participation, and clear, relevant reasoning.

3.2 Collective Lessons from the Cases

Collectively, these resource allocation cases bring out several important points. Separately, they raise other central issues. It is worth noting these general issues before commenting on the more specific problems raised by each case.

The first point the cases collectively make is that *efficiency* has ethical and not just economic importance (Daniels et al. 1996). If one health system is more efficient than another, it can meet more health needs per dollar spent than the less efficient one. If we want systems to meet more health needs, and we should, then we prefer more efficient health systems. Specifically, if we think we have obligations to meet more health needs, or if we think meeting more "does more good," and we ought to do as much good as we can with the resources we have, then we have an ethical basis for seeking more efficient health systems. The economic pursuit of efficiency should not, then, be dismissed as something that has no ethical rationale.

A second point the cases collectively make is that efficiency is not the only goal of health policy, for we have concerns about how health benefits are *distributed* as well as how they add up. Health policy is not only concerned with improving population health as a whole, but also with aiming to distribute that health fairly (Daniels 2008). That means many resource allocation decisions involve competing health policy goals.

The point about competing goals is illustrated by a problem often encountered in policy decisions: should we always favor getting the best outcome from the use of a resource, or should we give people "fair" chances to get a benefit if it is at least significant (Brock 1988)? For example, during an influenza pandemic, should we allocate ventilators to those with the best chance of survival, or should we give significant but lesser chances to a broader group?

Reasonable people often disagree about when the difference in expected benefits means we should favor best outcomes over fair chances, or even about what counts as a fair chance. Hence, a third point emerges from the cases taken collectively: *reasonable people often disagree* about the choice, and it is not possible to simply dismiss one side as irrational or insensitive to evidence and argument (Daniels and Sabin 2008). Indeed, reasonable people will disagree about how much priority to give to the sickest (or worst off) patients. They may think we have to weigh the seriousness of an illness against the potential benefit that we know how to deliver, they may disagree about how to trade off those considerations, or they may disagree about when modest benefits to larger numbers of people outweigh greater benefits delivered to fewer people. Together these "unsolved rationing" problems—the best outcome versus fair chances problem (when to prefer best outcomes to fair chances), the priorities problem (how much priority to give to those who are worst off), and the aggregation problem (when do modest benefits to more people outweigh significant benefits to fewer people)—mean that there is pervasive ethical disagreement underlying many resource allocation problems (Daniels 1993).

There are other common sources of disagreement. One of the most common sources of controversy in resource allocation decisions arises when a particular intervention is seen as the last chance to extend life by some—a necessity if we are to act compassionately—and when it is seen primarily as an unproven intervention by others that we have no obligation to provide it. Denials of such interventions in last-chance cases have been considered the "third rail" of resource allocation decisions (Daniels and Sabin 2008). Here we have two competing public values—compassion and stewardship—and most public officials would prefer to be seen by the public as committed to saving lives rather than as hard-nosed stewards of collective resources.

The cases taken collectively bring out one final point: our *main analytic tools for aiding resource allocation decision making are limited* in several ways, particularly by insensitivity to various ethical issues, especially issues of distribution. In short, these tools may take the first point, about the importance of efficiency, seriously, yet fail to help us with the second and third lessons the cases collectively bring out, that we are also interested in distributing efficiently produced health fairly, and that reasonable people disagree about how to do that. To see this, consider two widely used tools: comparative effectiveness research (CER), which has been given prominence as a research focus in the Patient Protection and Affordable Care Act of 2010, and cost-effectiveness analysis (CEA). Both help to answer policy-making questions. For example, a typical use of CER compares the effectiveness of two interventions (drugs, procedures, or even two methods of delivery), and policy makers may want to know if a new technology is more effective than older technologies.

Of course, they may also want to know if the new technology provides additional effectiveness at a reasonable cost, which points to a shortcoming of much CER in the United States, where considerations of cost are generally avoided. Similarly, if there is only one effective treatment for a condition, CER tells us nothing useful. It also tells us nothing about whether a more effective intervention is worth its extra cost. And, CER cannot help us compare intervention outcomes across different disease conditions, since it uses no measure of health that permits a comparison of effectiveness. Indeed, decision makers face many resource allocation questions that cannot be answered by CER, even if CER can help avoid wasteful investments in interventions that do not work or that offer no improvement over others.

In Germany, however, CER is combined with an economic analysis that takes cost into account and that allows the calculation of "efficiency frontiers" for different classes of drugs (Caro et al. 2010). Presumably, this method could be extended to different classes of public health interventions if they are grouped appropriately. To calculate an efficiency frontier, the effect of each drug in a class in producing some health outcome is plotted against its cost, and the curve is the efficiency frontier for that class of drugs.

It is then possible to calculate if a new intervention in that drug class improves effectiveness at a price more or less efficient than what is projected from the existing efficiency frontier. This use of CER allows German decision makers to negotiate the price of treatments with manufacturers, rejecting payments that yield inefficient improvements. German policy makers can then cover every effective intervention sold at a price that makes it reasonably efficient. Still, because German use of CER cannot make comparisons across diseases, it allows vast differences in efficiency across conditions.

CEA aims for greater scope than CER. It deploys a common unit for measuring health outcomes, either a disability-adjusted life year (DALY) or a quality-adjusted life year (QALY). This unit purports to combine duration with quality, permitting us to compare health states across a range of disease conditions. With this measure of health effects, we can construct a ratio (the incremental cost-effectiveness ratio, or ICER) of the change in costs that results from the new intervention with the change in health effects (as measured by QALYs or DALYs). We can then calculate the cost per QALY (or DALY) and arrive at an efficiency measure for a range of interventions that apply to different conditions.

Critics have noted problematic ethical assumptions in the construction of the health-adjusted life-year measures and in the use of CEA (Nord 1999; Brock 2004). To see some of these problems, consider the following table:

Rationing problem	CEA	Fairness
Priorities	No priority to worst off	Some priority to worst off
Aggregation	Any aggregation is OK	Some aggregations OK
Best outcomes/Fair chances	Best outcomes	Fair chances

CEA systematically departs from judgments many people will make about what is fair. The priorities problem asks how much priority we should give to people who are worse off. By constructing a unit of health effectiveness, such as the QALY, CEA assumes this unit has the same value, regardless of who gets it or wherever it goes in a life ("A QALY is a QALY" is the slogan). But intuitively, many people think that a unit of health is worth more if someone who is relatively worse off (sicker) gets it rather than someone who is better off (less sick) (Brock 2002). At the same time, people generally do not think we should give complete priority to those who are worse off. We may be able to do little for them, so giving them priority means we would have to forego doing more good for others. Few would defend creating a bottomless pit out of those unfortunate enough to be the worst off.

Similarly, CEA assumes that we should aggregate even small benefits. Then, if enough people get small benefits, it outweighs giving large benefits to a few. But intuitively, most people think some benefits are trivial goods that should not be aggregated to outweigh larger benefits to a few (Kamm 1993). Curing many people's colds, for example, does not outweigh saving a single life.

Finally, CEA favors putting resources where we get a best outcome, whereas people intuitively favor giving people a fair (if not equal) chance at a benefit. Locating an HIV/AIDS treatment clinic in an urban area may save more lives than placing a clinic in a rural area, but in doing so, we may deny many people a fair chance at a significant benefit (Daniels 2004).

In all three of these examples of rationing problems, CEA favors a maximizing strategy, whereas people making judgments about fairness are generally willing to sacrifice some aggregate population health to treat people fairly. In each example, whether it is giving some priority to those who are worse off, viewing some benefits as not worth aggregating, or giving people fair chances at some benefit, fairness deviates from the health maximization that CEA favors. Yet we lack agreement on principles that tell us how to trade off goals of maximization and fairness in these cases. People disagree about what trades they are willing to make, and this ethical disagreement is pervasive.

Determining priorities primarily by seeing whether an intervention achieves some cost/QALY standard is adopting a health maximization approach. This approach departs from widely held judgments about fairness, even where people differ in these judgments. Thus, the National Institute of Clinical and Health Excellence (NICE) in the United Kingdom has had to modify its more rigid practice of approving new interventions only if they met a cost/QALY standard in the face of recommendations from its Citizens Council. This council, intended to reflect representative social and ethical judgments among British citizens, has proposed relaxing NICE's threshold in various cases where judgments about fairness differed from concerns about health maximization. The judgments of the Citizens Council in this regard agree with what the social science literature suggests are widely held views in a range of cultures and contexts (Dolan et al. 2005; Menzel et al. 1999; Nord 1999; Ubel et al. 1999, 2001).

There are, of course, those who criticize departures from the NICE threshold of the sort that the Citizens Council recommended. Compromising the maximization of health that CEA promotes may be seen as a moral error, perhaps the result of elevating the rescue of an "identified" victim (say, a cancer patient whose life might be extended modestly by a new drug) over benefits to "statistical" lives (using the resources to provide greater benefits to others). The reasonable disagreement about how to proceed suggests that we should view CEA as an input into a discussion about resource allocation, not as an algorithm for making decisions. This "aid to decision making" role was proposed by the Public Health Service in its recommendations about the use of CEA (Gold et al. 1996). In short, controversial ethical positions are embedded in CEA, and using CEA uncritically commits one to these views, even though many disagree with them.

3.3 Specific Ethical Issues in Resource Allocation

We have already noted that the *efficiency* of a health system has ethical consequences. But what should we count as *efficiency*? Should we use our resources to generate more revenues for a unit of the health system—say, a hospital? Doing so would define efficiency the way most businesses do: other things being equal, an allocation that produces a greater return on investment is a more efficient use of stockholder or owner resources. Alternatively, we might narrow the range of effects to health effects on the covered population. Then we have greater efficiency when an allocation produces more positive health effects in that population than an alternative allocation.

The case Guzmán brings from Colombia raises this issue forcefully. Should hospitals, or a specific health plan, allocate resources favoring services (certain treatments) that raise more revenues than an alternative allocation (certain preventive measures)? Perhaps the gains from the treatments will involve fewer population health gains over time than those obtained by the preventive or health promotional measures, even if they show their improvement more quickly and so look better sooner. Which plan should the policy maker adopt?

This issue examines our purpose in designing a health system. Is it to meet the health needs of a population or is it to provide a good return on investment for those who invest in health services? We might think that this question is easier to answer in a system where health care delivery is seen largely as a public undertaking aimed at improving population health. In such a system, it might seem that there is only one purpose behind the health care system. Return on investment for the taxpayer funding such a system should be measured by how efficiently the system improves population health. In systems where resources are owned privately (and there are many of these), however, it seems we must consider at least two goals. Even if the private sector must in part seek to improve population health, which may be a requirement of state-imposed health care regulation or, in some people's opinions, a social responsibility of corporations, private health-care organizations still must deliver a reasonable return on investment for owners. Thus, policy makers within private health-care organizations have a dual task. Balancing return on investment with improvement in population health thus becomes the central issue in the Colombian case study.

The Chilean case written by Gómez and Luco raises a similar issue, but this case focuses on measurable differences in the cost effectiveness of certain services and in the severity of two conditions. If we consider only cost effectiveness, we view efficiency in one way—the best health outcomes in the aggregate for the population for an investment in health. If we take severity of condition into account, we might view this as an equity demand—in which case, we have an efficiency-equity conflict and must make a trade-off. Or, we might think of efficiency as a ranking of needs by severity of condition. In the latter, the resource allocation case turns on how we define efficiency. Specifically, the Chilean category of Guaranteed Health Interventions could include cataract surgery (the leading cause of blindness in the Chilean population), but not multiple sclerosis (MS) treatments, which might be viewed as maximizing efficiency in a standard sense. Or, the Guaranteed Health Interventions scheme could include the less cost-effective treatment of MS but not cataract surgery, since MS is viewed as a more severe condition (because it can be life threatening and lead to premature death), even if it is far less prevalent than cataracts. If this were the case, the more efficient system, in this nonstandard view, would rank treating more severe conditions as more efficient than treating less severe conditions. If budget limitations mean only one should be included in the Guaranteed Health Interventions program, either MS or cataract surgery, which should it be?

The cataract surgery intervention delivers a significant benefit in terms of QALYs to a larger part of the population than does the intervention package for MS, but the greater severity of premature death seems to be an important reason for favoring MS. If this reason is given priority over cost effectiveness and over the standard view of efficiency, then are less effective treatments for more severe conditions supposed to have priority over more effective and cost-effective treatments for less severe conditions? If so, what kind of a health system does that produce if all needs can not be met given resource limits? Alternatively, do we want a system that always weighs cost effectiveness more highly than the severity of a condition that some people have? That too seems problematic.

Suppose we think improving population health is a worthwhile and defensible goal of a health system, we favor improving population health over increasing revenues for the private sector (in the Guzmán case), and we also favor giving priority to cost effectiveness over severity of a condition (in the Gómez and Luco case). A conflict still remains between health maximization in the aggregate and concerns about equity, as illustrated in the Blacksher and Goold case (and arguably in the case about triage in pandemics by Smith and Viens).

In the case that Blacksher and Goold describe, the task is to decide whether to reallocate resources from a program focused on maternal-child health and reduction of black-white infant mortality disparities to a program that may get more health per dollar spent through other interventions. Infant mortality among blacks and whites has declined rapidly in the United States; and in absolute terms, the decline has been more rapid for blacks. Still, the ratio of black infant mortality to white infant mortality has increased. Because the public health department is in a highly segregated city, this shift in program focus might seem to require viewing the remaining black-white health disparities as morally acceptable (especially given the high rate of improvement that past programs gave to black infant mortality rates). When should we view health disparities as morally acceptable? When should we weigh reducing health disparities as more important than some aggregate gains in health that we know how to produce in a population? If public health has two goals—improving population health and distributing that health fairly—how should we weigh the goals when they conflict?

One important feature of the Blacksher and Goold case, namely the opinions within the community whose inequalities are at issue, is really a feature to which nearly all cases warrant attending. People affected by a policy ought to have some influence in determining that policy. Some people might believe this is what democracy requires. A difficulty this view of democracy faces, however, is that those who speak for the community may not appropriately represent the community affected by the decision. Nevertheless, the opinions of a broader range of stakeholders may improve deliberation (depending on how those opinions are managed). It may also improve the acceptance of the decisions, which arguably enhances the legitimacy of the decision-making process.

Resistance to including a broader range of stakeholders in decision making about health priorities may come from a concern that they bring with them "partiality." This resistance may come from the view that greater impartiality leads to better deliberation. Arguably, this concern about partiality ignores the positive gains that partiality often brings to deliberation, especially if we know how to manage such deliberation so that we minimize the risks that partiality sometimes brings. We need such management skills in any case since partiality is unavoidable in most contexts. Rather than banning what cannot be eliminated, managing partiality in deliberations is the best way to improve decision making in contexts of reasonable disagreement.

The conflict between improving population health and treating people fairly can arise in other contexts. Arguably, the problem raised by Smith and Viens about the principle that should govern triage in pandemics can be viewed as a conflict between health maximization, in this case, saving the most lives, versus recognizing the claims that the sickest people have on us for assistance. Ordinarily, health systems give some priority to those who are sickest, but should that priority disappear in favor of saving lives when scarce resources, such as ventilators, are allocated in pandemic conditions? If we allocate our ventilators to the sickest patients, we may save fewer lives than if we allocate them to those whose lives we can better expect to save. Even if we think we should give priority to those worst off, do we ordinarily think that concern for them should govern triage policy in pandemics? If we believe saving the most lives trumps concerns about helping those who are sickest in pandemics, can we justify why the priority we give to the sickest should be revised in pandemics?

Suppose we have an acceptable way of measuring the burden of disease in a population, and according to this measure, mental illness is not given the priority it ought to have. That is, it contributes more to the burden of disease than is normally recognized in standard health systems, which provide too few services to meet mental health needs. This is the problem upon which Rentmeester et al.'s case focuses. Specifically, some mental health conditions require significant resources for what Medicaid terms as "behavioral management," which is seen as a social support service not a medical treatment. As a result, these services, to the extent they are provided, fall to state-funded social service budgets. The services place a burden on state finances that would be diminished if they were instead included in Medicaid budgets (50 % of which are financed by each state). Arguably, the stigma that attaches to mental health issues is one important reason for this underprovision of social supports for people with mental health issues. In Nebraska, the political opposition to expanded Medicaid coverage through the Affordable Care Act adds to the burden on state budgets and the potential under-servicing of these mental-health induced needs.

It takes resources to meet public health needs. Suppose we can increase the resources to meet some of those needs by accepting a public-private partnership that improves a compromised private partner's image? Should we meet health needs at this price?

That is the issue posed by the Hernández-Aguado case from Spain. Specifically, should public health authorities put their stamp of approval, in the form of their logo, on flu epidemic notices printed on soft drink labels? The inclusion of the logo is a requirement of the private entities that are willing to donate space on the labels of their products. Obviously, this provides a form of public support for soft drinks that arguably contribute to obesity in a population and thus to the prevalence of noncommunicable diseases associated with obesity. But in view of the low budgets available for flu warnings, is this a price worth paying? What would the decision maker have to know about the effects of such labels to decide this case, or is the decision something that can be made independently of the specific payoffs of implementing the warning system? Is there a way to consider the cost and assess whether the outcome of the warning is worth this price? Is this simply an efficiency calculation about the cost effectiveness of reducing a disease burden in this way?

3.4 Decision-Making Process

One final crosscutting issue lurks behind all the cases in the resource allocation chapter (perhaps all the cases in the volume)—namely, the nature of the decision-making process that addresses the issues they raise. Public health decisions about resource allocation—judging from the cases on that topic in this volume—face reasonable ethical disagreement. That is because the tradeoffs involved in the two main goals of public health policy—improving population health and distributing health fairly—are trade-offs about which people often reasonably disagree. How can public health decisions be made in real time, given these ethical disagreements, in ways that enhance their legitimacy and are arguably fair to all parties?

One approach to the problem is to construct a fair process for making those decisions and to rely on the outcomes of such a process. People will judge the outcomes of a fair process to be fair (Daniels and Sabin 2008). What conditions should such a decision-making process meet if it is to be considered fair? Four conditions are arguably necessary (even if some may think they are not sufficient and want to add others): *(1)* The decisions and the rationales for them should be made *public*. *(2)* They should be based on reasons all think are *relevant*. *(3)* They should be *revisable* in light of new evidence and arguments. And *(4)*, these conditions should be *enforced* so that the public can see that they obtain. Some explanation is needed for these conditions.

The publicity condition is widely embraced, even if it is fairly strong. It calls for the grounds for decisions—not just the content of the decisions—to be transparent. People have a right to know why decisions that affect their health are made the way they are. Moreover, making the reasoning for such decisions public is a way of exposing them to scrutiny so errors in reasoning or evidence can be detected and decisions improved. Even though we may not be able to be explicit in advance about all criteria we use to decide such cases, that is, we may work out our reasons through deliberation, we can explain on what we base our decisions. And that gives people affected by our decisions the knowledge they have a right to possess.

The search for reasons that all consider relevant to making a reasonable public health decision about resource allocation can narrow disagreement considerably. Even if people can agree on what reasons they think are relevant—in the spirit of finding mutually justifiable grounds for their decisions—they may not agree about the weight they give these reasons. One way to test the relevance of such reasons is to subject them to scrutiny by an appropriate range of stakeholders. What counts as appropriate may vary with the case. Who should be heard in deliberations is itself worthy of deliberation. Stakeholders raise different arguments that should be heard, and including their voices improves buy-in to decisions. Since stakeholders may not in many instances be elected representatives, we may be skeptical about whether the democratic process is improved by including them, but, if the deliberation is well managed, the quality of the discussion may improve greatly.

The revisability condition, requiring that decisions be modifiable in light of new evidence and argument, is also widely embraced and not considered controversial. Decisions are made on the basis of evidence and arguments, and better evidence and arguments may emerge that require revisiting some decisions. Some decisions can then be modified, though it may be too late for others, and our consolation is that we made the best choices we could, given the evidence and arguments.

The intent of the enforcement condition is to ensure that the other, more substantive, conditions are met. Sometimes enforcement is a matter of state regulation. Sometimes it can be the result of voluntary conformance with a process.

Since ethical disagreements abound in resource allocation decisions, we need a process that enhances legitimacy. But can we claim that a decision-making process that is fair yields fair outcomes? One view is that we may ultimately become persuaded by a good argument that fairness requires a different decision than one that emerged from a fair process. We can in this way defeat the fairness we might ordinarily attribute to the outcome of a fair process. Does the prospect of defeating the fairness of a decision emerging from a fair process mean that we should not attribute fairness to the outcomes? Alternatively, we can admit that the fairness that comes from a deliberation is only "defeasible" fairness, but it is the fairest conclusion we can reach at the time.

References

Brock, D. 1988. Ethical issues in recipient selection for organ transplantation. In *Organ substitution technology: Ethical, legal, and public policy issues*, ed. D. Matheiu, 86–99. Boulder: Westview Press.

Brock, D. 2002. Priority to the worst off in health care resource prioritization. In *Medicine and social justice*, ed. M. Battin, R. Rhodes, and A. Silvers, 362–372. New York: Oxford University Press.

Brock, D. 2004. Ethical issues in the use of cost effectiveness analysis for the prioritization of health care resources. In *Handbook of bioethics: Taking stock of the field from a philosophical perspective*, ed. G. Khushf, 353–380. Dordrecht: Kluwer Academic Publishers.

Caro, J.J., E. Nord, U. Siebert, et al. 2010. The efficiency frontier approach to economic evaluation of health-care interventions. *Health Economics* 19(10): 1117–1127.

Daniels, N. 1993. Rationing fairly: Programmatic considerations. *Bioethics* 7(2/3): 224–233.

Daniels, N. 2004. *How to achieve fair distribution of ARTs in "3 by 5": Fair process and legitimacy in patient selection*. Geneva: World Health Organization/UNAIDS.

Daniels, N. 2008. *Just health: Meeting health needs fairly*. New York: Cambridge University Press.

Daniels, N., and J. Sabin. 2008. *Setting limits fairly: Learning to share resources for health*, 2nd ed. New York: Oxford University Press.

Daniels, N., D. Light, and R. Caplan. 1996. *Benchmarks of fairness for health care reform*. New York: Oxford University Press.

Dolan, P., R. Shaw, A. Tsuciya, and A. Williams. 2005. QALY maximization and people's preferences: A methodological review of the literature. *Health Economics* 14: 197–208.

Gold, M.R., J.E. Siegal, L.B. Russell, and M.C. Weinstein. 1996. *Cost-effectiveness in health and medicine*. New York: Oxford University Press.

Kamm, F. 1993. *Morality, mortality: Death and whom to save from it*, vol. I. New York: Oxford University Press.

Menzel, P., M. Gold, E. Nord, L. Pinto-Prades, J. Richardson, and P. Ubel. 1999. Toward a broader view of values in cost-effectiveness analysis in health care. *Hastings Center Report* 29(3): 7–15.

Nord, E. 1999. *Cost value analysis in health care: Making sense out of QLAYs*. Cambridge: Cambridge University Press.

Patient Protection and Affordable care Act (PPACA). 2010. http://www.gpo.gov/fdsys/pkg/PLAW-111publ148/html/PLAW-111publ148.htm. Accessed 8 June 2015.

Ubel, P.A., J. Richardson, and J.L. Pinto-Prades. 1999. Life saving treatments and disabilities: Are all QALYs created equal? *International Journal of Technology Assessment in Health Care* 15: 738–748.

Ubel, P.A., J. Baron, and D.A. Asch. 2001. Preference for equity as a framing effect. *Medical Decision Making* 21: 180–189.

3.5 Case 1: Priority Setting and Crisis of Public Hospitals in Colombia

María del Pilar Guzmán Urrea
Department of Community Medicine
El Bosque University
Bogotá, Colombia
e-mail: mapiguzmanu@gmail.com

This case is presented for instructional purposes only. The ideas and opinions expressed are the author's own. The case is not meant to reflect the official position, views, or policies of the editors, the editors' host institutions, or the author's host institution.

3.5.1 Background

During the 1990s, many Latin American countries began reforming their health systems according to a neoliberal development model that emphasizes free markets (Homedes and Ugalde 2005; Stocker et al. 1999). Approved in 1993, health reform in Colombia was supposed to overcome problems such as low coverage, inequality in access and use of health care services, and inefficiency in the allocation and distribution of resources. But the reform also hoped to encourage more focus on illness prevention and health promotion and more community participation in health decision-making processes. The reformers advocated predominantly for neoliberal values like efficiency, free choice, universality, and quality. Although they were also committed to the communitarian values of solidarity, equity, and social participation.

The Colombian health reform was one of the first examples of implementing managed competition in the developing world (Plaza et al. 2001). To stimulate competition among insurers and health service providers, both public and private, health reformers applied the theory of managed competition (Enthoven 1993). According to this theory, competition achieves efficiency and reduces cost, making health care services responsive to consumer needs (Londoño and Frenk 1997). Hospitals become responsive when they are able to sell services and become financially sustainable. To achieve sustainability, supply subsidies (direct transfers from the state to hospitals) had to replace demand subsidies (transfers directed to the poor through a subsided security plan).

The Colombian reform established a General Social Security System in Health that featured two insurance plans: *(1)* The Contributory Plan, financed by mandatory contributions (formal employees and employers from the public and private sectors). *(2)* The Subsidized Plan, funded by resources from the Contributory Plan and from taxes and other sources, which covered people unable to pay (Vargas et al. 2010). The actors of the system are the insurance companies, the health service providers, and the state regulatory organizations. Insurance companies contract with health service providers, and the regulatory organizations control compliance with the defined basic health packages.

To optimize resources, the reform placed controls on medical practitioners and established explicit priority criteria based on clinical guidelines that defined benefit packages. From 1993, some adjustments to the reform have been introduced, such as the creation, in 2012, of the Institute for Health Technology Assessment to provide an evidence base for health decisions. The Institute recommends which medical technologies should be paid with public resources on the basis of which technologies optimally improve the quality and cost effectiveness of medical care. To determine these technologies, it conducts health outcomes research that guides technology development, evaluation, and use (Giedion et al. 2012).

Nevertheless, 20 years later, the promise of reform lies unfulfilled and many patients still experience high out-of-pocket costs, long wait times, or denial of services. To access health services, frustrated citizens are turning to the legal system as a last resort and, by so doing, congesting the courts (Defensoría del Pueblo 2012). Physicians are responding to economic incentives and penalties by restricting hospitalization time and decreasing the use of expensive diagnostic tests and specialist referrals (Abadía and Oviedo 2009). To further reduce labor costs, service providers have increased the workload of health professionals and the number of patients seen per day, while reducing the time spent with each patient (Defensoría del Pueblo 2007).

Insurance companies often take a long time to pay health service providers, and they also contract their own service network (a process known as vertical integration), so many public hospitals are in serious financial difficulties. Meanwhile, hospital workers frequently disrupt the normal operation of hospitals as they strike to improve work conditions and have their paychecks issued more promptly. Should hospitals fail—40 % of the 968 public hospitals in Colombia are classified as being at medium or high financial risk—nearly ten million people could be left without health service (Ministerio de Salud y Protección Social 2012; Quintana 2002). Add to that, the reforms have increased inequity, as more affluent patients can more easily access quality health care services than can low-income patients (Vargas et al. 2010).

The described problems reflect a complex situation that requires profound structural reform. As one way to address the immediate problems of efficiency and quality, Colombia in 2012 instituted public hospital accreditation. Accreditation requires hospital directors to reach goals in service delivery related to financial viability, quality, and efficiency. Hospital boards can now fire directors who fail to meet these goals within a specified period (Rodríguez 2012). Given the imbalances between budgets, service demands, and ongoing costs, hospital directors face enormous challenges and ethical dilemmas in formulating and executing their management plans.

3.5.2 Case Description

You are a director of a public hospital that focuses on health promotion and prevention activities, such as general practice, dentistry, clinical laboratory, hospitalization, and emergency care. In developing your management plan, you must make decisions about which services to prioritize. If you prioritize services that represent higher revenues and lower costs as a way of conserving resources, you may have to reduce priority for some services. To guide your decision making, you conducted a retrospective study of service billing in the past 2 years and learned that the clinical laboratory and external medical consultation yielded higher incomes. The lowest yielding programs in the short term—vaccination, educational programs to improve lifestyles, and provision of micronutrient supplements to children and pregnant women—were associated with the best long-term health results.

Taking seriously your fiduciary responsibilities, you try to guarantee financial sustainability by containing labor costs, restricting consultation times, and shortening hospital stays. Your challenge is to do these things without diminishing the quality of patient care. But because you compete with other institutions, you must also assure sufficient reserves to maintain and update medical equipment that will improve the "sale of services." Knowing that every management decision you make will affect the population you serve, you begin to reflect on the factors affecting your hospital management plan.

3.5.3 Discussion Questions

1. Who are the major stakeholders in this case and what are their interests, values, and moral claims? Between which of them are there ethical conflicts or tensions?
2. Which of these interests, values, and moral claims should be prioritized? How would you justify your priorities?
3. Would you prioritize programs that in the short term brought in needed revenues or those programs that had highest impact long term?
4. How can tensions between the goals of efficiency, financial viability, and quality be resolved? What weight should be assigned to each goal by the hospital board when evaluating your performance?
5. At least in the short run, the new reforms seem to be prioritizing efficiency, viability, and quality over equity. Should a health system attain the former goals before tackling the problem of equity, or should it insist on equity from the start?
6. Can equity in health care be achieved without doing something about wealth inequity and other social determinants of health?
7. Should you justify your decisions by emphasizing solidarity with other hospital directors and seeking community support?
8. How could collaborations between public health, communities and the health care system begin to address neoliberal concerns with efficiency, viability, and quality?

References

Abadía, C.E., and D.G. Oviedo. 2009. Bureaucratic itineraries in Colombia: A theoretical and methodological tool to assess managed-care health care systems. *Social Science & Medicine* 68(6): 1153–1160.

Defensoría del Pueblo, Colombia. 2007. *Autonomía Médica y su Relación con la Prestación de los Servicios*. http://www.defensoria.gov.co/red/anexos/publicaciones/aut_med.pdf. Accessed 30 Apr 2013.

Defensoría del Pueblo, Colombia. 2012. La Tutela y el Derecho a la Salud 2011: 20 Años del Uso Efectivo de Tutela 1992–2011. http://www.federacionmedicacolombiana.com/index.php?option=com_content&view=article&id=1335:la-tutela-y-el-derecho-a-la-salud-2011&catid=58:libros&Itemid=104. Accessed 30 Apr 2013.

Enthoven, A. 1993. The history and principles of managed competition. *Health Affairs* 12(suppl 1): 24–48.

Giedion, U. A., Muñoz, and A. Ávila. 2012. *Serie de Notas Técnicas Sobre Procesos de Priorización de Salud: Introducción a la Serie de Priorización Explicita en Salud.* http://www.iadb.org/en/publications/publication-detail,7101.html?id=42686%20&dcLanguage=es&dcType=All. Accessed 30 Apr 2013.

Homedes, N., and A. Ugalde. 2005. Why neoliberal health reforms have failed in Latin America. *Health Policy* 71: 83–96.

Londoño, J.L., and J. Frenk. 1997. Structured pluralism: Towards an innovative model for health system reform in Latin America. *Health Policy* 41: 1–36.

Ministerio de Salud y Protección Social, Colombia. 2012. *Informe de Rendición de Cuentas.* https://www.minsalud.gov.co/Documentos%20y%20Publicaciones/Audiencia%20P%C3%BAblica%20Minsalud%202012.pdf. Accessed 4 May 2013.

Plaza, B., A.B. Barona, and N. Hearst. 2001. Managed competition for the poor or poorly managed competition? Lessons from the Colombian health reform experience. *Health Policy and Planning* 16(suppl 2): 44–51. http://heapol.oxfordjournals.org/content/16/suppl_2/44.long. Accessed 30 Apr 2013.

Quintana, S. 2002. *Los Actores e Intermediarios del Sistema de Salud en Colombia.* Médicos sin fronteras. http://www.disaster-info.net/desplazados/informes/msf/accesointermediarios.htm. Accessed 30 Apr 2013.

Rodríguez, C. 2012. *Gerentes de Hospitales Públicos y Acreditación en Salud.* http://www.elhospital.com/eh/secciones/EH/ES/MAIN/IN/ESTUDIOS_CASO/doc_89824_HTML.html?idDocumento=89824. Accessed 30 Apr 2013.

Stocker, K., H. Watzkin, and C. Iriart. 1999. The exportation of managed care to Latin America. *New England Journal of Medicine* 340(14): 1131–1136.

Vargas, I., M.L. Vásquez, A.S. Mogollón-Pérez, and J.-P. Unger. 2010. Barriers of access to care in a managed competition model: Lessons from Colombia. *BMC Health Services Research* 10: 297. http://www.biomedcentral.com/1472-6963/10/297. Accessed 30 Apr 2013.

3.6 Case 2: Intersection of Public Health and Mental Health: Meeting Family Needs

Christy A. Rentmeester
AMA Journal of Ethics
American Medical Association
Chicago, IL, USA
e-mail: christy.rentmeester@ama-assn.org

Sarah Ann Kotchian
Education and Early Childhood Policy
Holland Children's Movement and the Holland Children's Institute
Omaha, NE, USA

Sherry Fontaine
Department of Management
University of Wisconsin-La Crosse
La Crosse, WI, USA

This case is presented for instructional purposes only. The ideas and opinions expressed are the authors' own. The case is not meant to reflect the official position, views, or policies of the editors, the editors' host institutions, or the authors' host institutions.

3.6.1 Background

The Global Burden of Disease (GBD) compares disease burdens based on epidemiological measures of prevalence, mortality, disability, and associated costs. The GBD for mental illness amounts to 14 % of the world's total disease burden (World Health Organization 2005). In the United States alone, every fifth child suffers from a mental disorder (Perou et al. 2013). Although mental illness clearly causes disabilities (Prince et al. 2007), underservice to those with mental illness is commonplace. Lack of access to mental health services counts as the first of many hurdles facing families who have a child with a mental illness. Stigma and the lack of parity in health coverage for physical and mental illness are other hurdles for these families. Not surprisingly, these hurdles can critically affect the development of children with mental illness.

Lack of access to mental and behavioral health services for children 5 years and younger especially threatens their development. Rapid brain growth occurs in the first 5 years of life, which lays the foundation for cognitive, emotional, and moral development. Exposure to chronic stress can prompt the release of hormones in the brain that can have enduring consequences for how the adult brain is organized and how it functions (Shonkoff and Phillips 2000). Because poor health can show up in children as developmental delay, access to mental and behavioral health services is critical. Longitudinal studies demonstrate positive and long-acting effects of early childhood interventions, such as environmental enrichment programs, on a range of cognitive and noncognitive skills, social behaviors, academic achievement, and adult job performance (Heckman 2008). The estimated annual rate of return on investment from targeted early childhood development programs is 7 %, and early intervention reduces the predictable need for higher, more costly levels of care in later life (Heckman et al. 2010).

In the United States, Medicaid is a government-funded program that provides health coverage to people with certain disabilities and to low-income adults and their children. The Federal Medicaid Act (FMA) requires states participating in Medicaid programs to provide *medically necessary* treatment to eligible children.

Under federal Medicaid law, states must provide "early and periodic screening, diagnostics, and treatment," also known as EPSDT services, to eligible Medicaid recipients under age 21 (U.S.C. § 1396d(a)(4)(B)). The definition of EPSDT includes *necessary health care*, diagnostic services, treatment, and other measures described in the Medical Assistance subchapter for the United States Code (42 U.S.C. § 1396d (a)) (2012) that correct or ameliorate defects and physical and mental illnesses and conditions discovered by the screening services, regardless of whether such services are covered under the state plan (42 U.S.C. § 1396d (r)(5)) (2013). The *medical necessity* standard, which is based on clinical standards of care, refers to interventions that may be justified as reasonable, necessary, or appropriate. States must comply with the FMA standard to cover all treatments for a Medicaid-eligible child's physical or mental condition, even if service coverage is optional for adults covered by Medicaid. FMA also bars states from arbitrarily denying or reducing the amount, duration, or scope of a required service to an otherwise eligible recipient solely because of the diagnosis, illness, or condition (Nebraska Legislature 2012).

Despite the provisions of FMA, the U.S. Department of Health and Human Services, which oversees the Medicaid program, excludes certain behavioral health treatments for children with developmental disabilities and autism (National Health Law Program 2012; Autism Society of Nebraska 2012). In addition, some states' Medicaid contracts allow insurers more freedom than other states to deny payment for services. States also vary in who—the claimant or the insurer—must prove whether coverage provisions are adequate or fall short of federal Medicaid legal standards (Rosenbaum and Teitelbaum 1998). Differences among states in approval of payment for specific treatments, including mental and behavioral health treatment, illustrate the need for more consistency in Medicaid coverage provisions and the lack of parity between mental and physical health coverage. Mental health benefits must be offered at parity with medical services to newly eligible recipients as part of the 2010 Patient Protection and Affordable Care Act (ACA), and Medicaid expansion controversy is clear evidence that parity is a work in progress (Mental Health America 2013; U.S. Department of Labor 2008).

Because of inadequate coverage for mental and behavioral health services for Medicaid-eligible children, some parents have no option other than to surrender their child to the child welfare system so that the child will receive full coverage for necessary mental and behavioral health care services. This results in significant cost-shifting from Medicaid to the state's child welfare system. That is, when a state provides federally mandated services to Medicaid-eligible children, it receives a financial match from the federal government to pay the costs. When a state denies federally mandated Medicaid services and a family surrenders a child to state custody so the child can receive care, the state pays the expense of the previously denied Medicaid costs plus the expense of entitlements the child acquires as a ward of the state.

The ACA Medicaid expansion offers a window of opportunity to increase coverage for behavioral health treatment for children with mental illnesses. Although the federal government will bear the primary financial burden of Medicaid expansion, some states have elected, for political reasons, not to participate in this expansion. For participating states, ACA Medicaid expansion will replace state and local mental health services funds with federal Medicaid money that will cover a wider range of home and community-based services for mental illness treatment (Bazelon Center for Mental Health Law 2012).

Public health agencies and leaders often provide input for the Medicaid system, helping to develop protocols, criteria, and rules about which treatments are defined as *medically necessary*. Such decisions about medical necessity affect clinicians, patients, and families because they determine which treatments get recommended at the clinical level and influence which treatments insurers cover.

3.6.2 Case Description

You are the Medicaid director of a state with the country's highest percentage of children in the child welfare system. Twenty-five percent of children in the state's foster care system are there not because of abuse or neglect, but because of behavioral problems and mental illnesses. As a state official, you are aware that this results in significant cost-shifting from Medicaid to the state's child welfare system.

Recently, the case of 4-year-old Sam has come to your attention. Sam's family cannot afford mental and behavioral health care for Sam, although he is Medicaid-eligible and insured through Magiscare (a private company with a state contract to administer Medicaid for mental and behavioral health services). Sam's parents are considering surrendering their boy to become a state ward to get him the mental health services he needs.

Sam, you learn, eats random objects and dirt, throws tantrums, bangs his head on the ground, hits and bites himself and others, and often runs away. Recently diagnosed by his physician as having autism, Sam was referred to a psychologist who recommended outpatient behavioral therapy. Both the physician and the psychologist expect this therapy to be covered through the family's Magiscare plan.

Magiscare denied the psychologist's requests for payment on the grounds that, for children of Sam's age, behavioral management is not covered under state law because it is not "medically necessary." Magiscare substantiated their denial of payment because Sam's behaviors primarily reflect developmental disabilities related to autism, which are not covered under their contract with the state. When you ask the Magiscare executive director about this case, she suggests that Sam's parents could attend therapy sessions to help them cope with their son's behaviors, but she reasserts that behavioral management is not covered for children as young as Sam under state law because it is not medically necessary.

Members of the state legislature and child mental health advocacy groups are trying to expand access to home-based and community-based mental health services. They have asked you to support their efforts. You also consider that your governor, who is your boss, has publically stated his firm opposition to ACA Medicaid expansion, thus denying the state the opportunity to expand coverage for children's mental and behavioral health treatment through the ACA. At present, you know that your state is offering limited mental and behavioral health services and that narrow definitions of *medical necessity* are used to limit access to those services.

As the state Medicaid director, which steps should you take?

3.6.3 Discussion Questions

1. Who are the main stakeholders in this case, and what are their primary interests?
2. "Passing" the expense of coverage denied by Medicaid to other components of public service, such as the child welfare system, has fiscal and social implications.
   (a) What are some of these implications?
   (b) How should prevalence, mortality, disability, and cost be factored into thinking about ways to balance short- and long-term risks and benefits to individuals and to the public in this case?
3. Suppose a policy advisor warns that expanding behavioral health care for children will strain the Medicaid budget and require cuts in services for adults or reduce their eligibility.
   (a) How should you respond?
   (b) Which considerations or priorities would guide your funding allocations?
4. What role should ethical principles such as *stewardship*, *public health leadership*, and *moral courage* play in this case?
5. *Medical necessity* implies an acute care model of health service delivery and reflects a clinical perspective. How well does this idea apply to a public health prevention model of health service delivery? Are there better alternatives?
6. Parity in insurance coverage for mental health is federally mandated for private insurers, which covers most citizens, but has proven to be an elusive goal for people who do not have private insurance or do not have enough coverage. Medicaid is a public (government funded) insurance program, not a private one. Although Medicaid beneficiaries receive coverage for medically necessary mental health services, each state defines *medical necessity* uniquely.
   (a) Should a federal mandate define *medical necessity* for mental and behavioral services?
   (b) What financial implications would such a mandate have from a state perspective and from an overall perspective?
7. The term *principle-policy gap* can be used to characterize situations in which most people support health coverage in principle; but in practice, they are unable to pay for coverage or unwilling to take the political, social, cultural, or fiscal risks necessary to enable such coverage. What do such gaps tell us about which values the majority favors, and how might the term *principle-policy gap* help us understand the dynamics in this case? What roles should public health leaders play in responding to principle-policy gaps?

Acknowledgements The authors thank student Chelsea Williams for her assistance in assembling the facts of the case. We also thank Creighton University's Center for Health Policy & Ethics.

References

Autism Society of Nebraska. 2012. *Nebraska Appleseed—Cases of denial of behavioral health coverage for children are needed.* http://www.autismnebraska.org/2012/06/13/nebraskaappleseed-cases-of-denial-of-behavioral-health-coverage-for-children-are-needed/. Accessed 6 Nov 2012.

Bazelon Center for Mental Health Law. 2012. *Take advantage of new opportunities to expand medicaid under the Affordable Care Act: A guide to improving health coverage and mental health services for low-income people, following the Supreme Court ruling on the Affordable Care Act.* http://www.bazelon.org/LinkClick.aspx?fileticket=cwAuDZLEmQI%3D&tabid=619. Accessed 3 June 2013.

Heckman, J.J. 2008. Schools, skills, and synapses. *Economic Inquiry* 46(3): 289–324.

Heckman, J.J., S.H. Moon, R. Pinto, P.A. Savelyev, and A. Yavitz. 2010. The rate of return to the High/Scope Perry Preschool Program. *Journal of Public Economics* 94(1–2): 114–128.

Mental Health America. 2013. *Medicaid expansion fact sheet.* http://www.mentalhealthamerica.net/go/action/policy-issues-a-z/healthcare-reform/fact-sheet-medicaid-expansion/fact-sheet-medicaid-expansion. Accessed 23 May 2013.

National Health Law Program. 2012. *Lawsuit fi led to protect the rights of Nebraska children with autism and development disability.* http://www.conntact.com/component/content/article/121-press-release/13284-lawsuit-fi led-to-protect-the-rights-of-nebraska-children-with-autism-anddevelopmental-disabilities.html. Accessed 6 Nov 2012.

Nebraska Legislature. 2012. *Floor debate on LB 1063.* http://www.legislature.ne.gov/FloorDocs/102/PDF/Transcripts/FloorDebate/r2day47.pdf. Accessed 1 Apr 2013.

Perou, R., R.H. Bitsko, S.J. Blumberg, et al. 2013. Mental health surveillance among children – United States, 2005–2011. *Morbidity and Mortality Weekly Report* 62(2): 1–35.

Prince, M., V. Patel, S. Saxena, et al. 2007. No health without mental health. *Lancet* 370: 859–877.

Rosenbaum, A., and J.B. Teitelbaum. 1998. *Coverage decision-making in Medicaid managed care: Key issues in developing managed care contracts.* Washington, DC: The Center for Health Services Research and Policy, George Washington University Medical Center, School of Public Health and Health Services. http://sphhs.gwu.edu/departments/healthpolicy/CHPR/downloads/behavioral_health/bhib-1.pdf. Accessed 1 Apr 2013.

Shonkoff, J.P., D.A. Phillips, and Committee on Integrating the Science of Early Childhood Development; Board on Children, Youth, and Families; Institute of Medicine; Division of Behavioral and Social Sciences and Education (eds.). 2000. *From neurons to neighborhoods: The science of early childhood development.* Washington, DC: National Academy Press.

United States Code. 2012, 2013. *Title 42: Public health and welfare.* 42 U.S.C.A § 1396d(a)(4)(B) (West 2012) and 42 U.S.C. § 1396d (r)(5) (suppl 2013). http://www.gpo.gov/fdsys/pkg/USCODE-2010-title42/pdf/USCODE 2010 title42-chap7-subchapXIX-sec1396d.pdf. Accessed 29 May 2013.

U.S. Department of Labor. 2008. *The Mental Health Parity and Addiction Equity Act of 2008: Fact sheet.* Pub L 110–343. http://www.dol.gov/ebsa/newsroom/fsmhpaea.html. Accessed 23 May 2013.

World Health Organization (WHO). 2005. *Mental health: Facing the challenges, building solutions.* Report from the WHO European Ministerial Conference. Copenhagen: WHO Regional Office for Europe.

3.7 Case 3: Public-Private Partnerships: Role of Corporate Sponsorship in Public Health

Ildefonso Hernández-Aguado and Blanca Lumbreras
Department of Public Health, History of Science and Gynecology
Universidad Miguel Hernández and CIBER de Epidemiología y Salud Pública
San Juan, Alicante, Spain
e-mail: ihernandez@umh.es

This case is presented for instructional purposes only. The ideas and opinions expressed are the authors' own. The case is not meant to reflect the official position, views, or policies of the editors, the editors' host institutions, or the authors' host institutions.

3.7.1 Background

Public health systems are usually underfunded in comparison with health care systems. In fact, the Organisation for Economic Co-operation and Development (OECD) countries allocate on average only 3 % of their health spending to public health and prevention activities (OECD 2011). This low funding of public health programs hinders the capacity to implement effective public health policies (Robert Wood Johnson Foundation 2011).

Population health challenges, such as influenza pandemics, are increasingly complex, and tackling them involves urgently executing a wide array of public health measures to prevent disease transmission. In the case of influenza pandemics, measures can vary from border quarantine, social distancing, provision of antivirals and vaccines, and personal hygiene strategies. Recommendations often need to be made quickly even when knowledge about the seriousness and potential health and social effects are incomplete. The target for preventive interventions is the entire population. However, resources for intense and sustained health campaigns through mass communications are expensive. In addition, the social determinants of the disease must be understood and considered (Crowcroft and Rosella 2012). This typically involves the need for policies that engage the health and non-health sectors, such as educational policies and social or economic factors (Savoia et al. 2012). This complexity, together with decreasing funds and other factors, has contributed to increasing private sector involvement in health care.

According to the World Health Organization (WHO), a public-private partnership gathers a set of actors for the common goal of improving population health through agreed roles and principles. This may also be described as public sector programs with private sector participation (WHO 2013). WHO has described several types of partnerships, including philanthropic, transactional, and transformational. Sponsorship is a form of a public-private partnership defined as "any form of monetary or in-kind payment or contribution to an event, activity, or individual that directly or indirectly promotes a company's name, brand, products, or services" (Kraak et al. 2012). In this sense, sponsorship is a commercial transaction, not type of philanthropy.

Public-private partnerships have become increasingly common for public health campaigns. Some transnational companies and their corporate foundations collaborate with public institutions, such as United Nations agencies and governments, to tackle complex public health problems, such as treatment of diarrhea in developing countries (Torjesen 2011), tuberculosis, and malaria (Ridley et al. 2001). These collaborations have been encouraged by international institutions and experts as a way to mobilize resources and expertise, which could complement the public sector. WHO has also encouraged using public-private partnerships to deliver health services for a range of health problems, including HIV infection, malaria, tuberculosis, trachoma, and vaccine-preventable diseases (Buse and Walt 2000a, b). However, corporations' increasing role in public health has been criticized as jeopardizing the mission of public health and its commitment to population health (Hastings 2012; Ludwig and Nestle 2008). Some corporations have used tactics that discredit public health actions, such as distorting scientific information and using financial tactics and political influence to avoid unfavorable regulations (Wiist 2011).

Public health professionals, public health agencies, and governments often must decide whether to collaborate with the private sector to improve population health. These decisions are increasingly frequent as health department budgets shrink and public-private partnerships are seen as a way to secure funds for core public health programs. Ethical considerations can help us decide whether and when to form such partnerships. However, the available public health ethics frameworks (e.g., Public Health Leadership Society 2002; Nuffield Council on Bioethics 2007; Kass 2001) do not specifically discuss public-private partnerships. Only the Public Health Leadership Society provides guidance for such collaborations. Principle 10 proposes that, "Public health institutions and their employees should engage in collaborations and affiliations in ways that build the public's trust and the institution's effectiveness." Continued discussion about the ethical implications of private-public partnerships is needed.

3.7.2 Case Description

Top health officials in an industrialized country have declared a public health emergency due to an influenza pandemic. The head of the country's health department receives a call from the president of a multinational company that produces sugary, high-calorie drinks. The company president expresses his concern about the pandemic and wants to collaborate with the government to prevent the spread of flu. The company offers the health department a considerable amount of space, one third of each can, on its star product (a soft drink) free of charge, to include messages on flu prevention. The company insists that the health department logo be included on the can along with the preventive messages. For them, the association between the health department (through the logo) and their product is essential for the collaboration as it would be an acknowledgement by the health department of the company's social responsibility.

The head of the health department arranges a meeting with several health authorities and officials to consider the offer. On one side, some members of the group support the proposal because of the need to carry out far-reaching public health campaigns to limit the impact of pandemic flu. At that stage, the incidence of pandemic flu is increasing quickly and the number of new outbreaks in schools is worrying the health authorities and the population. There have been recent budget cuts to the health department, and some officials argue the company's contribution may be the best option to ensure a far-reaching campaign on prevention measures to benefit the population. They see sponsorship as a form of social responsibility because the company does not have any apparent economic interest in flu-related activities. They also note that there are no other companies offering a similar collaboration.

But other officials say the company's soft drink products contribute to the obesity and diabetes epidemic and that the company's use of the health department logo would label it a pro-health industry with the backing of the highest health authority in the country. They also raise concerns about risking the independence of the health department in future regulatory action on sugar-rich beverages.

As the head of the health department, you must decide if you should collaborate with the company.

3.7.3 Discussion Questions

1. What considerations should the health department director weigh when deciding whether to collaborate with the beverage company?
2. Who are the major stakeholders the health department should consider, and what values might each of these stakeholders bring to this decision?
3. In making your decision, what values should be prioritized?
4. What positive or negative impacts would displaying the health department logo on the soft drink cans have on health department operations?
5. How might sponsorship by a company that produces sugary beverages affect public trust in the health department and the institution's effectiveness?
6. Would the decision be different if the company produced healthy foods and the department's logo was placed on a healthy product?
7. Would community involvement facilitate decision making and the consideration of the ethical questions? What ethical criteria or guidance should be established to accept or reject a future donations or sponsorship of a public health program by a company?

Acknowledgements We thank Mr. Jonathan Whitehead for language editing.

References

Buse, K., and G. Walt. 2000a. Global public-private partnerships: Part I—A new development in health? *Bulletin of the World Health Organization* 78: 549–561.

Buse, K., and G. Walt. 2000b. Global public-private partnerships: Part II—What are the health issues for global governance? *Bulletin of the World Health Organization* 78: 699–709.

Crowcroft, N.S., and L.C. Rosella. 2012. The potential effect of temporary immunity as a result of bias associated with healthy users and social determinants on observations of influenza vaccine effectiveness; Could unmeasured confounding explain observed links between seasonal influenza vaccine and pandemic H1N1 infection? *BMC Public Health* 12: 458.

Hastings, G. 2012. Why corporate power is a public health priority. *British Medical Journal* 345: e5124.

Kass, N.E. 2001. An ethics framework for public health. *American Journal of Public Health* 91(11): 1776–1782.

Kraak, V.I., P.B. Harrigan, M. Lawrence, P.J. Harrison, M.A. Jackson, and B. Swinburn. 2012. Balancing the benefits and risks of public-private partnerships to address the global double burden of malnutrition. *Public Health Nutrition* 15(3): 503–517.

Ludwig, D.S., and M. Nestle. 2008. Can the food industry play a constructive role in the obesity epidemic? *JAMA* 300(15): 1808–1811.

Nuffield Council on Bioethics. 2007. *Public health: Ethical issues*. London: Nuffield Council on Bioethics. http://nuffieldbioethics.org/wp-content/uploads/2014/07/Public-health-ethicalissues.pdf. Accessed 22 May 2015.

Organisation for Economic Co-operation and Development (OECD). 2011. Health at a glance 2011. In *OECD indicators*. OECD Publishing. http://www.oecd.org/els/healthsystems/49105858.pdf. Accessed 22 May 2015.

Public Health Leadership Society. 2002. *Principles of the ethical practice of public health*. http://phls.org/CMSuploads/Principles-of-the-Ethical-Practice-of-PH-Version-2.2-68496.pdf. Accessed 22 May 2015.

Ridley, R.G., J. Lob-Levyt, and J. Sachs. 2001. A role for public-private partnerships in controlling neglected diseases? *Bulletin of the World Health Organization* 79(8): 771–777.

Robert Wood Johnson Foundation. 2011. *Investing in America's health: A state-by-state look at public health funding and key health facts*. http://healthyamericans.org/report/83/. Accessed 22 May 2015.

Savoia, E., M.A. Testa, and K. Viswanath. 2012. Predictors of knowledge of H1N1 infection and transmission in the U.S. population. *BMC Public Health* 12: 328.

Torjesen, I. 2011. Coca-Cola supply chain helps bring diarrhoea treatments to developing world. *British Medical Journal* 343: d5825.

Wiist, W.W. 2011. The corporate play book, health and democracy: The snack food and the beverage industry's tactics in context. In *Sick societies: Responding to the global challenge of chronic diseases*, ed. D. Stuckler and K. Siegel, 206–216. New York: Oxford University Press.

World Health Organization (WHO). 2013. *Public-private partnerships for health*. http://www.who.int/trade/glossary/story077/en/. Accessed 22 May 2015.

3.8 Case 4: Black-White Infant Mortality: Disparities, Priorities, and Social Justice

Erika Blacksher
Department of Bioethics and Humanities
University of Washington
Seattle, WA, USA
e-mail: eb2010@u.washington.edu

Susan D. Goold
Department of Internal Medicine and Department of Health Management and Policy Center for Bioethics and Social Sciences in Medicine
University of Michigan
Ann Arbor, Michigan, USA

This case is presented for instructional purposes only. The ideas and opinions expressed are the authors' own. The case is not meant to reflect the official position, views, or policies of the editors, the editors' host institutions, or the authors' host institutions.

3.8.1 Background

Preterm births, the leading cause of infant mortality, are increasing annually worldwide (World Health Organization 2012). The United States shares company with Nigeria, India, and Brazil among the top ten countries with the highest numbers of preterm births and ranks 31st among Organisation for Economic Co-operation and Development (OECD) nations in infant mortality (OECD 2010). Within the United States, racial and ethnic disparities in infant mortality remain entrenched and have increased (MacDorman and Mathews 2009). U.S. health policy leaders have made the elimination of health disparities a top public health priority (Centers for Disease Control and Prevention 2011; U.S. Department of Health and Human Services 2011). Infant mortality is an important area of focus for eliminating disparities, both in its own right and because the rate of infant mortality serves as an indicator of the nation's health due to its association with maternal health, social and economic conditions, racial discrimination, access to health care, and public health practices (MacDorman and Mathews 2009).

During the twentieth century, U.S. infant mortality declined 93 % (MacDorman 2011). In 1900, about 100 infants died per 1000 live births. By 2000, that number fell to 6.89. During the last half of the twentieth century, the rate of black infant mortality dropped dramatically. In 1950, black infant mortality was 43.9 deaths per 1000 live births compared with 26.8 deaths per 1000 live births among whites (Mechanic 2002). But by 1998 black infant mortality fell to 13.8 deaths per 1000 live births compared with 6.0 deaths per 1000 live births among whites. As these numbers show, both groups made significant absolute gains, with blacks gaining more in absolute terms—a reduction of 30.1 for blacks and 20.8 for whites. Yet, black infant mortality still remained about twice that of whites.

These disparities have persisted in the twenty-first century. In 2006, non-Hispanic black women experienced the highest rate of infant mortality, with 13.4 infant deaths per 1000 live births, while non-Hispanic white women had a considerably lower rate, with 5.6 infant deaths per 1000 live births. Citing a 2006 report from the National Healthy Start Association, MacDorman and Mathews (2009) report that programmatic efforts to reduce disparities in black-white infant mortality have had some successes at local levels, but eliminating the disparities is difficult.

The U.S. Centers for Disease Control and Prevention and the U.S. Department of Health and Human Services have prioritized both the elimination of health disparities and improvement in overall population health. These twin goals—one distributive, the other aggregative—are separate and sometimes conflict (Anand 2004). Increases in health disparities often accompany advances in aggregate gains in population health (Mechanic 2007). Although this case is specific to the United States, the dilemma is not. Data show that significant progress on child mortality has been made in many countries but that this overall success is often coupled with increased inequalities between advantaged and disadvantaged groups (Chopra et al. 2012). In China and India, for example, disparities in mortality persist between boys and girls younger than 5 years, a function of entrenched gender discrimination (You et al. 2010). These examples raise challenging questions about how ethically to assess such cases and set priorities for the allocation of scarce public health resources.

3.8.2 *Case Description*

You serve as the director for the local health department in a racially segregated urban city in the Midwest with one of the greatest concentrations of African Americans in the United States. The city has a long history of civil rights activism that led to protests and marches that ultimately empowered and mobilized black communities and organizations. Your health department has a history of prioritizing maternal-child health and the elimination of black-white disparities in infant mortality in its programs, an investment of resources affirmed by the city residents through the department's community outreach program and planning processes.

Chronic underfunding of public health, made worse by the economic downturn, has resulted in drastic and unprecedented reductions in the public health budget. In consultation with your staff and community board of health, you have raised the possibility of redirecting resources from maternal-child health into other programs based on a number of practical and ethical considerations. As with national statistics, the city has seen significant declines in black infant mortality, even as black-white disparities remain. You note that although the maternal-child health programs are cost-effective, their impact on reducing black-white disparities seems to have stalled. Other programs appear to meet targets more consistently. To help support these other programs, you note that allocating resources to more effective programs provides more "health" per dollar, thus meeting the utilitarian demand to maximize overall health, which many view as the primary goal of public health and health policy (Powers and Faden 2006). In addition, although black-white disparities in infant mortality persist, blacks have made significant gains, declining more than whites in some decades. You note that remaining inequalities could be deemed ethically acceptable by some standards of equity, such as the "maximin" principle. Although this distributive principle is subject to interpretation (Van Parijs 2003), it is generally understood to require that social and economic inequalities work to benefit society's least advantaged groups. Thus, inequalities (even significant ones) are morally acceptable as long as the least advantaged have significantly benefited (Powers and Faden 2006).

The director of community outreach proposes that the health department not make this decision unilaterally, but instead listen to community opinions on these questions of priorities and fairness. He suggests that the health department collaborate with community partners to host a series of public forums. He insists that a topic of such historic and contemporary concern to the community must be subject to public deliberation. Despite having a history of supporting community discussions, you are concerned about the cost of community forums, noting that they will drain resources from an already slim budget.

3.8.3 Discussion Questions

1. Have local health departments met their ethical obligations when community health improves overall, but health disparities persist? If not, why not? If so, on what grounds?
2. Is there something about infant mortality that makes it special in considerations of fairness? If so, what is it?
3. Should the role of race and racism in infant mortality shape priority setting and the allocation of resources in public health? If so, why?
4. On what grounds and how should you as the local health department director make resource allocation decisions? What standards—evidence, principles of justice, public opinion—should influence priority setting?
5. Should the community have a role in identifying community health priorities or, more specifically, in providing input into allocation decisions that directly affect them? If so, how should the community be involved and who represents the community?

References

Anand, S. 2004. The concern for equity in health. In *Public health, ethics, and equity*, ed. S. Anand, F. Peter, and A. Sen, 15–20. New York: Oxford University Press.

Centers for Disease Control and Prevention. 2011. *About CDC's Office of Minority Health & Health Equity (OMHHE)*. http://www.cdc.gov/minorityhealth/OMHHE.html. Accessed 29 Apr 2013.

Chopra, M., H. Campbell, and I. Rudan. 2012. Understanding the determinants of the complex interplay between cost-effectiveness and equitable impact in maternal and child mortality reduction. *Journal of Global Health* 2(1): 1–10.
MacDorman, M.F. 2011. Infant deaths—United States, 2000–2007. *MMWR Supplement* 60: 49–51.
MacDorman, M.F., and T.J. Mathews. 2009. The challenge of infant mortality: Have we reached a plateau? *Public Health Reports* 124(5): 670–681.
Mechanic, D. 2002. Disadvantage, inequality, and social policy. *Health Affairs* 21(2): 48–59.
Mechanic, D. 2007. Population health: Challenges for science and society. *The Milbank Quarterly* 85(3): 533–559.
Organisation for Economic Co-operation and Development (OECD). 2010. *OECD health data: Infant mortality.* https://data.oecd.org/healthstat/infant-mortality-rates.htm. Accessed 25 May 2015.
Powers, M., and R. Faden. 2006. *Social justice: The moral foundations of public health and health policy.* New York: Oxford University Press.
U.S. Department of Health and Human Services. 2011. *HHS action plan to reduce racial and ethnic health disparities.* http://www.minorityhealth.hhs.gov/npa/templates/content.aspx?lvl=1&lvlid=33&ID=285. Accessed 25 May 2015.
Van Parijs, P. 2003. Difference principles. In *The Cambridge companion to Rawls*, ed. S. Freeman, 200–240. Cambridge: Cambridge University Press.
World Health Organization (WHO). 2012. *Born too soon: The global action report on preterm birth.* http://whqlibdoc.who.int/publications/2012/9789241503433_eng.pdf. Accessed 29 Apr 2013.
You, D., G. Jones, T. Wardlaw, and M. Chopra. 2010. Levels and trends in child mortality, 1990–2009. *Lancet* 376(9745): 931–933.

3.9 Case 5: Priority Setting in Health Care: Ethical Issues

M. Inés Gómez and Lorna Luco
Centro de Bioética, Facultad de Medicina
Clínica Alemana–Universidad del Desarrollo
Santiago, Chile
e-mail: migomezb@gmail.com

This case is presented for instructional purposes only. The ideas and opinions expressed are the authors' own. The case is not meant to reflect the official position, views, or policies of the editors, the editors' host institutions, or the authors' host institutions.

3.9.1 Background

The Chilean System of Guarantees in Health—created by law in 2004—aims to establish guaranteed health care interventions in health promotion, disease and injury prevention, diagnosis and treatment, rehabilitation and palliative care (Ministerio de Salud 2004). The law mandates that public and private insurers provide the resources needed to protect the public against excessive health-related spending and guarantee timely and universal access to authorized interventions based on standards of care.[1]

National health objectives, established by the Ministry of Health, determine the list of guaranteed interventions. This list, however, is reviewed every 3 years and amended as new scientific and health information emerges. As of 2013, the System of Guarantees in Health included interventions for 80 health-related conditions (Ministerio de Salud 2013), accounting for almost 60 % of the Chilean burden of disease. The System of Guarantees in Health is a priority system based on acknowledged criteria, namely scientific evidence and socially shared values. For the system to be effective, the criteria must be transparent, publicly accepted, and open to review and modification.

The law that created the System of Guarantees in Health also mandated a procedure for selecting the guaranteed interventions (Ministerio de Salud 2004). The procedure factors in public opinion research to identify social consensus on health priorities, studies to identify effective interventions that prolong and improve quality of life, and assessments of interventions' cost effectiveness (Burrows 2008). The procedure determines priorities with an algorithm that includes these factors and information on disease burden and health system capacity (Missoni and Solimano 2010). After choosing the health interventions, the health ministry elaborates on a package of interventions related to specific health conditions and develops clinical guidelines for such interventions.

3.9.2 Case Description

You direct a team within the Ministry of Health that is responsible for recommending priorities for guaranteed health interventions. The priority ranking system emphasizes the selection of cost-effective interventions for conditions with the greatest burden. However, the health ministry also has authorized including expensive interventions that are less effective or treating health conditions with low prevalence, if that condition or those interventions significantly impact health. Because of budget reductions, a number of interventions are under review. Your team has been asked to recommend funding interventions for two health conditions—cataract (a common condition with highly effective treatment) and multiple sclerosis (a less prevalent condition but one with significant health and social impact).

[1] Law 19.966 for the System of Guarantees in Health includes the following definitions for guarantees: *Guaranteed Access*—Public and private health insurers must grant the resources to provide guaranteed interventions; *Guaranteed Opportunity*—Guaranteed interventions must be delivered within a deadline established in the protocols elaborated by the Ministry of Health; *Guaranteed Quality:* Interventions must be delivered by registered and accredited health care providers; *Financial Protection*—A maximum copayment is established to avoid the insured falling into financial insolvency.

Cataract, the main cause of blindness, primarily affects people over 40. This health problem has a high impact as measured by quality-adjusted life years (QALYs) (Ministerio de Salud 2007). Its surgical treatment is effective for 80–95 % of patients. The package of guaranteed interventions includes diagnostic confirmation within 180 days after suspected diagnosis and surgical treatment 90 days after confirmation. In 2013, it was expected that 48,424 cataract surgeries would be performed in Chilean public hospitals and 416 in private institutions.

Multiple sclerosis, an autoimmune inflammatory disease leading to demyelination in the central nervous system, produces a progressive deterioration of health and quality of life. It represents a minimal disease burden at the population level, mainly due to premature death. In Chile, it is estimated that 385 patients are treated for multiple sclerosis each year. The package of guaranteed interventions includes diagnostic confirmation within 60 days; confirmed cases must receive treatment within 30 days. Treatment includes pharmacological therapy and physiotherapy.

3.9.3 Discussion Questions

1. What are some of the ethical, scientific, and social considerations that should be weighed in deciding if interventions for both cataract and multiple sclerosis should be covered by the System of Guarantees in Health?
2. Is there an obligation for health systems to cover all health problems affecting a population? Are there limits?
3. How should health problems be prioritized and who should have the authority to make these decisions? Which criteria should receive the most weight in ranking priorities?
4. How should resources be distributed among health conditions affecting many people versus health conditions affecting few people?
5. How should resources be distributed among procedures that are preventive versus treatments for existing conditions?
6. How does taking a public health perspective versus a clinical medicine perspective affect your thinking about including these two conditions in the System of Guarantees in Health?
7. What role should transparency play in the selection procedure?

References

Burrows, J. 2008. Inequalities and healthcare reform in Chile: Equity of what? *Journal of Medical Ethics* 34: e13.

Ministerio de Salud. 2004. *Establece un Régimen General de Garantías en Salud.* Ley No. 19.966. http://www.leychile.cl/Navegar?idNorma=229834. Accessed 8 June 2015.

Ministerio de Salud. 2007. *Estudio Carga Enfermedad y Carga Atribuible.* http://epi.minsal.cl/epi/html/invest/cargaenf2008/Informe%20final%20carga_Enf_2007.pdf. Accessed 27 June 2013.

Ministerio de Salud. 2013. *Decreto Supremo No. 4. Aprueba Garantías Explícitas en Salud del Régimen General de Garantías en Salud.* http://web.minsal.cl/portal/url/item/d6924d33612dd5e6e040010164015e8f.pdf. Accessed 8 June 2015.
Missoni, E., and G. Solimano. 2010. *Towards universal health coverage: The Chilean experience*, Background paper, no. 4. Geneva: World Health Organization. http://www.who.int/healthsystems/topics/financing/healthreport/4Chile.pdf. Accessed 27 June 2013.

3.10 Case 6: Critical Care Triage in Pandemics

Maxwell J. Smith
Dalla Lana School of Public Health and the Joint Centre for Bioethics
University of Toronto
Toronto, ON, Canada
e-mail: max.smith@utoronto.ca

A.M. Viens
Centre for Health, Ethics and Law, Southampton Law School
University of Southampton
Southampton, UK

This case is presented for instructional purposes only. The ideas and opinions expressed are the authors' own. The case is not meant to reflect the official position, views, or policies of the editors, the editors' host institutions, or the authors' host institutions.

3.10.1 Background

Infectious diseases such as pandemic influenza and severe acute respiratory syndrome (SARS) have attuned the attention of policy makers and health practitioners to the importance of protecting and promoting the public's health in the face of increased care needs and extreme resource scarcity. In particular, acute care needs for the critically ill and discussions of treatment priorities have been the subject of much debate in pandemic planning (Hick et al. 2007; Melnychuk and Kenny 2006; Uscher-Pines et al. 2006). This is not surprising, as it has been estimated that more than 700,000 Americans may require mechanical ventilation during a pandemic, far outnumbering available ventilators (Rubinson et al. 2010; U.S. Department of Health and Human Services 2005). Additionally, shortages of hospital beds, personnel, and other equipment can be expected during a pandemic, which may limit the ability to meet an expected increase in patient volume (World Health Organization 2008).

Prudentially planning for the public's increased care needs during a pandemic requires assessing surge capacity, especially in critical care units (CCU). However, as pandemics increase in severity, they can overwhelm critical care capacity and contingency arrangements. To make the best use of resources and personnel (even in the absence of a pandemic), patients are triaged—evaluated to determine the type and priority of care to be received. While medical information informs the development of triage criteria, ethical considerations about triage goals—whether explicit or implicit—also play a role. For public health emergencies that overwhelm capacity, some propose adjusting critical care triage criteria to emphasize certain public health goals, like saving the most lives possible (Christian et al. 2006; Silva et al. 2010).

Some contend that utilitarian reasoning should predominate in critical care triage, based on the intuition that, when resources are scarce, allocation decisions should produce the greatest good for the greatest number (Charlesworth 1993; Childress 2004). Critics of utilitarianism reply that it requires coercion or covertness to succeed, because the public will not voluntarily sacrifice their lives or their loved ones for the greater good (Baker and Strosberg 1992). Utilitarian triage may be unpalatable to the public on the further ground that it quantifies and judges the value of one life over another, which could disproportionally impact particular population groups (Hoffman 2009). Others therefore would base triage decisions on egalitarian considerations, for instance, by giving everyone an equal chance at obtaining a scarce good, an approach for which historical precedent exists (Baker and Strosberg 1992).

Whatever approach is adopted, prior arrangements between policy makers, practitioners, and the public based on thoughtful, transparent deliberation about the most ethical approach to CCU triage usually will improve the legitimacy of decisions. Those who promote an approach based on fairness and equity need to consider that, during public health emergencies, the goal of saving lives may force a retreat to utilitarian ethics (Kirkwood 2010; Veatch 2005). While not necessarily unethical in itself, a retreat that overturns prior arrangements lays itself open to charges of illegitimacy.

Variability in the frameworks used to allocate public health resources illustrates the importance of reflecting upon the values that undergird policy decisions and individual practices, like critical care triage. Appealing spontaneously in the heat of the moment to values that have not been adequately reflected upon or discussed in a transparent and deliberative manner may lead to undesirable outcomes and accusations of unethical practices. While discussions of CCU triage criteria ultimately concern institutional clinical policy and practice, they reflect a larger discussion about the overarching public health goals in the face of large-scale, widespread public health emergencies, like pandemics.

3.10.2 Case Description

An outbreak of a novel influenza virus has progressed to the point that the World Health Organization has declared a pandemic. In the pandemic's first wave, hospital capacities were sufficient to handle the influx of pandemic influenza patients, whose morbidity and mortality rates mirrored rates for seasonal influenza. However, despite a vaccination campaign and other measures, such as ensuring surge capacity, rates of morbidity and mortality associated with the virus have increased drastically during the pandemic's second wave.

The resulting increased number of patients needing hospital beds has overwhelmed even the surge capacity of the CCUs of a metropolitan city's tertiary care hospitals. To meet this challenge, a teleconference has been scheduled between several members of the hospitals' administration, the CCU directors from each hospital, and public health officials involved in leading the jurisdiction's pandemic response. As a public health official who played a central role in developing the pandemic plan for your jurisdiction, you have been included on the call to provide guidance for the pandemic response.

During the meeting, a number of CCU directors report that their physicians and nurses are concerned about the type of patients being admitted into the CCU. Some of the directors see a trend that they suggest is ultimately undermining the efficiency of the pandemic response. They argue that, as the severity of the pandemic continues to increase, their triage criteria should be modified so as to use CCU resources to save the most lives possible. They worry that admitting those who present with the most need is preventing treatment of those who will benefit most from CCU admission. "So long as our triage scheme saves the most lives, it is ethically justifiable" a number of them declare.

The group takes up the proposal of a CCU director to triage according to Sequential Organ Failure Assessment (SOFA) scores—which are derived using a tool that determines a patient's organ function and failure rate to predict outcomes (Vincent et al. 2000). Were the pandemic's severity to increase, the group suggests that, in addition to the CCU director's proposal to use SOFA criteria, even more inclusion, exclusion, and priority criteria could be added with the goal of saving as many lives as possible. They've proposed exclusion criteria for CCU admittance that include patients with a poor prognosis, patients with other known health issues, and some mention of age cut-offs, to name a few.

Others involved in the teleconference question whether this is the right approach to take. They argue that, by aiming to save the most lives possible, those who may benefit less from CCU admission, like older adults or individuals with disabilities, will be unfairly affected. They say, "we should not just aim to save lives, but rather save lives *fairly*." As you and your public health colleagues are leading the pandemic response, the hospital administrators and CCU directors look to you for a recommendation or decision about how to proceed.

3.10.3 Discussion Questions

1. Ensuring that the CCU has surge capacity is a common strategy to accommodate an influx of patients who have been infected with pandemic influenza.

   (a) Does surge capability require alternative critical care triage criteria?
   (b) If the population's health needs exceed contingency arrangements, should alternative critical care triage criteria be used?
   (c) How should these decisions be made?
   (d) What principles, values, or processes should influence these decisions?

2. What considerations might exist during a pandemic that do not exist in everyday critical care and critical care triage that do or do not support the modification of triage criteria? If pandemic critical care triage requires a unique conceptual framework, what principles ought to be valued in such a framework (e.g. need, equality, utility, efficiency)?
3. Would the severity of a pandemic ever warrant the use of a utilitarian scheme for critical care triage, given that the public generally finds it unpalatable and carrying out such a plan could require coercion? How could an adverse public reaction to coercive or covert measures be mitigated?
4. In a pandemic, the most seriously ill patients with the lowest probability of being saved might be left untreated because their care would require too many resources with little prospect of recovery. This illustrates a conflict between the common good and the best interests of individual patients. What other conflicts might arise when triaging in a pandemic?
5. Triage can be used to maximize the number of lives saved with available resources. Should we aim to maximize the number of lives or, alternatively, the number of life years saved? This can also give rise to questions about the quality of those lives and years lived. Is it ever appropriate to make allocation decisions based on quality of life or life years?

Acknowledgements MJS is supported by a Canadian Institutes of Health Research Frederick Banting and Charles Best Canada Graduate Scholarship and the Canadian Institutes of Health Research Douglas Kinsella Doctoral Award for Research in Bioethics. AMV is supported by the Faculty of Medicine, Ruhr-University Bochum.

References

Baker, R., and M. Strosberg. 1992. Triage and equality: An historical reassessment of utilitarian analyses of triage. *Kennedy Institute of Ethics Journal* 2(2): 103–123.
Charlesworth, M. 1993. *Bioethics in a liberal society.* New York: Cambridge University Press.

Childress, J. F. 2004. Disaster triage. *Virtual Mentor* 6(5). http://journalofethics.ama-assn.org/2004/05/ccas2-0405.html (accessed on 20 Nov 2015).

Christian, M.D., L. Hawryluck, R.S. Wax, et al. 2006. Development of a triage protocol for critical care during an influenza pandemic. *Canadian Medical Association Journal* 175(11): 1377–1381.

Hick, J., L. Rubinson, D. O'Laughlin, and J. Farmer. 2007. Allocating ventilators during largescale disasters—Problem, planning, and process. *Critical Care* 11(3): 217–226.

Hoffman, S. 2009. Preparing for disaster: Protecting the most vulnerable in emergencies. *UC Davis Law Review* 42: 1491–1547.

Kirkwood, K. 2010. In the name of the greater good? *Emerging Health Threats Journal* 2(E12): 1–3.

Melnychuk, R.M., and N.P. Kenny. 2006. Pandemic triage: The ethical challenge. *Canadian Medical Association Journal* 175(11): 1393–1394.

Rubinson, L., F. Vaughn, S. Nelson, et al. 2010. Mechanical ventilators in US acute care hospitals. *Disaster Medicine and Public Health Preparedness* 4(3): 199–206.

Silva, D.S., J.X. Nie, K. Rossiter, S. Sahni, and R.E. Upshur. 2010. Contextualizing ethics: Ventilators, H1N1 and marginalized populations. *Healthcare Quarterly* 13(1): 32–36.

U.S. Department of Health and Human Services. 2005. *HHS pandemic influenza plan.* http://www.flu.gov/planning-preparedness/federal/hhspandemicinfluenzaplan.pdf. Accessed 7 Jan 2013.

Uscher-Pines, L., S.B. Omer, D.J. Barnett, T.A. Burke, and R.D. Balicer. 2006. Priority setting for pandemic influenza: An analysis of national preparedness plans. *PLoS Medicine* 3(10): 1721–1727.

Veatch, R.M. 2005. Disaster preparedness and triage: Justice and the common good. *The Mount Sinai Journal of Medicine* 72(4): 236–241.

Vincent, J.L., F. Ferreira, and R. Moreno. 2000. Scoring systems for assessing organ dysfunction and survival. *Critical Care Clinics* 16(2): 353–366.

World Health Organization (WHO). 2008. *Addressing ethical issues in pandemic influenza planning: Discussion papers.* http://www.who.int/csr/resources/publications/cds_flu_ethics_5web.pdf. Accessed 2 July 2013.

Chapter 4
Disease Prevention and Control

Michael J. Selgelid

4.1 Introduction

Ethical issues surrounding public health policy and practice regarding disease prevention and control often involve conflicting rights and values. Such conflicts partly arise from tension between individual and community interests or tension involving cultural beliefs and practices. This chapter outlines how such conflicts and tensions arise in the context of disease prevention and control by exploring ethical issues associated with mandatory treatment and vaccination, disease screening and surveillance, diseases prone to stigma, access to care, health promotion incentives, and emergency response.

4.2 Mandatory Treatment and Vaccination

In standard biomedical ethics (as opposed to public health ethics) discourse, the patient's right to informed consent to medical intervention is often considered sacrosanct. A primary aim of informed consent is to avoid medical paternalism, such as coercing a patient to do something for his or her own benefit. The transition in clinical practice from medical paternalism to informed consent was largely based on the ideas that (1) a well-informed patient is better placed than the doctor to determine which actions are in the patient's best interests (Goldman 1980) and (2) that a patient's autonomy should, in any case, be respected.

The opinions, findings, and conclusions of the author do not necessarily reflect the official position, views, or policies of the editors, the editors' host institutions, or the author's host institution.

M.J. Selgelid, MA, PhD (✉)
Centre for Human Bioethics, Monash University, Melbourne, Australia
e-mail: michael.selgelid@monash.edu

D.H. Barrett et al. (eds.), *Public Health Ethics: Cases Spanning the Globe*, Public Health Ethics Analysis 3, DOI 10.1007/978-3-319-23847-0_4

In public health, however, treatment and vaccination may, in addition to the health of the individual, be important to population health. As such, individual patients are not the only stakeholders whose interests must be considered. In the context of tuberculosis (TB), coercive treatment is common—in so far as, in many jurisdictions, patients with active TB are required to undergo (often directly observed) treatment under threat of confinement if they refuse. While TB treatment usually benefits those subjected to this kind of coercion, the primary motive for such policies is the protection of public health rather than paternalism. Because patients with untreated active TB remain contagious, their treatment is essential to prevent infection of others. Though objections to paternalism are not as relevant to mandatory treatment in this context, ethical issues remain. Because mandatory treatment (aimed at protection of others) conflicts with individual liberty, there is a conflict between legitimate values—i.e., individual liberty versus public health. There are also conflicting rights—i.e., the right of coerced individuals to autonomy versus the rights of others to health (or their rights not to be harmed by being infected). Each of these values and rights is legitimate; and, arguably, none should be given absolute priority over the others. A key ethical question about mandatory treatment is, thus, how great the threat to others (and public health in general) would need to be in order for mandatory treatment to be justified.[1] It is noteworthy that TB is relatively exceptional—i.e., there are not many other cases of infectious diseases for which treatment is routinely required.

Similar issues arise in the context of vaccination. While vaccination usually benefits the vaccinated, it also benefits others via contribution to herd immunity (Verweij and Dawson 2004). Mandatory vaccination is also more common than mandatory treatment. In some jurisdictions, for example, vaccination of children is required for school attendance. The case presented by Simón-Lorda et al. considers the scenario of a measles outbreak, resulting from a low rate of vaccination uptake, at a school in Spain. In the scenario, the conflicting rights associated with mandatory medical intervention again come into play. The suggestion that unvaccinated children should not be permitted to attend school, for example, is initially rejected by health authorities on the grounds that this would conflict with their right to education. Unvaccinated children's right to education, thus, conflicts with the rights of other children not to be infected. How should such a conflict of rights be resolved? In the case presented by Simón-Lorda et al., the outbreak finally becomes so widespread that mandatory vaccination is called for as an emergency measure. Assuming such a decision would be legitimate in the scenario under consideration, it might be grounded on the belief that public health outweighs individual liberty when the stakes are sufficiently high (rather than the belief that the value of public health outweighs the value of liberty in general).

A complicating factor regarding mandatory vaccination is that when one unvaccinated child ends up becoming infected with a disease (such as measles) and then goes on to infect others, it could be argued that those others who become infected do not in fact have their rights violated because they could have avoided infection

[1] With respect to the public health ethics framework discussed in Chap. 1, the question here is what, exactly, the proportionality requirement should be thought to consist in. For further discussion of this issue, see Selgelid (2009).

by getting vaccinated themselves. It would usually be parents, rather than children, however, who make decisions about childhood vaccination. This raises the question of who (e.g., parents or the government) should have authority to make decisions about children's health and well-being—and vaccination in particular. Assuming that parents should usually retain decision-making authority about childhood vaccination, the relevance of cultural differences to public health ethics is highlighted by the fact that some parents may refuse vaccination of their children for what are ultimately cultural reasons (e.g., religious beliefs). This leads to questions (also raised by other cases presented in this chapter) about whether, and to what extent, cultural beliefs and practices should influence public health policy and practice.

4.3 Disease Screening and Surveillance

As in the cases of treatment and vaccination, informed consent to diagnostic testing is usually considered essential in standard biomedical ethics discourse regarding doctor-patient relationships. In public health, however, diagnostic testing is sometimes required, for example as a condition of employment (such as tuberculin skin testing of restaurant and hospital employees) or immigration (for which both TB and HIV testing are common). Testing of tissues or other biological samples also sometimes takes place, for research or surveillance purposes, without patients' or donors' awareness or consent (e.g., testing of stored sputum samples to determine TB drug resistance prevalence). Cases such as these may pose conflict between the goal to promote public health, on the one hand, and the goals to respect individual autonomy and privacy, on the other. As with mandatory treatment and vaccination, however, such practices are arguably justifiable in cases where public health benefits are sufficiently high (which is not to say that public health generally trumps autonomy and privacy).

As with vaccination, questions about parental authority in decision making regarding childhood health arise in the context of disease screening. The case presented by Nicholls et al., raises such issues. Bloodspot screening is commonly used to test newborns for numerous serious health conditions, and stored bloodspots are sometimes later used for research and surveillance that lead to important public health benefits. Given the potential importance of such practices for a child's health, and to public health more generally, to what extent is parental informed consent to bloodspot screening or secondary use of stored bloodspots essential? The case presented by Nicholls et al. raises the worry that more parents, out of privacy concerns, might refuse newborn bloodspot screening if a thoroughgoing informed consent process (as opposed to the current opt-out model) were required, and that this could have adverse effects for both newborns and, given the benefits of research and surveillance with stored bloodspots, public health more generally. Among other important questions, Nicholls et al. ask, "How should clinically actionable results [of secondary investigations involving bloodspots] be dealt with?" When surveillance testing of stored bloodspots or other stored tissues leads to identification of not-previously-recognized disease (or predispositions thereto), for example, to what extent do investigators have duties to track down and inform individuals from whom bloodspots or other stored tissues were originally obtained? Like research, surveillance raises ethical issues about standards of care (Selgelid 2012).

Ethical issues concerning testing and surveillance are also highlighted in the case presented by Bhattacharya. In this case, the criminalization of HIV transmission and mandatory name-based reporting requirements (in the case of HIV diagnosis) are portrayed as deterrents to sex workers' seeking of HIV testing. In the case of criminalized transmission, the disincentive to testing is that criminal penalties associated with prostitution are greater (in some jurisdictions) for those who have tested HIV positive. Among other things, criminalizing HIV makes it difficult for public health workers to promote HIV testing of sex workers (who are an especially vulnerable group, and for whom testing is especially important—for their own sake and for public health more generally) while adhering to mandatory reporting requirements. This challenge is further exacerbated by socio-economic and cultural factors that promote prostitution to begin with.

This case also raises more general issues about the criminalization of infectious disease transmission. Many argue that there is a moral obligation to avoid infecting others, based on a duty not to harm others (Harris and Holm 1995). Criminalizing infectious disease transmission involves the legal enforcement of such a moral duty. Given that HIV transmission usually involves consenting adults knowingly taking risks, one might question whether criminalization of HIV transmission, in particular, is necessary. It should be noted, however, that it is usually *intentional* transmission of HIV that is criminalized. In any case, criminalization of HIV transmission raises questions about the extent to which intentional transmission of other diseases should also be criminalized and whether, or why, *negligent* transmission (of HIV or other diseases) should also be subject to legal penalties.

The case by Bhattacharya also raises ethical questions about name-based reporting, which is legally required upon positive diagnosis of numerous diseases of public health importance (Fairchild et al. 2007). As a surveillance measure, the purpose of name-based reporting pertains to contact tracing and, among other issues, estimations of disease incidence or prevalence, which are used to inform public health policy and practice (Lee et al. 2010). While mandatory name-based reporting may have important public health benefits, it conflicts with privacy and informed consent. It may also have adverse effects upon public health if it ends up driving epidemics underground, when those especially in need of testing and treatment are reluctant to seek care due to concerns about privacy or lack of trust in health care providers. What the overall public health consequences of name-based reporting actually are, with any reportable disease, is ultimately an empirical question.

4.4 Stigma

Related to the privacy issues considered above is the problem of disease stigmatization, which can lead to discrimination and other abuses of those known (or, perhaps wrongly, believed) to be affected. The extent and nature of disease stigmatization, and the effects thereof, are often largely related to cultural factors or misunderstanding of the diseases in question. The unjust discrimination and abuse commonly associated with disease stigmatization are especially problematic because they make matters worse for those who are already badly off (by virtue of health status). As in the case considered above, stigma can also deter those in need from seeking testing or health care to begin with. The problem of stigma could be reduced via better public education about the nature of stigmatized diseases and better legal protections against unjust discrimination and other abuses associated with stigma.

Ways in which stigmatization can interfere with individual and public health is illustrated in the case presented by Henning and Nair. While risks of vertical HIV transmission from infected mother to newborn can be reduced by replacing breastfeeding with formula and providing antiretrovirals to the mother, in some southern African countries HIV is so heavily stigmatized that women may be reluctant to pursue such measures in fear they will suffer violence or be abandoned by their husbands (if such measures reveal, or raise suspicions about, their HIV status). In the case presented by Henning and Nair, such fears on the part of a mother create a dilemma for her doctor, who, based on best medical practice and concern for the baby (and public health), would presumably want to encourage such measures, but, based on concern for the mother's privacy and well-being, might not want to insist on them. While there is no obvious answer to the question of what the doctor should immediately do in this poignant case presented by Henning and Nair, the long-term solution to this kind of problem would presumably require cultural change involving reduction of HIV stigma via public engagement and awareness-raising, and greater empowerment and protection of women in general.

4.5 Access to Care

It is commonly believed that there is a universal human right to health and/or health care, and such rights are enshrined by the *Universal Declaration of Human Rights* and other human rights instruments (Selgelid and Pogge 2010). In addition to being a matter of human rights and justice, access to care is also important for public health. In the context of infectious diseases, for example, lack of access to care results in perpetuation of epidemics when those left untreated remain contagious. This is one reason the burden of infectious disease is more heavily shouldered by impoverished developing nations, where access to care is limited, largely due to resource constraints. When such diseases run rampant in developing countries, this poses threats to global health more generally—because infectious diseases show no respect for international borders. This points to self-interested reasons, in addition to egalitarian and human rights reasons, for wealthy countries to do more to promote health care improvement in developing countries.

Although the right to health care is widely recognized (if not always well respected and protected) it is questionable whether such a right should be considered absolute. Some means of health care may be too expensive, even in wealthy countries, to be routinely provided. In other cases, providing health care to individual patients might itself have adverse effects on public health. When patients fail to complete a full course of antimicrobial treatment, for example, this promotes emergence of drug resistance (which increases danger to others who might be infected). Luco et al. present a case involving a TB patient who repeatedly fails to complete his prescribed course of medication and ends up with drug-resistant TB as a result. In light of this patient's history of noncompliance, his adherence to further courses of treatment might be considered unlikely. The patient nonetheless pleads for a new course of treatment and promises to adhere to the prescribed regimen. Whether providing additional treatment in a case like this would be warranted depends at least partly on whether there is a decent chance the treatment will succeed (assuming the patient does in fact adhere) in light of the current level of drug resistance. If the patient's TB is already resistant to all available treatments, then further treatment (even if the patient adheres) might at best be futile or at worst lead to greater drug resistance.

If, on the other hand, the patient's TB remains susceptible to treatment then deciding whether to provide additional medication might partly depend on the likelihood that the patient will comply with treatment in the future. One might argue that a doctor's decision to withhold treatment based on predictions about continued noncompliance would involve unjust discrimination based on the doctors' judgment of the patient's character, and that doctors, in general, have no special expertise for making such judgments or predicting patients' behavior in the first place (World Health Organization [WHO] 2010). If the patient is left untreated, then this would arguably infringe on his right to health care and threaten public health (i.e., if the patient remains infectious and at large in the community). On the other hand, based on past experience, there appears to be a legitimate concern that providing care (or respecting the patient's right to care) may conflict with others' right to health and public health more generally (i.e., as continued noncompliance may lead to increased drug resistance). Consideration of this case motivates further reflection on mandatory treatment (discussed above) because if treatment compliance was better enforced to begin with, then dilemmas posed by cases like this might be avoided.

4.6 Health Promotion Incentives

Public health policies often involve incentivizing health promoting behaviors (e.g., provision of financial benefits to parents when children are vaccinated) and/or disincentivizing unhealthy behavior (e.g., heavy taxation of things like cigarettes and alcohol). While such policies might be considered manipulative or paternalistic in spirit, they do not rely on outright coercion if people are still ultimately free to behave as they wish, and so autonomy is largely respected. Their legitimate aim is health improvement. Such policies, however, may sometimes involve tension with cultural beliefs and practices. In the case presented by Bhati, for example, cash incentives are used to encourage childbirth in health care institutions in India, where homebirth remains traditional. This situation leads to a tragic conclusion in the case of a mother who resists her in-laws' pressure (apparently based on monetary motive) toward institutional delivery. She ends up losing her child due to delivery complications while traveling to her home village where she planned to give birth and is then faced with "the wrath of her husband and in-laws." While the cash incentive aims to promote the health of mothers and children, and public health more generally, the point of this case is to show how this kind of health promotion incentive might exacerbate pressures on women who, in the cultural milieu of India, already suffer diminished autonomy. The warning is that, despite good intentions, health promotion incentives can backfire if they lack adequate cultural sensitivity.

4.7 Emergency Response

Emergencies are extreme situations (Viens and Selgelid 2012) where threats to public health can be exceptionally severe. Examples include epidemics, other natural disasters (e.g., floods, hurricanes, earthquakes), and manmade disasters (e.g., war, terrorism, severe environmental damage). As noted in cases previously discussed, public health policies and practices often give rise to conflicts between the rights and liberties of individuals, on the one hand, and the goal to promote public health, on the other. It has also been repeatedly suggested (above) that the importance of public health protection is more likely (than would otherwise be the case) to outweigh the importance of protecting/respecting individual rights and liberties in cases where the magnitude of threat to public health is especially great. During emergencies, therefore, it may be more necessary than in other contexts to resort to liberty infringing measures. In the case of a severe epidemic, for example, social distancing measures such as isolation and quarantine might be justified despite the fact that they interfere with one of the most basic human rights, freedom of movement.

Emergencies also often put unprecedented pressure on limited resources and thus require difficult ethical decisions regarding resource allocation. Given the spectre of a future severe influenza pandemic, for example, there has been much debate about who should be given priority for resources like antivirals, vaccines, and ventilators if (as may be expected) need outstrips supply (Verweij 2009).

Emergencies, finally, also often call for urgent action. So, decisions must be made quickly, and other time-saving measures may be needed to mitigate harm. While urgent research might be needed to understand and control an epidemic caused by a novel pathogen, for example, it has been argued that the usual procedures for ethical clearance of research (which can be very slow) might need to be altered in the case of emergency research in particular (WHO 2009).

The issue of urgency is well illustrated by the case presented by Peacock and colleagues. In the event of a major bioterrorist attack involving anthrax, it might be necessary to vaccinate large numbers of people quickly. Administration of vaccine shortly after exposure is important because anthrax vaccine provides prophylactic protection. Because anthrax vaccine has not been tested in children, however, its use in children would require informed consent of parents according to U.S. law. In a scenario where huge numbers of children would need to be vaccinated quickly, however, going through usual informed consent processes might take too much time (and perhaps lead to unrest among those waiting to be vaccinated). This motivates examination of possible ways to hasten the consent process, for example, via group information sessions rather than the usual one-on-one consent process. While group consent procedures may facilitate more timely vaccination of children, the question is whether, or the extent to which, group sessions would ultimately compromise informed consent and whether such compromise would be justified by public health benefits. As with other cases presented in this chapter, the case presented by Peacock et al. illustrates how cultural factors may pose special difficulties. For example, quick consent would be especially challenging in cases where children's parents do not speak English. Quick consent (to a vaccine that has not been studied in children) may likewise be difficult in cases where parents are generally skeptical about vaccine safety.

The case presented by Viens and Smith explores a range of ethical challenges associated with mass evacuation that might be called for in an emergency scenario involving a major hurricane. Among other issues, this case raises questions about when evacuation should be voluntary or mandatory (while the latter, like isolation and quarantine, would involve interference with freedom of movement); whether, or how, mandatory evacuation should be enforced; whether there are duties to rescue those who refuse to comply with calls for evacuation; whether such people should be financially sanctioned if they are in fact rescued; who should be given special assistance with evacuation efforts, and how those in need of assistance should be prioritized; whether it might be acceptable to abandon unstable patients who cannot be moved (or for whom movement would be excessively expensive); whether compensation might be due to those who suffer financial (or other) loss as a result of compliance with calls for voluntary or mandatory evacuation; and whether there should be legal protections against price gouging of commodities like gasoline.

4.8 Conclusion

This chapter has illustrated ways in which ethical issues associated with disease prevention and control involve conflicting rights and values, tensions between individual and community interests, and tensions involving cultural beliefs and practices. While the cases discussed in this chapter provide a good overview of many of the most important and difficult ethical issues associated with disease prevention and control, the discussion above reveals that their resolution would require resolution of both empirical questions (about the extent to which alternative values would likely be promoted or compromised by one practice or policy or another) and philosophical questions (about how to balance legitimate values in cases of conflict). It is also important to recognize that resolution of any of the specific issues in the cases discussed above would not necessarily imply resolution of the more general issues raised by these cases. Resolving the question of whether or not there should be mandatory measles vaccination in Spain, for example, would not resolve the question of whether there should be mandatory vaccination of measles in other countries, or whether there should be mandatory vaccination against other diseases (in Spain or elsewhere). A virtue of case studies is that context is crucial to the empirical questions that ethical issues (partly) turn on.

References

Fairchild, A.L., R. Bayer, and J. Colgrove. 2007. *Searching eyes: Privacy, the state, and disease surveillance in America*. Berkeley: University of California Press.

Goldman, A. 1980. *The moral foundations of professional ethics*. Totowa: Rowman and Littlefield.

Harris, J., and S. Holm. 1995. Is there a moral obligation not to infect others? *British Medical Journal* 311: 1215–1217.

Lee, L.M., S.M. Teutsch, S.B. Thacker, and M.E. St. Louis (eds.). 2010. *Principles and practice of public health surveillance*. New York: Oxford University Press.

Selgelid, M.J. 2009. A moderate pluralist approach to public health policy and ethics. *Public Health Ethics* 2(2): 195–205.

Selgelid, M.J. 2012. Case discussion in response to obesity surveillance in school children. In *Population and public health ethics: Cases from research, policy, and practice*, 26–31. Toronto: University of Toronto Joint Centre for Bioethics.

Selgelid, M.J., and T. Pogge. 2010. *Health rights*. Farnham: Ashgate.

Verweij, M. 2009. Moral principles for allocating scarce medical resources in an influenza pandemic. *Journal of Bioethical Inquiry* 6(2): 159–169.

Verweij, M., and A. Dawson. 2004. Ethical principles for collective immunisation programmes. *Vaccine* 22(23–24): 3122–3126.

Viens, A.M., and M.J. Selgelid. 2012. *Emergency ethics*. Farnham: Ashgate.

World Health Organization (WHO). 2009. *Research ethics in international epidemic response*. Geneva: World Health Organization. http://www.who.int/ethics/gip_research_ethics_.pdf. Accessed 5 Nov 2013.

World Health Organization (WHO). 2010. *Guidance on ethics of tuberculosis prevention, care and control*. Geneva: World Health Organization. http://whqlibdoc.who.int/publications/2010/9789241500531_eng.pdf. Accessed 5 Nov 2013.

4.9 Case 1: Mandatory Vaccination in Measles Outbreaks

Pablo Simón-Lorda
Primary Health Care Centre Chauchina
UGC Santa Fe, Granada, Spain

Department of Health and Social Welfare–Regional Government of Andalusia
Granada, Spain
e-mail: psimoneasp@gmail.com

Isabel Marin-Rodríguez
Provincial Office of Health and Social Welfare of Granada
Department of Health and Social Welfare–Regional Government of Andalusia
Granada, Spain

Juan Laguna-Sorinas
Department of Epidemiological Surveillance, Provincial Office of Health and Social Welfare of Granada

Department of Health and Social Welfare–Regional Government of Andalusia
Granada, Spain

Maite Cruz-Piqueras and Maribel Tamayo-Velázquez
Andalusian School of Public Health
Granada, Spain

Miguel Angel Royo-Bordonada
National School of Public Health
Madrid, Spain

This case is presented for instructional purposes only. The ideas and opinions expressed are the authors' own. The case is not meant to reflect the official position, views, or policies of the editors, the editors' host institutions, or the authors' host institutions.

4.9.1 Background

In 2005, the European Regional Office of the World Health Organization (WHO-EUR), which includes 53 countries, set the goal of eliminating measles in Europe in 2010 (WHO 2005). The Pan American Health Organization (PAHO) declared the WHO Region of the Americas free from endemic measles in 2002 (Castillo-Solorzano et al. 2011). Nevertheless, that region has continued to experience periodic outbreaks, probably due to importation of measles from other parts of the world. In 2008, WHO's Executive Board (EB) began to determine whether to extend the goal of eradicating measles to the rest of the world (WHO 2010a).

The decrease in measles cases after a vaccine was introduced in the 1980s made the WHO-EUR goal of eliminating measles in Europe realistic. However, in 2006–2007, the vaccine coverage rates remained below 90 % in many European countries, and although the number of cases continued to fall, epidemic outbreaks still occurred periodically (Muscat et al. 2009). At the end of 2009, an explosion of outbreaks was recorded and the number of cases began to increase sharply. This upward trend continued throughout 2010, when 30,639 measles cases were reported (WHO 2011). This forced WHO-EUR to postpone its eradication goal until 2015 (WHO 2010b).

The increase in measles cases can be attributed to the inability to achieve appropriate levels of vaccine coverage (>90 %) either because people cannot access health services, or because they hold personal beliefs against vaccination (Muscat 2011). The latter group includes members of the anti-vaccination movement, which makes extensive use of the Internet and social networks to share ideas (Kata 2010). After rumors spread about an association between measles vaccination and autism, vaccine coverage rates decreased in countries such as the United Kingdom, where "anti-vaccination" sentiment has gradually grown during the past 10 years (Flaherty 2011).

Measles is a notifiable disease in the 53 WHO-EUR countries, all of which employ a two-dose regimen for immunization. However, measles vaccination is not mandatory in all WHO-EUR countries. A study of 29 of the 53 WHO EUR member countries showed that, in 2010, vaccination against measles was only obligatory for children in 8 of the 29 (Haverkate et al. 2012). Within the 21 remaining countries, vaccination was recommended but voluntary. The debate about which of the two positions, voluntary or compulsory vaccination, is better from an ethical point of view, remains open (Moran et al. 2008; Schröder-Bäck et al. 2009).

Spain is one of the European countries where measles has reappeared. The first childhood immunization schedule (CIS) was introduced in Spain in 1975. In 1978, Spain began to vaccinate against measles (one dose at 15 months) which beginning in 1981 was administered as a measles-mumps-rubella (MMR) vaccine. Starting in 1990, a second dose at 11 years of age was introduced. In 2004, the age at which the second dose was administered was revised to 8 years of age. As a result, the illness almost disappeared over the course of a 20-year period: 220,096 cases in 1986, but only 17 cases in 2005. However, since that time, cases have increased, with periodic local outbreaks: 2006 (349 cases), 2007 (260 cases), 2008 (305 cases), 2009 (43 cases), 2010 (285 cases) and 2011 (3507 cases) (WHO 2012). In 2011, an infected person died.

In contrast with countries such as the United States, Spain has made childhood vaccination voluntary and not a requirement for attending school (Colgrove 2006; Stadlin et al. 2012). However, the average vaccine coverage rates are high (>90 %) (Masa et al. 2010). This can be attributed largely to the public health system's primary care teams, distributed throughout the country and composed of family doctors, pediatricians and nurses. Even so, there are still places where coverage is less extensive, particularly in poor parts of large cities with low levels of socioeconomic development.

In Spain, health professionals document administration of childhood vaccines in handwriting in a paper booklet maintained by the parents. They also register this information in the child's medical record, which is commonly computer based. However, discrepancies can occur between the two vaccine registration systems.

4.9.2 *Case Description*

You are the chief public health officer in a province of Spain. One day, a pediatrician tells you about a 13-year-old who is suspected to have measles. The child and his family attended a wedding the week before. Within 10 days, six more people who also attended the wedding were diagnosed with measles and nine secondary cases are confirmed. Of the secondary cases, seven were thought to have been exposed at school and two were in the hospital emergency ward.

All cases occurred in a historic quarter of the city with a large degree of cultural, economic, religious, ethnic, and social diversity. This multicultural identity diverges from the relative homogeneity of the rest of the city.

The public primary school of the historic quarter is now the focal point of the outbreak. There are 216 students enrolled in the school. You order two initial public health measures outlined in the regional health ministry's Alert Protocol for Measles: (1) that a letter be sent to parents asking them to bring their child's vaccination booklet to the school, and (2) that a meeting be held with the parents to have health professionals inform them about the disease and the immunization process.

As a result of the letter, the parents of 137 children take the vaccine booklet to the school, which shows a low degree of measles vaccine coverage (60 %). Those children not immunized are then vaccinated with their parents' consent. However, the parents of 79 children fail to bring the vaccine booklet to the school.

In the parent meeting, some of the parents express their support for the anti-vaccination movement. They express sentiments such as "the disease is a natural process, so we prefer to organize measles parties;" "risk of measles is very low, but vaccines are toxic poisons;" "a lot of hidden complications of vaccines exist, for example, autism;" and "Big Pharma and politicians are looking out for profits, not for the welfare of our kids." They also allege, "vaccination is not obligatory in Spain, and we have a right to educate our children in accordance with our values." These remarks generated a heated dispute between parents for and against vaccination. The majority of parents seem misinformed about the risks and benefits of vaccination and do not even know the immunization status of their own children.

The next day, the measles outbreak at the school comes to the attention of the local and national media. Alarmist messages and negative stories about anti-vaccination groups grab headlines. There are stories that seem to blame the outbreak on the cultural diversity of the historic quarter. You worry that the negative media reports may stigmatize the people living in this quarter or, even more worrisome, blame specific religious or ethnic groups.

Therefore, you consider adopting additional public health measures such as maximizing surveillance in the city, controlling emergency rooms to decrease (or eliminate) transmission, and vaccinating health professionals and children under 6 months. You also consider having unvaccinated children stay home, but health authorities reject the idea, alleging it would violate the right to education. Little by little, a number of parents consent to having their children vaccinated, or the children are stricken and become immune.

Nevertheless, new cases linked to the school continue to occur. In the regional health ministry, attention is turned to the possibility of requiring vaccination via a court order, citing a fundamental law that enables such exceptional actions in public health emergencies.

Finally, a request is put to the judge to authorize the enforced vaccination of 35 children. He does and you inform the parents. Two nurses, accompanied by a police officer, visit the houses one by one. The majority of the parents give consent to the vaccination. Ten days later, only nine children remain unvaccinated as a result of the refusal of their parents. You inform the judge that the number is so low that the situation of special risk generated has now been overcome. You suspend compulsory vaccinations.

Since the first case was diagnosed, 10 months have elapsed. A total of 308 cases have been confirmed, 96 in minors younger than 1 year old. And 71 patients required hospitalisation (23 %), including five adults.

4.9.3 Discussion Questions

1. What are the values, ethical principles, and rights that come into conflict in this case? If it is not possible to respect all of them, how should they be prioritized?
2. Is the decision to allow unvaccinated children to attend the school justified?
3. Think of a solution that adequately balances the freedom of choice of parents who are against vaccination with the protection of the health of a community where vaccination is not compulsory.
4. Was there sufficient epidemiological risk to justify the court order? Were there other possible solutions? Once the judicial measure had been adopted, why was it not pursued to its conclusion? Does the argument to suspend administering vaccines provide sufficient grounds for this decision?
5. Once the outbreak has subsided, what measures should be introduced to avoid further outbreaks? If the vaccination rate in the country later falls and new outbreaks occur, should the government consider mandatory vaccination?

Acknowledgements The authors would like to acknowledge the EuroPubHealth Consortium (www.europubhealth.org) for funding the academic stay of Pablo Simón as visiting scholar at the Mailman School of Public Health, Columbia University, New York (USA), during October through November 2012. This support made his preparation of the case possible.

References

Castillo-Solorzano, C.C., C. Ruiz-Matus, B. Flannery, C. Marsigli, G. Tambini, and J.K. Andrus. 2011. The Americas: Paving the road toward global measles eradication. *Journal of Infectious Diseases* 204(suppl 1): S270–S278.

Colgrove, J. 2006. *State of immunity: The politics of vaccination in twentieth-century America*. Berkeley: University of California.

Flaherty, D.K. 2011. The vaccine-autism connection: A public health crisis caused by unethical medical practices and fraudulent science. *The Annals of Pharmacotherapy* 45(10): 1302–1304.

Haverkate, M., F. D'Ancona, C. Giambi, K. Johansen, P.L. Lopalco, and V. Cozza, et al. 2012. Mandatory and recommended vaccination in the EU, Iceland and Norway: Results of the VENICE 2010 survey on the ways of implementing national vaccination programmes. *Euro Surveillance* 17(22): pii: 20183. http://www.eurosurveillance.org/ViewArticle.aspx?ArticleId=20183. Accessed 10 June 2015.

Kata, A. 2010. A postmodern Pandora's box: Anti-vaccination misinformation on the internet. *Vaccine* 28(7): 1709–1716.

Masa, J., T. Castellanos, and M. Terrés. 2010. *Annual report of the Spanish plan for the eradication of measles and rubella–2010*. Working Party of the Spanish Plan for the Eradication of Measles and Rubella of the National Center of Epidemiology – Carlos III Institute of Health. http://www.isciii.es/ISCIII/es/contenidos/fd-servicios-cientifico-tecnicos/fd-vigilancias-alertas/fd-enfermedades/fd-enfermedades-prevenibles-vacunacion/Informe-Anual-Plan-Eliminacion-del-Sarampion-Rubeola-y-Sindrome-de-Rubeola-Congenita-Espana-2010.pdf. Accessed 10 June 2015.

Moran, N.E., S. Gainotti, and C. Petrini. 2008. From compulsory to voluntary immunisation: Italy's national vaccination plan (2005–2007) and the ethical and organisational challenges facing public health policy-makers across Europe. *Journal of Medical Ethics* 34(9): 669–674.
Muscat, M. 2011. Who gets measles in Europe? *The Journal of Infectious Diseases* 204(suppl 1): S353–S365.
Muscat, M., H. Bang, J. Wohlfahrt, S. Glismann, K. Mølbak, and EUVAC.NET Group. 2009. Measles in Europe: An epidemiological assessment. *Lancet* 373(9661): 383–389.
Schröder-Bäck, P., H. Brand, I. Escamilla, J.K. Davies, C. Hall, K. Hickey, et al. 2009. Ethical evaluation of compulsory measles immunisation as a benchmark for good health management in the European Union. *Central European Journal of Public Health* 17(4): 183–186.
Stadlin, S., R.A. Bednarczyk, and S.B. Omer. 2012. Medical exemptions to school immunization requirements in the United States—Association of state policies with medical exemption rates (2004–2011). *The Journal of Infectious Diseases* 206(7): 989–992.
World Health Organization (WHO). 2005. *Eliminating measles and rubella and preventing congenital rubella infection: WHO European Region Strategic Plan 2005–2010*. http://www.euro.who.int/__data/assets/pdf_file/0008/79028/E87772.pdf. Accessed 10 June 2015.
World Health Organization (WHO). 2010a. Proceedings of the global technical consultation to assess the feasibility of measles eradication, 28–30 July 2010. *The Journal of Infectious Diseases* 204(suppl 1): S4–S13. doi:10.1093/infdis/jir100.
World Health Organization (WHO). 2010b. *Resolution: Renewed commitment to elimination of measles and rubella and prevention of congenital rubella syndrome by 2015 and sustained support for poliofree status in the WHO European Region*. Regional Committee for Europe (EUR/RC60/R12). http://www.euro.who.int/__data/assets/pdf_file/0016/122236/RC60_eRes12.pdf. Accessed 10 June 2015.
World Health Organization (WHO). 2011. Increased transmission and outbreaks of measles, European region, 2011. *Weekly Epidemiological Record* 86(49): 557–564.
World Health Organization (WHO). 2012. *Centralized information system for infectious diseases (CISID): Measles*. Geneva: World Health Organization. http://data.euro.who.int/cisid. Accessed 10 June 2015.

4.10 Case 2: Public Health Approaches to Preventing Mother-to-Child HIV Transmission

Margaret Henning
International Health Systems Program
Harvard T. H. Chan School of Public Health
Boston, MA, USA

Health Science
Keene State College
Keene, NH, USA
e-mail: mhenning@keene.edu

Indira Nair
Department of Engineering and Public Policy
Carnegie Mellon University
Pittsburgh, PA, USA

This case is presented for instructional purposes only. The ideas and opinions expressed are the authors' own. The case is not meant to reflect the official position, views, or policies of the editors, the editors' host institutions, or the authors' host institutions.

4.10.1 Background

> *The pursuit of global public health takes place in an unjust world, demanding that its practitioners judge when and to what extent to compromise their ideals and standards in order to remain effective.* (Wikler and Cash 2009)

Mother-to-child transmission (MTCT)—also known as vertical transmission—is the primary cause of HIV infection in children under 10 years of age (Interagency Coalition on AIDS and Development 2011). Each year, more than 600,000 infants become infected with HIV from prenatal transmission during pregnancy, labor and delivery, or breastfeeding, primarily in under-resourced countries (Centers for Disease Control and Prevention 2012; Interagency Coalition on AIDS and Development 2011; Mnyani and McIntyre 2009).

For women who are HIV-negative, breastfeeding is the preferred child survival strategy. It is linked to a lower risk of various health problems for babies, including a reduction in the risk of death from diarrhea and malnutrition (World Health Organization 2007; O'Reilly et al. 2012). However, the risk of an HIV-positive woman transmitting the virus to her baby in the absence of any intervention ranges from 15 to 45 % (De Cock et al. 2000; World Health Organization 2015). Avoidance of breastfeeding (use of replacement feeding) reduces the risk of neonatal transmission to 20 % (Interagency Coalition on AIDS and Development 2011). Modified feeding, also known as mixed feeding (liquids or solids), results in a risk of transmission of about 30–35 % (Coutsoudis et al. 1999). The safety of replacing breastfeeding depends on access to clean water, a reliable supply of formula, and availability of instruction. Thus, use of mixed feeding techniques can be a challenge in many middle- or low-income countries (World Health Organization 2007; O'Reilly et al. 2012).

To help reduce the risk of babies becoming infected with HIV and to ensure quality services across the different levels of the health system, the World Health Organization (WHO) released revised guidelines in 2010 for use by managers of national HIV and AIDS programmers, as well as local managers and health care providers. The guidelines emphasize treatment for pregnant, HIV-infected women. Those with stage 3 or stage 4 disease (CD4 count $\leq$350 cells/μL) require lifelong three-drug antiretroviral therapy (ART) to treat their own HIV infections and for prevention of mother-to-child transmission of HIV (PMTCT). For women with less-advanced disease, WHO recommends a country- or program-level choice between Option A (maternal zidovudine during pregnancy and infant nevirapine [NVP] throughout breastfeeding), and Option B (maternal three-drug ART regimens throughout pregnancy and breastfeeding) (WHO 2010). Mutations of the virus can occur when the required course of treatment is not followed (Interagency Coalition on AIDS and Development 2011).

In many countries, social stigma, fear of the risk of discrimination, rejection, and violence can thwart a woman's intention to have an HIV test, take antiretroviral drugs, or substitute breast milk (Interagency Coalition on AIDS and Development 2011). Such obstacles arise in part from traditional beliefs and values and from unfamiliarity with the practice of biomedicine. In some cultures, a woman is viewed as responsible for her own HIV infection and that of her child, and she may suffer emotional or physical abuse at the hands of her family if her HIV status is discovered.

However, it can be important for her family to be aware of her HIV status, as they are often the ones who advise her on child feeding practices. Dealing with a woman's fear of being exposed as an HIV-positive mother is a challenge inherent in programs that focus on PMTCT.

4.10.2 Case Description

In a sub-Saharan African country, Dr. Charles directs a rural health clinic that an international organization funds. Funding requires the clinic to follow new WHO guidelines for the PMTCT. The guidelines specifically recommend using antiretroviral drugs throughout the breastfeeding period by HIV-positive women (WHO 2010). The district health office is also requiring Dr. Charles to develop guidance for his clinical staff on how to carry out the guidelines in a way that takes the values and beliefs of the community into account. Implementing the guidelines poses a major challenge for Dr. Charles because of the country's weak health infrastructure, the small number of paid staff in his clinic, and an inadequate facility with limited general supplies. However, his facility boasts a lab, and he has received some funding to support the PMTCT program.

Recently, a woman in labor came to the clinic and told Dr. Charles she was HIV positive. She wanted to know how she could breastfeed without awakening suspicions of her HIV status. She was worried that if neighbors or family found out, her husband would abandon her, and she would have to support herself and the child in a hostile environment.

4.10.3 Discussion Questions

1. How should this patient's plight influence Dr. Charles as he helps his clinic carry out the WHO guidelines? From a public health perspective, what conflicts does Dr. Charles have in meeting his patient's needs?
2. Who are the stakeholders Dr. Charles should consider as he develops his guidance and what information does he need to ensure success in reducing mother-to-child transmission of HIV in this community?
3. What procedures can he put in place to decrease the risk of HIV-positive women being stigmatized by their partners, family, or community?
4. How should the infant's well-being be balanced with maintaining the mother's health, social welfare, and survival?
5. To what extent should Dr. Charles consider the culture of his community in which family decision making and traditions about infant feeding often hamper mothers' efforts to decrease the risk for HIV transmission? How can public health programs build flexibility that anticipates cultural diversity in beliefs, values, and practice?
6. Instead of just focusing on his patients, should Dr. Charles consider holding structured conversations with people in the community to influence social norms or with village elders as a way to influence social norms counterproductive to program aims?

References

Centers for Disease Control and Prevention. 2012. *HIV for women.* http://www.cdc.gov/HIV/risk/gender/women/facts/index.html. Accessed 23 May 2013.

Coutsoudis, A., K. Pillay, E. Spooner, L. Kuhn, and H.M. Coovadia. 1999. Influence of infant-feeding patterns on early mother-to-child transmission of HIV-1 in Durban, South-Africa: A prospective cohort study. *Lancet* 354(9177): 471–476.

De Cock, K.M., M. Fowler, E. Mercier, et al. 2000. Prevention of mother-to-child HIV transmission in resource-poor countries: Translating research into policy and practice. *JAMA* 283(9): 1175–1182. doi:10.1001/jama.283.9.1175.

Interagency Coalition on AIDS and Development. 2011. *HIV/AIDS: Mother-to-child transmission.* http://www.icad-cisd.com/. Accessed 23 May 2013.

Mnyani, C., and J. McIntyre. 2009. Preventing mother-to-child transmission of HIV. *BJOG: An International Journal of Obstetrics & Gynaecology* 116(suppl 1): 71–76.

O'Reilly, C.E., P. Jaron, B. Ochieng, et al. 2012. Risk factors for death among children less than 5 years old hospitalized with diarrhea in rural western Kenya, 2005–2007: A cohort study. *PLoS Medicine* 9(7): e1001256. doi:10.1371/journal.pmed.1001256.

Wikler, D., and R. Cash. 2009. Ethical issues. In *Global public health: A new era*, ed. R. Beaglehole and R. Bonita, 249–266. Oxford: Oxford University Press.

World Health Organization (WHO). 2007. *HIV transmission through breastfeeding: A review of available evidence.* http://whqlibdoc.who.int/publications/2008/9789241596596_eng.pdf. Accessed 1 May 2013.

World Health Organization (WHO). 2010. *Antiretroviral drugs for treating pregnant women and preventing HIV infection in infants.* http://www.who.int/hiv/pub/mtct/guidelines/en/. Accessed 1 May 2013.

World Health Organization (WHO). 2015. *Mother-to-child transmission of HIV.* http://www.who.int/hiv/topics/mtct/en/. Accessed 1 June 2015.

4.11 Case 3: Newborn Bloodspot Screening: Personal Choice or Public Health Necessity? Storage and Ownership of Newborn Bloodspots

Stuart G. Nicholls
School of Epidemiology, Public Health and Preventive Medicine
University of Ottawa
Ottawa, ON, Canada
e-mail: snicholl@uottawa.ca

Jennifer Milburn
Newborn Screening Ontario
Children's Hospital of Eastern Ontario
Ottawa, ON, Canada

Daryl Pullman
Division of Community Health and Humanities, Faculty of Medicine
Memorial University
St. John's, NL, Canada

This case is presented for instructional purposes only. The ideas and opinions expressed are the authors' own. The case is not meant to reflect the official position, views, or policies of the editors, the editors' host institutions, or the authors' host institutions.

4.11.1 Background

Newborn bloodspot screening (NBS) is the process in which a small blood sample is collected from the heel of a newborn, sent to a laboratory, and tested for serious and life-limiting conditions. If diseases are detected in the newborn period, treatment can begin immediately. NBS is conducted on almost 100 % of the newborn population in North America, roughly four million infants per year in the United States (Botkin et al. 2012). Screening panels have steadily increased the number of conditions tested, with upward of 40 conditions included in some NBS programs. This momentum to include more conditions in screening panels reflects a transition away from an 'emergency' model to a 'public health service' model. In the emergency model, testing identifies conditions amenable to treatment or associated with catastrophic morbidity or mortality. In contrast, a key goal of the public health service model is to inform decision making or avoid a "diagnostic odyssey" (Bailey et al. 2006; Buchbinder and Timmermans 2011; Metcalfe et al. 2012). Advances in newborn screening have increased our ability to detect previously unidentifiable conditions. However, they have also raised a number of ethical challenges about how to best use the information. For example, testing can now reveal someone's carrier status (i.e., the person carries a recessive copy of a genetic disorder without being affected by the condition). Knowing a child's carrier status can inform future reproductive decision making but may induce anxiety, lead to potential stigma, or reveal non-paternity (Hayeems et al. 2008).

Newborn screening is a routine practice in many states. In the U.S. state of Nebraska, for example, screening is mandatory without exception (Schweers 2012; Foral 2006). In other U.S. states, screening proceeds on an opt-out basis, although studies indicate that often parents are not afforded the opportunity to consent or are poorly informed about the opt-out option (Botkin et al. 2012). This may even be the case where screening proceeds in an ostensibly informed choice manner, such as in the United Kingdom (Nicholls 2012; Nicholls and Southern 2012).

Dried bloodspot samples are often stored for a number of years after collection, but the length of storage varies by jurisdiction (Botkin et al. 2012). Samples are retained for various reasons including repeat testing, quality control of testing procedures, or as part of diagnosis. In addition, samples also may be used (anonymously) for external quality assurance and research. While there is no consensus, a recent expert panel recommended a minimum storage period of about 3 months to allow for quality assurance, and indefinite storage when initial positive (i.e., disease suspected) results are confirmed by diagnostic testing (Botkin et al. 2012). In five U.S. states, a parent has the legal right to request destruction or release of dried bloodspot samples, and in three states children may do so when they reach the age of majority (Lewis et al. 2011). A number of other jurisdictions have followed suit with similar procedures (Newborn Screening Ontario 2011). In most cases, release or destruction of the bloodspot requires a signed formal request by a parent or legal guardian.

Research to date has provided important findings for both clinical decision making and public health. For example, studies exploring childhood leukemia have used bloodspots to identify whether genetic changes are present at birth, or have accumulated over time, helping to clarify how the disease is caused. Others have considered the effects of public health policies, such as the removal of perfluorinated compounds, and examined the levels of these in bloodspot samples, noting significant declines in analyte levels following the phasing out of these compounds (Spliethoff et al. 2008). As such, bloodspots may provide a useful resource for evaluating public health policy. Bloodspot samples may also be requested by the coroner's office or be used in forensic investigations as was proposed, for example, in the Netherlands following an explosion at a fireworks factory (Couzin-Frankel 2009; Douglas et al. 2012).

However, there has been a great deal of media discussion regarding the retention, storage, and use of dried bloodspots due to public concerns about privacy (Couzin-Frankel 2009; Muchamore et al. 2006; Bombard et al. 2012). In particular, there has been debate regarding the secondary use of stored bloodspots for research, which are seen as having tremendous research value (Tarini 2011). This has culminated in several lawsuits in the United States and Canada (Lewis et al. 2012; Armstrong 2010) that have led to changes in storage policy and the destruction of millions of dried bloodspot samples (Lewis et al. 2012).

4.11.2 Case Description

As manager of a newborn screening program, you are responsible for the daily operations of the program, as well as risk and resource management, program evaluation, and quality improvement initiatives. Your program screens approximately 150,000 newborns annually for 28 conditions. Each year, on average, 140 babies are identified as affected by at least one of the screened conditions.

Your program publishes a leaflet and hosts a website that provides information for parents regarding the screening process, the conditions for which screening is conducted, and about storage. Your jurisdiction's regulations recommend that bloodspot samples be stored for a minimum of 5 years. Parents have the legal right to request destruction or release of a bloodspot sample at any time. To do so, the parents or legal guardian must complete a request form.

While parents are informed of the screening process and retention of bloodspots, consent is not required, and screening proceeds on an 'opt-out' basis (i.e., screening proceeds unless parents explicitly object). There is no distinction between decisions for screening and decisions regarding retention of bloodspots.

The recent debate regarding the secondary use of stored bloodspots for research has increased researcher awareness of bloodspots as a resource and has put increased pressure on your office to facilitate research requests. At the same time, you have also received political pressure from the health ministry to review storage and consent policy due to public concerns about privacy.

In light of increasing media and researcher interest and political pressure, the health ministry has asked the standing advisory committee on newborn screening to convene a working group to review your jurisdictions' policy on the retention of newborn bloodspots and the information provided to parents. You have been charged with advising the committee regarding potential policy changes and the potential impacts of these on the screening program.

You are aware of the potential conflict between public health benefits and parental consent to the secondary use of bloodspots for research. However, you are concerned that providing too much information or raising concerns with parents may decrease uptake of what is an important population screening program.

4.11.3 Discussion Questions

1. Newborn bloodspot screening is both a public health program and a tool for individual clinical care. How should the public health gains from newborn screening weigh against individual privacy concerns?
2. Given expressed concerns, how should participation in newborn screening be managed? Should the current opt-out policy be retained or would an informed consent model be ethically more justifiable? Should screening be distinguished from secondary use? If so, how should these two elements be handled?
3. To what extent, if any, should the screening program attempt to persuade parents to withdraw their requests for return or destruction of bloodspots?
4. Studies indicate that anonymized research data might be de-anonymised via surname inference using genealogy databases (Gymrek et al. 2013) or based on date of birth, gender, and 5-digit ZIP code (Sweeney et al. 2013). Should parents have the right to consent or opt out of studies even in cases where only anonymised data is used, and which may provide improvements to population health?
5. Should residual dried bloodspots ever be made available to researchers? How should clinically actionable results be dealt with?
6. One option is the indefinite storage of residual bloodspots. Is this permissible, and if so, should the consent of the child be sought when they reach the age of majority?

References

Armstrong, J. 2010. Storage of newborns' blood samples raises privacy concerns. *The Globe and Mail*, May 11. http://www.theglobeandmail.com/news/british-columbia/storage-of-newborns-blood-samples-raises-privacy-concerns/article4318768/. Accessed 30 May 2013.

Bailey Jr., D.B., L.M. Beskow, A.M. Davis, and D. Skinner. 2006. Changing perspectives on the benefits of newborn screening. *Mental Retardation and Developmental Disabilities Research Reviews* 12(4): 270–279. doi:10.1002/mrdd.20119.

Bombard, Y., F.A. Miller, R.S. Hayeems, et al. 2012. Citizens' values regarding research with stored samples from newborn screening in Canada. *Pediatrics* 129: 239–247. doi:10.1542/peds.2011-2572.

Botkin, J.R., A.J. Goldenberg, E. Rothwell, et al. 2012. Retention and research use of residual newborn screening bloodspots. *Pediatrics* 131(1): 1–8. doi:10.1542/peds.2012-0852.

Buchbinder, M., and S. Timmermans. 2011. Newborn screening and maternal diagnosis: Rethinking family benefi t. *Social Science & Medicine* 73(7): 1014–1018. doi:10.1016/j.socscimed.2011.06.062.

Couzin-Frankel, J. 2009. Newborn blood collections. Science gold mine, ethical minefield. *Science* 324(5924): 166–168.

Douglas, C., C. van El, M. Radstake, S. van Teeffelen, and M.C. Cornel. 2012. The politics of representation in the governance of emergent 'secondary use' biobanks: The case of dried blood spot cards in the Netherlands. *Studies in Ethics, Law, and Technology* 6(1): Article 4. doi:10.1515/1941-6008.1178.

Foral, F.E. 2006. Necessity's sharp pinch: Parental and states' rights in conflict in an era of newborn genetic screening. *Journal of Health & Biomedical Law* 11(1): 109–128.

Gymrek, M., A.L. McGuire, D. Golan, and Y. Erlich. 2013. Identifying personal genomes by surname inference. *Science* 339(6117): 321–324. doi:10.1126/science.1229566.

Hayeems, R.Z., J.P. Bytautas, and F.A. Miller. 2008. A systematic review of the effects of disclosing carrier results generated through newborn screening. *Journal of Genetic Counseling* 17(6): 538–549. doi:10.1007/s10897-008-9180-1.

Lewis, M.H., A. Goldenberg, R. Anderson, E. Rothwell, and J. Botkin. 2011. State laws regarding the retention and use of residual newborn screening blood samples. *Pediatrics* 127(4): 703–712. doi:10.1542/peds.2010-1468.

Lewis, M.H., M.E. Scheurer, R.C. Green, and A.L. McGuire. 2012. Research results: Preserving newborn blood samples. *Science Translational Medicine* 4(159): 1–3.

Metcalfe, S.A., A.D. Archibald, and A.L. Atkinson, et al. 2012. *Conflicting views on newborn and infant genetic screening: Perspectives of relatives of children with genetic conditions causing developmental delay and parents of healthy children.* Paper presented at the 62nd annual meeting of the American Society of Human Genetics, San Francisco, CA, 6–10 November.

Muchamore, I., L. Morphett, and K. Barlow-Stewart. 2006. Exploring existing and deliberated community perspectives of newborn screening: Informing the development of state and national policy standards in newborn screening and the use of dried blood spots. *Australia and New Zealand Health Policy* 3: 14. doi:10.1186/1743-8462-3-14.

Newborn Screening Ontario. 2011. *Storage and secondary use of the newborn screening samples.* Ottawa. http://www.newbornscreening.on.ca/data/1/rec_docs/434_Storage_and_Secondary_Use_of_the_Newborn_Screening_Samples.pdf. Accessed 28 Jan 2014.

Nicholls, S.G. 2012. Proceduralisation, choice and parental reflections on decisions to accept newborn bloodspot screening. *Journal of Medical Ethics* 38: 299–303. doi:10.1136/medethics-2011–100040.

Nicholls, S.G., and K.W. Southern. 2012. Informed choice for newborn blood spot screening in the United Kingdom: A survey of parental perceptions. *Pediatrics* 130(6): e1527–e1533. doi:10.1542/peds.2012-1479.

Schweers, R.L. 2012. Newborn screening programs: How do we best protect privacy rights while ensuring optimal newborn health? *DePaul L Rev* 61: 869.

Spliethoff, H.M., L. Tao, S.M. Shaver, et al. 2008. Use of newborn screening program blood spots for exposure assessment: Declining levels of perfluorinated compounds in New York State infants. *Environmental Science & Technology* 42(14): 5361–5367.

Sweeney, L., A. Abu, and J. Winn. 2013. *Identifying participants in the personal genome project by name.* Cambridge, MA: Harvard University Data Privacy Lab, White Paper 1021–1. http://privacytools.seas.harvard.edu/files/privacytools/fi les/1021 1.pdf. Accessed 30 May 2013.

Tarini, B.A. 2011. Storage and use of residual newborn screening blood spots: A public policy emergency. *Genetics in Medicine* 13(7): 619–620. doi:10.1097/GIM.0b013e31822176df.

4.12 Case 4: Decoding Public Health Ethics and Inequity in India: A Conditional Cash Incentive Scheme—Janani Suraksha Yojana

Divya Kanwar Bhati
World Health Organization Collaborating Centre for District Health System Based on Primary Health Care
Indian Institute of Health Management Research University
Jaipur, Rajasthan, India
e-mail: bhatidivyak@gmail.com

This case is presented for instructional purposes only. The ideas and opinions expressed are the author's own. The case is not meant to reflect the official position, views, or policies of the editors, the editors' host institutions, or the author's host institution.

4.12.1 Background

The domestic sphere of home and family defines the lives of most women in India, where they assume the role of caregiver, either as wife or mother. Overall, age and sex govern the household's hierarchy of authority, older over younger, men over women. Women, especially those living in northern India, experience decreased autonomy and increased inequalities in all areas of life (Iyengar et al. 2009; Bloom et al. 2001). Limited autonomy harms women's maternal health outcomes, restricting their ability to choose safe childbirth options. In India, most births still occur in the home; less than 41 % occur in an institutional setting (International Institute for Population Sciences 2007).

Worldwide, more than half a million women die each year from complications during pregnancy and childbirth (UNICEF 2009). About 99 % of these deaths occur in developing countries. Based on maternal mortality trends from 1990 to 2008, developing countries, especially India, contribute about 18 % of the global burden of maternal deaths (Dikid et al. 2013). Data during 2007 through 2009 indicated that India's maternal mortality ratio (MMR) was 212 per 100,000 live births (Registrar General of India 2011). Regional differences in MMR are found in India; during 2007 through 2009 the MMR in northern states was 308/100,000 compared with 207/100,000 in the southern states.

India has had a long history of redistributive poverty-reduction programs, but few programs provide direct cash assistance to the needy (Mehrotra 2010). Cash incentive programs started in the 1990s predominantly in Latin America where their success led to adoption in other parts of the world (Powell-Jackson et al. 2009b). These programs vary in size and scope; examples include programs that address vaccinations, education, health care, safe childbirth, sterilization, and poverty. An example from an Asian country is the Safe Delivery Incentives Programme (SDIP), which was started in

2005 in Nepal with funds from the U.K. Department of International Development and the Nepalese government (Powell-Jackson et al. 2009a; Karki 2012). The program provided cash incentives to women who gave birth in health facilities and to health providers for each attended delivery (either in the woman's home or in a facility). The program implementers or administrators expected that the cash incentive would reduce transportation barriers and delays in maternal care seeking (Bhandari and Dangal 2012). The program was most effective in changing health care-seeking behavior wherever women's groups highlighted the importance of effective communication of the policy to the public (Powell-Jackson et al. 2008). Women exposed to the program were 24 % more likely to deliver in government health institutions, 5 % less likely to deliver at home, and 13 % more likely to have their delivery attended by a skilled health worker. Deliveries in government health institutions went from 34 % in the first year (2005/2006) to 59 % in the third year (2007/2008). Overall, the program was well received, however certain aspects of the policy were not accepted, including a condition that limited receipt of the cash incentive to women who had no more than two living children (Powell-Jackson et al. 2008).

India's conditional cash transfer program, Janani Suraksha Yojana (JSY), is one of the largest programs of its kind in the world (Lim et al. 2010). JSY is funded through the central government, provides welfare to women living in indigent families, and includes efforts to empower women to choose institutional childbirth rather than home delivery.

JSY represents a novel and useful way to ensure the social welfare of women by integrating cash assistance with childbirth delivery and post delivery care. The program focuses on poor pregnant woman, especially those living in states with high MMRs and low institutional delivery rates. These low-performing states include Uttar Pradesh, Uttaranchal, Bihar, Jharkhand, Madhya Pradesh, Chhattisgarh, Assam, Rajasthan, Orissa, and Jammu and Kashmir (Tiwari 2013). An important component of this program is its focus on monitoring, evaluating, and providing, health care for the mother and her baby (Lim et al. 2010). District-level household surveys have documented a decline in the proportion of home deliveries, which dropped from 59 % in the 2002–2004 survey (International Institute for Population Sciences 2006) to 52 % in the 2007–2008 survey (International Institute for Population Sciences 2010).

Despite indicators of success, the JSY program has raised a number of concerns. One of the aims of JSY is equity in addition to coverage; the JSY program does not include private health care providers. The increased deliveries (from 35 % to 65 %) in public health care facilities may raise issues in the quality and standards of health care (MacDonald 2011). Another concern is that the lack of comprehensive emergency obstetric care at many institutions compromises the safety of institutional deliveries (International Institute for Population Sciences 2010). A final concern is that socioeconomic status, caste, and education create large inequities in access to the program's cash incentives, while women who do gain access lack financial control over the cash incentives (Gopichandran and Chetlapalli 2012).

4.12.2 Case Description

A 19-year-old woman from a poor area in India is pregnant for the first time and only weeks from her delivery date. Wearing a long pardah to cover the lower half of her face and traditional maang tikka jewelry on her forehead to indicate married status, her attire reflects the traditional values embedded in her culture. She wants to deliver her baby in her home village, which is an overnight's journey away. But her husband and in-laws have other ideas. They have just learned of a government program that provides a cash payment of 1000 rupees to women who opt for institutional delivery over home delivery. Her mother-in-law insists that the delivery take place in their district institution. The woman's parents, believing the in-laws to be driven purely by greed, support their daughter. With encouragement from her parents, the woman disobeys her husband and in-laws to travel to her parent's home, but goes into labor on the road and loses her child due to complications in the delivery. The young woman not only is disconsolate over the loss of her child, she must now face the wrath of her husband and in-laws.

This is a poignant case, but only one in a dossier full of similar cases that you, as the state director for the maternal cash incentive program, have read that involve clashes between traditional ways and the incentive program. As a result, you have decided to convene an expert panel to consider recommendations to smooth not only the cultural friction the program is causing, but also the program's impact on the quality and safety of care, as well as access to it.

4.12.3 Discussion Questions

1. Who are the main stakeholders in the case of the 19-year-old woman and what values and cultural perspectives does each stakeholder bring to this situation?
2. How should you consider the issues about this and similar cases when deciding whether to revise the cash incentive program?
3. What are the pros and cons of cash incentive programs from a public health perspective?
4. What role should government play in improving the public's health?
5. In the context of inequities based on socioeconomic status, caste, and education, to what extent should you attempt to ensure that a woman's autonomy is not violated? Should the same notion of autonomy be applied in India or other unique contexts as prevails in European and North American countries?
6. Due to a financial downturn, the state government is thinking about eliminating the maternal cash benefit program. How can an ethical analysis assist in making this decision? What factors should be considered as part of this ethical analysis?

References

Bhandari, T.R., and G. Dangal. 2012. Maternal mortality: Paradigm shift in Nepal. *Nepal Journal of Obstetrics and Gynecology* 7(2): 3–8.

Bloom, S.S., D. Wypij, and M. Das Gupta. 2001. Dimensions of women's autonomy and the influence on maternal health care utilization in a north Indian city. *Demography* 38: 67–78.

Dikid, T., M. Gupta, M. Kaur, S. Goel, A.K. Aggarwal, and J. Caravotta. 2013. Maternal and perinatal death inquiry and response project implementation review in India. *Journal of Obstetrics and Gynaecology of India* 63(2): 101–107.

Gopichandran, V., and S.K. Chetlapalli. 2012. Conditional cash transfer to promote institutional deliveries in India: Toward a sustainable ethical model to achieve MDG 5A. *Public Health Ethics* 5(2): 173–180.

International Institute for Population Sciences (IIPS). 2006. *District Level Household Survey (DLHS-2), 2002–04: India.* Mumbai: IIPS. http://www.rchiips.org/PRCH-2.html. Accessed 29 May 2013.

International Institute for Population Sciences. 2010. *District Level Household Survey (DLHS-3), 2007–08: India.* Mumbai: IIPS. http://www.rchiips.org/pdf/INDIA_REPORT_DLHS-3.pdf. Accessed 29 May 2013.

International Institute for Population Sciences and Macro International. 2007. *National Level Household Survey (NFHS-3), 2005–06: India: Volume I.* Mumbai: IIPS. http://www.rchiips.org/nfhs/nfhs3_national_report.shtml. Accessed 29 May 2013.

Iyengar, S.D., K. Iyengar, and V. Gupta. 2009. Maternal health: A case study of Rajasthan. *Journal of Health, Population, and Nutrition* 27(2): 271–292.

Karki, A. 2012. *Safe delivery incentive program under maternal health financing policy of Nepal: A case of Kailali district in Nepal.* Dhaka: North South University. Accessed 29 May 2013.

Lim, S.S., L. Dandona, J.A. Hoisington, S.L. James, M.C. Hogan, and E. Gakidou. 2010. India's Janani Suraksha Yojana, a conditional cash transfer programme to increase births in health facilities: An impact evaluation. *Lancet* 375(9730): 2009–2023.

MacDonald, R. 2011. Janani Suraksha Yojana—The Indian way of improving maternal and child health. *PLOS Medicine Community Blog.* http://blogs.plos.org/speakingofmedicine/2011/12/19/janani-suraksha-yojana-%E2%80%94-the-indian-way-of-improving-maternal-and-child-health/. Accessed 29 May 2013.

Mehrotra, S. 2010. *Introducing conditional cash transfers in India: A proposal for five CCTs.* Institute of Applied Manpower Research, Planning Commission. http://www.google.com/url?sa=t&rct=j&q=&esrc=s&frm=1&source=web&cd=1&ved=0CCYQFjAA&url=http%3A%2F%2Fwww.ids.ac.uk%2Ffiles%2Fdmfile%2FConditionalCashTransfersforDevChange2.doc&ei=MBrpUpbqN5C_sQTo74G4Bg&usg=AFQjCNHUgH8o22hjaLX1SNVgsjwK8Ww_YQ&bvm=bv.60157871,d.cWc. Accessed 29 May 2013.

Powell-Jackson, T., B.D. Neupane, S. Tiwari, J. Morrison, and A. Costello. 2008. *Evaluation of the safe delivery incentive programme: Final report of the evaluation.* Nepal: Support to Safe Motherhood Programme. http://s3.amazonaws.com/zanran_storage/www.safemotherhood.org.np/ContentPages/2469459188.pdf. Access 29 May 2013.

Powell-Jackson, T., J. Morrison, S. Tiwari, B.D. Neupane, and A.M. Costello. 2009a. The experiences of districts in implementing a national incentive programme to promote safe delivery in Nepal. *BMC Health Services Research* 9: 97. http://www.biomedcentral.com/content/pdf/1472-6963-9–97.pdf. Accessed 29 May 2013.

Powell-Jackson, T., B.D. Neupane, S. Tiwari, K. Tumbahangphe, D. Manandhar, and A.M. Costello. 2009b. The impact of Nepal's national incentive programme to promote safe delivery in the district of Makwanpur. *Advances in Health Economics and Health Services Research* 21: 221–249.

Registrar General of India. 2011. *Maternal and child mortality and total fertility rates: Sample registration system.* New Delhi: Registrar General of India. http://censusindia.gov.in/vital_statistics/SRS_Bulletins/MMR_release_070711.pdf. Accessed 29 May 2013.

Tiwari, D. 2013. *Role of national rural health mission in promoting institutional delivery services in rural Uttar Pradesh, India: An assessment of Janani Suraksha Yojana*. Paper presented at the 2013 annual meeting of the Population Association of America, New Orleans, 10–13 April.

UNICEF. 2009. *The state of the world's children 2009: Maternal and newborn death*. http://www.unicef.org/sowc09/docs/SOWC09-FullReport-EN.pdf.

4.13 Case 5: HIV Criminalization and STD Prevention and Control

Dhrubajyoti Bhattacharya
Department of Population Health Sciences, School of Nursing and Health Professions
University of San Francisco
San Francisco, CA, USA
e-mail: dbhattacharya@usfca.edu

This case is presented for instructional purposes only. The ideas and opinions expressed are the author's own. The case is not meant to reflect the official position, views, or policies of the editors, the editors' host institutions, or the author's host institution.

4.13.1 Background

About 34.0 million people live with HIV worldwide, with 1.1 million residing in the United States (Centers for Disease Control and Prevention 2010). The lack of a cure, coupled with the ailment's debilitating and potentially fatal consequences, has prompted governments to enact structural interventions that, although well-intentioned, may be ineffective in preventing and controlling the spread of HIV.

HIV-specific criminal statutes are one example of a structural intervention used in at least 63 countries, including the United States. In the United States, the initial federal response to HIV included potential criminal prosecution for people aware of their HIV-positive status who knowingly engaged in sexual activity with the intent to expose others to HIV. Under the original text of the Ryan White Care Act of 1990, no federal grant would be issued to a state unless it had criminal laws under which to prosecute an HIV-infected person who knowingly engaged in sexual relations, donated blood (or semen or breast milk), or injected himself with a needle and provided the needle to another, with the intent to expose the other person to HIV (Public Law 101–381 1990). The Ryan White Care Act of 1990 became a template for many states, leading to the passage of laws that included a determination of guilt for HIV-infected individuals who engaged in sexual activity or shared drug paraphernalia. Consent was a defense so long as the uninfected person knew of the partner's HIV-positive status and provided informed consent before engaging in the activity (i.e., sexual or drug-related) (Public Law 101–381, 1990). Although the provision to award grants on the condition of having an HIV-criminal law in place was repealed in 2000, more than 33 states currently have one or more HIV-specific criminal laws in effect.

While the merits of using criminal law to prevent HIV transmission remains questionable, there has not been enough thought given to the related effect of laws criminalizing commercial sex work that, coupled with HIV-criminalization laws, poses unique challenges for women and public health professionals. Together, these laws disproportionately affect women by virtue of their voluntary participation in—or coercion into—prostitution, and the harsher sentencing that may ensue upon conviction. In the state of Florida, for example, prostitutes who test positive for HIV before committing a crime have their sentence increased from a misdemeanor (serving a term of imprisonment not exceeding 1 year) to a felony (serving a term of imprisonment not exceeding 5 years) (Fl. Stat. Ann. § 796.08(4)(2010)). Notably, a person convicted of prostitution in Florida must undergo mandatory HIV testing. Consequently, the specter of criminal prosecution and up to 5 years imprisonment may deter many women from getting tested in the first place, increasing the risk of acquiring and transmitting the virus.

Globally, women are at heightened risk of contracting HIV because of social, economic, and cultural factors stemming from human rights violations, gender inequality, and inadequate forums to pursue legal redress (Murthy and Bhattacharya 2010). An estimated 60 % of people infected with HIV in sub-Saharan Africa are women; and females ages 15–24 years make up 75 % of those afflicted with the virus. Moreover, "male-to-female transmission during sex is about twice as likely to occur as female-to-male transmission, if no other sexually transmitted infections are present" (Joint United Nations Programme on HIV/AIDS [UNAIDS] 2004). For commercial sex workers, this disproportionate risk of exposure is exacerbated. Researchers have found that among female sex workers 15–49 years old, the prevalence of HIV infection is 13.5 times higher than the prevalence among the general population of women (Kerrigan et al. 2013).

Public health practitioners are faced with a dilemma of promoting HIV testing and simultaneously adhering to mandatory reporting requirements. All states in the United States have enacted laws or regulations requiring laboratory reporting of HIV infection, with 32 states (and the District of Columbia) also enacting laws requiring reporting of CD4 levels (white blood cells that protect against infection) and viral loads of people who test positive (Centers for Disease Control and Prevention 2013). Nonexistent or inadequate surveillance of commercial sex workers, however, may prevent researchers from understanding the evolving nature of HIV and the burden it poses on this particular population. For example, a recent study found that a common CD4 gene variant (i.e. alteration of the gene sequence) is associated with an increased risk of HIV-1 infection in Kenyan female commercial sex workers (Oyugi et al. 2009). The researchers suggest that the effect of this variant on the epidemic in Africa could be dramatic.

For many human rights activists, laws criminalizing sex work discriminate against women and deny them their right to work. For others, prostitution is inherently exploitative, with all commercial sex workers being victims who are denied legitimate (i.e., alternative) forms of employment. In most countries, however, the law does not discriminate between these types of women or their reasons for engaging in commercial sex work, compelling many women to avoid HIV testing altogether (UNAIDS 2012a). By contrast, where voluntary counseling and testing have been extended to commercial sex workers, the results have been far more promising. A recent study found that voluntary counseling and treatment among a cohort of 421 commercial sex workers in Guinea resulted in 92 % of participants returning for their results (Aho et al. 2012).

The 35th anniversary of the international Convention on the Elimination of All Forms of Discrimination against Women (CEDAW) affords an opportunity for governments to affirm that extending HIV services to commercial sex workers and promoting public health are not mutually exclusive endeavors. As the only treaty that rejects sex-discrimination in employment and in health care access, CEDAW helps women show the link between health and human rights, and particularly the right to health and employment. The CEDAW Committee, which oversees the treaty's execution, has advocated for the decriminalization of prostitution, in countries like China, where women are disproportionately prosecuted in lieu of the traffickers and pimps; and encourages governments to focus on rehabilitating and reintegrating women into society, enhancing opportunities, and providing support to ensure that their civil liberties are not violated (CEDAW 1981, Committee on the Elimination of Discrimination Against Women 2006). As of 2013, 187 countries are parties to CEDAW, but the United States has not ratified it (United Nations 2013).

4.13.2 Case Description

You are the sexually transmitted infections (STI) program manager of the Communicable Disease Control Unit in a public health department in a large city. A recent news story of an HIV-positive commercial sex worker has prompted public concern. While reviewing the county's HIV surveillance report for the last period of data collection, you note that the department does not conduct official surveillance of commercial sex workers. Studies have found that the HIV infection rate among female prostitutes has been as low as 12 % in Atlanta and as high as 57 % in northern New Jersey (Elifson et al. 1999). You are also aware of a UNAIDS report that found "where health and social services are provided and sex workers are actively engaged in efforts to provide universal access to HIV prevention, treatment, care and support, HIV incidence declines" (UNAIDS 2012b). Therefore, you are eager to start an intervention program that encourages commercial sex workers to undergo HIV testing. You recall that an intervention in a neighboring state used caseworkers to offer prostitutes testing for STIs, including HIV. However, a number of challenges abound.

Prostitution is illegal in your state, with penalties ranging from a Class A misdemeanor (punishable by up to a year in prison) for first-time offenders, to a Class 4 felony (punishable by 1–3 years in prison) for repeat offenders. Moreover, state law requires that health care providers report to the Department of Health the names of patients who test HIV-positive.

As an STI program manager, you are aware of the role of social determinants of health and the need to think broadly about possible interventions and collaborations with other agencies. You have been influenced by a study on 222 commercial sex workers from the Center for Impact Research (2002) that found the following:

- 72 % of young commercial sex workers had run away from home and were likely to have used drugs or alcohol growing up;
- 60 % reported domestic violence in the household;
- 25 % had completed a high school education or passed a general educational development (GED) test;
- More than 50 % grew up in a household in which prostitution took place;
- 87 % had someone suggest they engage in prostitution while they were growing up;
- 22 % reported they were HIV-positive;
- 21 % indicated being raped more than 10 times;
- 50 % of women worked on behalf of another person (i.e., pimp), with 75 % reporting they believed the other person would harm them if they discontinued their services;
- More than 90 % increased their drug or alcohol use after becoming commercial sex workers;
- Almost 75 % of them had been arrested at least once, with close to 50 % of them reporting that the arrest took place before age 18; and
- More than 50 % were homeless.

Your health department provides services related to homeless prevention and substance abuse treatment, yet eligibility is dependent on an ability to meet monetary obligations (rent, utilities, etc.) after the assistance has been granted based on current or anticipated income. It is unlikely that commercial sex work would satisfy this criterion.

You consider all of these issues as you think about how to begin an intervention program for commercial sex workers to encourage them to undergo HIV testing.

4.13.3 Discussion Questions

1. Who are the main public and private stakeholders in this case?
2. How should the criminal nature of commercial sex work influence the intervention you develop to encourage commercial sex workers to undergo HIV testing? Should your intervention also target other risk factors for illness, such as homelessness, unemployment, and substance abuse?
3. Are you obligated to seek help from law enforcement to carry out your intervention?
4. What standard should you use to evaluate your intervention's success? How would you treat empirical findings alongside issues of equity and discrimination?

5. Given the many social determinants implicated by prostitution and its attendant health effects, what other agencies should you collaborate with and what other services should you consider providing along with, or instead of, HIV testing?
6. Does the threat of prison ever get in the way of promoting healthy behaviors? If so, what criteria should be used to determine which activities and behaviors merit criminalization? Does reducing the number of women engaged in commercial sex work or their incidence of HIV—or both—satisfy these criteria?
7. Should the public health department conduct surveillance of the incidence of HIV among commercial sex workers? What challenges exist for the department in undertaking this task?
8. Do you think ratification of international laws like CEDAW can improve the health of commercial sex workers?

References

Aho, J., V.K. Nguyen, S.L. Diakité, A. Sow, A. Koushik, and S. Rashed. 2012. High acceptability of HIV voluntary counselling and testing among female sex workers: Impact of individual and social factors. *HIV Medicine* 13(3): 156–165.

Center for Impact Research. 2002. *Sisters speak out: The lives and needs of prostituted women in Chicago. A research study.* http://www.healthtrust.net/sites/default/files/publications/sisters-speakout.pdf. Accessed 1 June 2015.

Centers for Disease Control and Prevention. 2010. *HIV in the United States: At a glance.* http://www.cdc.gov/hiv/statistics/basics/ataglance.html. Accessed 29 May 2013.

Centers for Disease Control and Prevention. 2013. *State laboratory reporting laws: Viral load and CD4 requirements.* http://www.cdc.gov/hiv/law/states/laboratory.htm. Accessed 1 June 2015.

Committee on the Elimination of Discrimination Against Women. 2006. *Concluding comments of the committee on the elimination of discrimination against Women: China.* http://www.un.org/womenwatch/daw/cedaw/cedaw36/cc/CHINA_advance%20unedited.pdf. Accessed 1 June 2015

Convention on the Elimination of All Forms of Discrimination Against Women (CEDAW). 1981. *Sex role stereotyping and prejudice.* Article 5(a)-(b), Sept. 3, 1981, 1249 U.N.T.S. 13. http://www.un.org/womenwatch/daw/cedaw/cedaw.htm. Accessed 1 June 2015.

Elifson, K.W., J. Boles, W.W. Darrow, and C.E. Sterk. 1999. HIV seroprevalence and risk factors among clients of female and male prostitutes. *Journal of Acquired Immune Deficiency Syndromes and Human Retrovirology* 20(2): 195–200.

Joint United Nations Programme on HIV/AIDS (UNAIDS). 2004. *Report on the Global AIDS epidemic.* http://www.unaids.org/sites/default/files/en/media/unaids/contentassets/documents/unaidspublication/2004/GAR2004_en.pdf. Accessed 25 June 2015.

Joint United Nations Programme on HIV/AIDS. 2012a. *Criminalisation of HIV non-disclosure, exposure and transmission: Background and current landscape.* http://www.unaids.org/en/media/unaids/contentassets/documents/document/2012/BackgroundCurrentLandscapeCriminalisationHIV_Final.pdf. Accessed 1 June 2015.

Joint United Nations Programme on HIV/AIDS. 2012b. *UNAIDS guidance note on HIV and sex work.* http://www.unaids.org/en/media/unaids/contentassets/documents/unaidspublication/2009/JC2306_UNAIDS-guidance-note-HIV-sex-work_en.pdf. Accessed 1 June 2015.

Kerrigan, D., A. Wirtz, S. Baral, et al. 2013. *The global HIV epidemics among sex workers.* Washington, DC: World Bank. http://www.worldbank.org/content/dam/Worldbank/document/GlobalHIVEpidemicsAmongSexWorkers.pdf. Accessed 1 June 2015.

Murthy, P., and D. Bhattacharya. 2010. Human rights and women's health. In *Rights-based approaches to public health*, ed. E. Beracochea, C. Weinstein, and D. Evans, 169–182. New York: Springer Pub. Co.

Oyugi, J.O., F.C. Vouriot, J. Alimonti, et al. 2009. A common CD4 gene variant is associated with an increased risk of HIV-1 infection in Kenyan female commercial sex workers. *Journal of Infectious Diseases* 199(9): 1327–1334.

Public Law 101–381. 1990. *Ryan White Comprehensive AIDS Resources Emergency Act of 1990.* Section 2647(a)(1)-(a)(2). http://history.nih.gov/research/downloads/PL101-381.pdf. Accessed 1 June 2015.

United Nations. 2013. *United Nations treaty collection: Chapter IV human rights (8) convention on the elimination of all forms of discrimination against women.* http://treaties.un.org/Pages/ViewDetails.aspx?src=TREATY&mtdsg_no=IV-8&chapter=4&lang=en. Accessed 1 June 2015.

4.14 Case 6: Ethics of Administering Anthrax Vaccine to Children

Georgina Peacock
Division of Human Development and Disability, National Center on Birth Defects and Developmental Disabilities
Centers for Disease Control and Prevention
Atlanta, GA, USA
e-mail: ghn3@cdc.gov

Michael T. Bartenfeld
Children's Preparedness Unit, Disability and Health Branch, Division of Human Development and Disability, National Center on Birth Defects and Developmental Disabilities, Centers for Disease Control and Prevention
Atlanta, GA, USA
e-mail: vdv4@cdc.gov

Cynthia H. Cassell
Birth Defects Branch, Division of Birth Defects and Developmental Disabilities, National Center on Birth Defects and Developmental Disabilities
Centers for Disease Control and Prevention
Atlanta, GA, USA

Daniel M. Sosin
Office of Public Health Preparedness and Response
Centers for Disease Control and Prevention
Atlanta, GA, USA

This case is presented for instructional purposes only. The ideas and opinions expressed are the authors' own. The case is not meant to reflect the official position, views, or policies of the editors, the editors' host institutions, or the authors' host institutions.

4.14.1 Background

Bacillus anthracis is a hardy, spore-forming bacterium that leads to anthrax disease upon infection. The organism has long been considered a likely agent for biological warfare. A weaponized form of the agent would likely result in widespread inhalation anthrax, a severe form of the disease that carries a high (>50 %) case fatality rate. *B. anthracis* spores can last inside the body for weeks before germinating to induce infection and can persist for years in the environment. Anthrax disease is preventable if antibiotics and vaccine are administered prophylactically before someone has symptoms.

The U.S. Centers for Disease Control and Prevention (CDC) and U.S. Department of Homeland Security are concerned about *B. anthracis* as an agent of biological terrorism due to its ease of dispersal, severe health impact, persistence in the environment, and the special public health response it requires (CDC 2013). The U.S. anthrax attacks in 2001 infected 22 people, 5 of whom died, all from inhalation anthrax. The U.S. Department of Health and Human Services prepares for a number of disaster scenarios, one of which is an aerosolized anthrax attack. In this scenario, *B. anthracis* spores are released into the air in a densely populated area, potentially infecting thousands of people.

Children (<18 years) are given special considerations in an anthrax attack scenario, one of which involves receiving the anthrax vaccine, Anthrax Vaccine Adsorbed (AVA). The U.S. Advisory Committee on Immunization Practices recommends giving AVA in conjunction with 60 days of antibiotics for post-exposure prophylaxis of the exposed population against anthrax (Wright et al. 2010). This 60-day antibiotic regimen covers the disease's incubation period and allows for protection before the vaccine takes effect. The vaccine is likely to protect people longer than antibiotics alone and potentially protects against multiple strains of anthrax disease, including bioengineered strains that are resistant to antibiotics (Joellenbeck et al. 2002).

While most of the U.S. population can receive the anthrax vaccine under an Emergency Use Authorization (EUA), children must receive the vaccine under an investigational new drug (IND) protocol as approved by the U.S. Food and Drug Administration. The IND protocol requires informed consent from parents, which is not required under an EUA. The informed consent requirement stems from the lack of safety or efficacy data for AVA in children. Also, due to a requirement under the IND, a subset of the children with IND consent will be asked to enroll in a research IND so that safety and immunogenicity data in children may be obtained during the emergency. The Presidential Commission for the Study of Bioethical Issues debated the study of AVA in children before the event, and has laid out a strict framework for approaching how best to ethically collect these data from a research perspective (Presidential Commission for the Study of Bioethical Issues 2013).

4.14.2 Case Description

A terrorist group has released an anthrax aerosol over a major city in the United States and in a country with a weak public health infrastructure. Of the more than 9 million people in the U.S. metropolitan area at the time, 1.39 million people are exposed, 329,430 of whom are children (Kyriacou et al. 2012). All 1.39 million people exposed will need the vaccine and a 60-day supply of antibiotics to protect them from developing disease. It is unclear what plans have been made to provide prophylaxis to the population living in the other country. In the United States, people thought to be exposed will receive antibiotics and vaccine at points of dispensing (PODs) run by local health departments. The dispensing of antibiotics, which must begin within the first 48 h and finish within 10 days, would require 20 sites providing medicine to 500 people per hour to achieve the goal for the exposed population. Vaccination routinely takes more time and involves additional staff and separate sites to care for the entire population. Additional steps will require more resources and time. Timeliness is essential to ensure those exposed are protected.

In the United States, children needing vaccine come to the vaccination clinic with their parents, slowing the lines to meet the informed consent requirements. Unaccompanied children also show up, slowing the lines to a crawl, as staff attempt to contact parents. The complexity of different vaccine needs for different people, especially those who do not speak English, is overwhelming vaccination staff. To keep lines moving, the staff has created a separate line for families with children, but the slow pace of this line is challenging the clinic's effort to achieve high vaccine coverage rates among children. Tempers flare as families watch adults without children move through the clinic quickly while the family lines grow ever longer. But the parents, who have lots of questions, cannot be rushed to provide their consent. They have been hearing disconcerting media stories highlighting issues related to anthrax vaccine side effects and the lack of testing and safety data. Many parents worry about immunizing their child with an untested vaccine never given to children and posing unknown risks. The vaccination clinic manager, who has had little time to plan, quickly devises the following scenarios to speed decision making:

- Provide parents with the informed consent document and have a public health nurse meet with them to answer questions and discuss concerns about risks and benefits.
- Discuss the informed consent document with a group of families, answering questions and working through concerns about risks and benefits in the larger group, but having a nurse on call to answer confidential questions and speak to families privately.
- Show a large group of families assembled in an auditorium a video produced by the local health department explaining the safety and efficacy profile of the vaccine in adults, and afterward have a nurse discuss with parents the information from the informed consent document and allow parents to ask questions.

4.14.3 Discussion Questions

1. Of the options listed above, which should you choose? Justify your answer in terms of the benefits gained, harms avoided, respect for parental autonomy, privacy and confidentiality, fairness, or other ethical values, such as trust and protecting vulnerable populations.
2. Consider how placing families with children in separate lines affects the distribution of vaccine. Is this the fairest or optimal way to distribute the vaccine? Are there innovative or better options for administering the IND that adhere to FDA rules and achieve maximum vaccination coverage for children? Are these options ethically justifiable?
3. If following the IND protocol for unaccompanied children makes vaccine coverage impossible, what should the vaccine clinic manager and staff do? How would you ethically justify your decision? Would this justification hold if the group in question were all children, not just unaccompanied children?
4. What roles will government trustworthiness and the public's trust in the government play in the vaccination campaign?
5. What ethical concerns are presented by collecting data for research purposes during such an event?
6. The other country under anthrax attack, which is resource poor and lacks public health infrastructure, has received vaccine from the United States, but is under no obligation to follow the mandated U.S. procedures through which antibiotics are administered. To ensure that vulnerable populations are protected against anthrax, what ethical principles, values, and concerns should this country consider? Do these ethical principles, values, and concerns differ from those in the United States? If yes, how? If no, why not?
7. A high percentage of the parents with young children do not speak English. Because the informed consent forms are only in English, translating them will take a lot longer, or an interpreter will need to be available. How would you balance the obligation to protect vulnerable populations with the obligation to maximize coverage?

References

Centers for Disease Control and Prevention (CDC). 2013. *Bioterrorism agents/diseases*. http://www.bt.cdc.gov/agent/agentlist-category.asp. Accessed 3 Jan 2013.

Joellenbeck, L., L.L. Zwanziger, J.S. Durch, and B.L. Strom (eds.). 2002. *The anthrax vaccine: Is it safe? Does it work?* Washington, DC: National Academy Press.

Kyriacou, D.N., D. Dobrez, J.P. Parada, et al. 2012. Cost-effectiveness comparison of response strategies to a large-scale anthrax attack on the Chicago metropolitan area: Impact of timing and surge capacity. *Biosecurity and Bioterrorism* 10(3): 264–279.

Presidential Commission for the Study of Bioethical Issues. 2013. *Safeguarding children: Pediatric medical countermeasure research*. http://bioethics.gov/sites/default/files/PCSBI_Pediatric-MCM_2.pdf. Accessed 2 June 2015.

Wright, J.G., C.P. Quinn, S. Shadomy, and N. Messonnier. 2010. Use of anthrax vaccine in the United States: Recommendations of the Advisory Committee on Immunization Practices (ACIP), 2009. *MMWR Recommendations and Reports* 59(6): 1–30.

4.15 Case 7: Non-adherence to Treatment in Patients with Tuberculosis: A Challenge for Minimalist Ethics

Lorna Luco and M. Inés Gómez
Centro de Bioética, Facultad de Medicina
Clínica Alemana–Universidad del Desarrollo
Santiago, Chile
e-mail: lornamuriel@gmail.com

M. Gabriela Doberti
Hospital Padre Hurtado, Facultad de Medicina
Clínica Alemana–Universidad del Desarrollo
Santiago, Chile

This case is presented for instructional purposes only. The ideas and opinions expressed are the authors' own. The case is not meant to reflect the official position, views, or policies of the editors, the editors' host institutions, or the authors' host institutions.

4.15.1 Background

In Chile, tuberculosis (TB) belongs to the list of "mandatory notification" diseases, a status that allows for the confidential registration and monitoring of cases. Mandatory notification, part of Chile's Communicable Disease Surveillances System, is legally authorized by the 1968 Sanitary Code of the Ministry of Health, specifically the Regulation on Notification of Communicable Diseases (Código Sanitario 1968). By the early 1970s, health authorities created the Program for Control and Eradication of Tuberculosis (PROCET), a model program in its technical conception and application of control measures. The program illustrates how to confront a public health care problem properly through systematically applied, adequate coverage and continuous quality evaluation (PROCET 2005).

Currently, TB prevalence is low in Chile, with the country significantly reducing the disease's mortality and morbidity rates in the closing decades of the twentieth century (Pan American Health Organization 2006). By 2000, this reduction had allowed Chile to cross the eradication threshold (i.e., to reduce the incidence rate below 20 cases per 100,000 people). Over the first decade of this century, however, the pace of reduction in the annual TB incidence rate slowed, decreasing from 7.5 % (1996–2000) to 4.2 % (2000–2005) to just 1.3 % (2005–2010).

This slowing resulted in a 2010 incidence rate of 13.2 cases per 100,000 people—still below the eradication threshold—but falling short of the official target of 10 cases per 100,000 people. To explain the slowing pace, researchers have studied a number of variables, most notably, the role of treatment procedures (Herrero et al. 2011).

To meet the target of 10 TB cases per 100,000 people, PROCET established the following goals: (1) 90 % recovery rate for treated cases, (2) <5 % withdrawals from treatment, and (3) <3 % mortality rate for those undergoing treatment. Achieving these goals requires a stringent treatment regimen that consists of health care workers delivering TB medication on an outpatient basis and directly observing patients while they take their medication. The medications are free for patients within the health care system, including those who have multidrug-resistant TB (MDR-TB).

Analysis of the treatment outcomes for the 2008–2010 cohort of TB patients indicates a recovery rate of 80 %, a withdrawal rate of 7 %, and a mortality rate of 10 % (Ministerio de Salud 2012). Although the latter two numbers are high, analysis reveals that TB treatment continues to be effective, given that the treatment failure percentage, less than 1 %, is quite small. However, the unsatisfactory withdrawal and mortality rates suggest PROCET needs to improve its performance in getting patients to adhere to treatment and in following up more quickly with patients to prevent mortality.

4.15.2 Case Description

Pedro is a 42-year-old divorced father of two. He is a mechanic, but is unemployed and living with his parents.

Diagnosed in 2009 with sputum-smear positive pulmonary TB, Pedro received first-line treatment at an outpatient primary care clinic in Santiago. In October 2009, he moved to the northern part of the country to work as a driver and withdrew from treatment for the first time. While up north, his sputum-smear again tested positive. However, after five attempts in 3 years, Pedro was unable to complete the daily phase of the treatment. As indicated by medical staff, he either refused to attend the local medical center for treatment or rejected the treatment and even verbally attacked staff when they tried to administer medicines.

In January 2012, he returned to Santiago seeking care at the same primary care clinic he had previously visited, continuing to test positive but now presenting respiratory symptoms. A final attempt at treatment, this time with second-line treatment, failed after 2 months due to his irregular attendance at the health care facility and failure to take the medication regularly.

Pedro acknowledged he understood the consequences of his behavior and the possibility of microbial mutations leading to antibiotic resistance, which would change his condition to incurable. Yet, when questioned about the reasons for his behavior, he refused to take responsibility, claiming, among other things, that TB drugs made him feel sick.

In October 2012, he again visited the primary care medical clinic, this time accompanied by his mother and claiming he wanted to "start over." He was feeling ill, having night sweats, losing weight, and had diminished functional capacity that prevented him from working. Because of his previous history, he was now referred to a specialized center, where the physician in charge of the TB program evaluated his case and wrote in his medical records, "The patient does not seem to understand his situation and the risk he is posing to his family…it seems to me that health care personnel are more concerned about patient's disease than the patient himself." The specialist concluded that the chance of the patient completing treatment after six failures was unlikely. The specialist therefore decided not to renew treatment "since this would cause even more microbial resistance. Disciplinary discharge would be more fitting for this patient," the physician added, "especially in view of the great demand for hospital care."

Pedro subsequently revisits the medical center demanding treatment, this time claiming he will not withdraw from therapy because he has joined a church and has had "an awakening of consciousness to the will of God, which is to serve and love your neighbor as yourself, and therefore, not to infect others."

Despite the earlier decision of the physician in charge of the TB program, doctors reevaluate the case and decide that he should receive further TB treatment. Doctors refer him to a social worker for a mental health assessment and the initiation of mental health treatment if needed as a condition of restarting TB treatment.

4.15.3 Discussion Questions

1. Do you agree with the doctors' decision to allow further TB treatment for the patient? Why or why not?
2. Can denial of treatment to a patient with a potentially curable disease be ethically justified, considering that this denial could lead to the patient's death? On what ethical basis should the decision to deny or not deny treatment be made?
3. Given that health resources are limited, what role does the principle of distributive justice play in determining whether patients should be allowed to start treatment after multiple episodes of noncompliance with previous treatment?
4. In view of the risk that the patient could infect his family with TB, should he be denied further treatment or should he be given another chance to complete it? How would you ethically justify your decision?
5. What role should social factors such as educational level, economic status, or family situation play in making such decisions?
6. When a patient could transmit a serious infectious disease, should there be legal enforcement of the requirement to get treated?

References

Código Sanitario. 1968. D.F.L. N° 725/67. *Publicado en el Diario Oficial de 31.01.68*. Gobierno de Chile. Ministerio de Salud. www.bcn.cl/leyes/pdf/actualizado/5595.pdf. Accessed 11 Feb 2014.

Herrero, M., A. Greco, S. Ramos, and S. Arrossi. 2011. From individual risk to social vulnerability: Factors associated with non-compliance with anti-tuberculosis treatment. *Rev Argent Salud Pública* 2(8): 36–42.

Ministerio de Salud. 2012. *Programa Nacional de Control y Eliminación de la Tuberculosis. Informe de Situación 2008 – 2011*. http://web.minsal.cl/sites/default/files/fi les/TB2008-2011.pdf. Accessed 11 Feb 2014.

Pan American Health Organization. 2006. *Tuberculosis: Regional plan for tuberculosis control, 2006–2015*. Washington, DC: PAHO. http://www.stoptb.org/assets/documents/global/plan/tb-reg-plan-2006-15%20AMRO.pdf. Accessed 11 Feb 2014.

Programa Nacional de Control y Erradicación de la Tuberculosis (PROCET). 2005. *Manual de Organización y Normas Técnicas*. Subsecretaría de Salud Pública, Departamento de Prevención y Control de Enfermedades, Ministerio de Salud de Chile. http://web.minsal.cl/portal/url/item/803048171acc60f8e04001011f0148e2.pdf. Accessed 11 Feb 2014.

4.16 Case 8: Mass Evacuation

A.M. Viens
Centre for Health, Ethics and Law, Southampton Law School
University of Southampton
Southampton, UK
e-mail: a.m.viens@soton.ac.uk

Maxwell J. Smith
Dalla Lana School of Public Health and the Joint Centre for Bioethics
University of Toronto
Toronto, ON, Canada

This case is presented for instructional purposes only. The ideas and opinions expressed are the authors' own. The case is not meant to reflect the official position, views, or policies of the editors, the editors' host institutions, or the authors' host institutions.

4.16.1 Background

Mass evacuation involves moving people (and sometimes their property and animals) to alternative locations to protect them from threats to their health and safety (Kemetzhofer and Weinstein 2012). Threats to public health can be direct or indirect. Direct threats include natural hazards (e.g., hurricanes, floods, earthquakes, wildfires) and human-caused hazards (e.g., release of hazardous materials, nuclear incident, bioterrorist attack). These threats can also negatively affect essential public services (e.g., water, sewage, electricity) or create conditions for the proliferation of waterborne and vectorborne diseases. Mass evacuation is an important public health response, but it raises practical and moral issues (Settles 2012; Kodama 2015).

The sudden and unpredictable nature of some threats limits opportunities to provide notice for safe, orderly, and rapid evacuation. Such threats often force large numbers of people with different capabilities to travel great distances. Given limited time, resources, and personnel, those requiring assistance in evacuating will need to be categorized according to method of evacuation (e.g., medevac, ambulance, bus) and in what order they should be evacuated.

Although evacuation aims to promote or protect the well-being of the population, its use also raises considerations of fairness. Because evacuation orders may negatively affect vulnerable and marginalized populations disproportionately (Morrow 1999), special attention needs to be paid to these populations (Van Willigen et al. 2002). Public health officials need to consider socioeconomic disparities that can disadvantage community members in ways that impede compliance with evacuation orders. For example, during the 2005 Hurricane Katrina in New Orleans, lack of access to transportation or to financial resources prevented many people from evacuating. To mitigate such disadvantages and deficiencies, evacuation policies and procedures must be established for vulnerable or marginalized populations.

Mass evacuation can be voluntary or mandatory. Most evacuations will be voluntary because most people will comply with the recommendation to evacuate. Nevertheless, implementation seldom occurs without complication, and predicting evacuation behavior of a population is inherently difficult (Baker 1991; Perry and Lindell 1991; Riad et al. 1999; Dash and Gladwin 2007). Evacuations are often ordered by different levels of government and carried out by local responders, requiring a high level of coordination among agencies. Mandatory evacuation adds further complications. Requiring people to leave their homes or work whether or not they consent raises moral questions, such as justifying liberty restrictions.

Whether evacuation is voluntary or mandatory, a small segment of the community will choose not to evacuate, even if they have the ability to do so. In all cases, efforts should be made to educate the public about the personal risks and societal costs of noncompliance with evacuation orders. Those who do not comply with evacuation orders raise the issue of whether they should be forced to evacuate and whether first responders have a moral obligation to go back and rescue them. Enforcement of evacuation orders illustrates how law might be used as a public health tool (e.g., a jurisdiction may criminalize failure to comply with an evacuation order) (Viens et al. 2013).

Attention also has to be paid to the process of returning evacuated populations to their communities. Here, too, both practical and ethical issues arise: the extent to which damaged property and infrastructure should be rebuilt, the level of compensation or restitution that could be paid to evacuees or first responders, and possible sanctions to be levied on nonevacuators later rescued.

4.16.2 Case Description

Your community is a large, metropolitan city under a category 5 hurricane warning. The hurricane, which has been forecasted to make landfall in 48–72 h, threatens massive flooding and property damage. A large number of people widely dispersed in the city will need to be evacuated. They speak many languages, have varying levels of access to transportation, and require various levels of care. Special needs and vulnerable populations (e.g., the disabled, ill and injured, homeless, and the incarcerated) will also need help to evacuate.

As a result of emergency preparedness incident-training simulations, some agencies have developed evacuation plans. These plans are not always easily accessible to all first responders and the lack of coordination between agencies has led to confusion. Responders are unclear about who should be given priority in evacuation assistance, which resources and personnel should be devoted to evacuation efforts, and when to halt evacuation and rescue efforts and shift to recovering bodies. Of particular concern are the number of high-rise commercial buildings and medical facilities in the city. Although these buildings and facilities have individual evacuation plans, most only make evacuation provisions for short-term events, such as power outages or fires. Worse, no central registry or database lists which community members will require help to evacuate.

In less affluent neighborhoods, some residents lack access to a car or sufficient money to transport their family outside the hurricane's path. Some of those unable to evacuate will be able to stay with friends or family. However, evacuees who cannot stay with people they know are quickly overwhelming the capacity of evacuation facilities in nearby towns. Decisions will need to be made about how to coordinate and efficiently use resources and personnel to maximize the number of people protected from the hurricane.

Officials managing the evacuation have realized that mass evacuation raises some logistical and ethical issues shared by public health measures involved in the movement or restriction of people (e.g., quarantine, isolation, social distancing). They have therefore asked you, an experienced public health official, to provide input on which groups of people should be evacuated, how, and in what order of priority. Your special concern in planning and coordinating with other agencies will be the health of the population, mitigating inequalities and the safety of the first responders.

4.16.3 Discussion Questions

1. What are the relevant ethical considerations for deciding who should be evacuated first and whether the evacuation order should be mandatory or voluntary? Of those to be evacuated, who should we evacuate first? How should decisions be made regarding who to evacuate when not all can be evacuated?

2. What role should community engagement play in determining the order of priority of groups to be evacuated?
3. How should authorities deal with those who do not comply with an evacuation order? What are the ethical implications of allowing people not to evacuate? Do authorities have obligations toward people who refuse to evacuate and later need to be rescued? Should people who had the ability to evacuate but failed to do so be blamed or punished in some way when they later need to be rescued?
4. What kind of legal protections are needed to protect people who are made more vulnerable by virtue of having to evacuate? For example, should there be provisions to prevent price gouging on gasoline or to keep extra police officers around to prevent looting?
5. Are those who comply with voluntary evacuation orders owed anything? To what extent must resources be provided for the evacuated population? How much effort should be put into keeping families together? Should compensation be paid when people are asked to evacuate with little time for protecting valuable items that end up getting lost, damaged, or destroyed? How would your answers to these questions change if the evacuation orders were mandatory?
6. In a clinical setting, some patients will be too unstable to be moved or, if movable, will require disproportionate medical care and resources. Would it ever be acceptable to abandon some patients? If so, under what conditions? Would it be morally required that a clinician or first responder stay within the evacuation area with such patients—at greater risk to themselves—to provide constant care until rescue can be provided at a later time?

Acknowledgements Maxwell J. Smith is supported by a Canadian Institutes of Health Research Frederick Banting and Charles Best Canada Graduate Scholarship and the Canadian Institutes of Health Research Douglas Kinsella Doctoral Award for Research in Bioethics.

References

Baker, E.J. 1991. Hurricane evacuation behavior. *International Journal of Mass Emergencies and Disasters* 9(2): 287–310.

Dash, N., and H. Gladwin. 2007. Evacuation decision making and behavioral responses: Individual and household. *Natural Hazards Review* 8: 69–77.

Kemetzhofer, P., and E.S. Weinstein. 2012. Evacuation. In *Oxford American handbook of disaster medicine*, ed. R.A. Partridge, L. Proano, and D. Marcozzi, 227–237. Oxford: Oxford University Press.

Kodama, S. 2015. Tsunami-tendenko and morality in disasters. *Journal of Medical Ethics* 41: 361–363.

Morrow, B.H. 1999. Identifying and mapping community vulnerability. *Disasters* 23: 1–18.

Perry, R.W., and M.K. Lindell. 1991. The effects of ethnicity on evacuation decision-making. *International Journal of Mass Emergencies and Disasters* 9: 47–68.

Riad, J.K., F.H. Norris, and R.B. Ruback. 1999. Predicting evacuation in two major disasters: Risk perception, social influence, and access to resources. *Journal of Applied Social Psychology* 29(5): 918–934.

Settles, T.L. 2012. Federalism, law and the ethics of disaster evacuations. In *Disasters, hazards and law*, Sociology of crime law and deviance, vol. 17, ed. M. Deflem, 65–81. Bingley: Emerald Group.

Van Willigen, M., B. Edwards, T. Edwards, and S. Hessee. 2002. Riding out the storm: The experiences of the physically disabled during hurricanes Bonnie, Dennis, and Floyd. *Natural Hazards Review* 3: 98–106.

Viens, A.M., J. Coggon, and A. Kessel (eds.). 2013. *Criminal law, philosophy and public health.* Cambridge: Cambridge University Press.

Chapter 5
Chronic Disease Prevention and Health Promotion

Harald Schmidt

5.1 Introduction

Chronic diseases include conditions such as heart disease, stroke, cancer, diabetes, respiratory conditions, and arthritis. In high-income countries, chronic diseases have long been the leading causes of death and disability. Globally, more than 70 % of deaths are due to chronic diseases, in the United States, more than 87 % (World Health Organization [WHO] 2011). Almost one in two Americans has at least one chronic condition (Wu and Green 2000). Aside from the cost in terms of human welfare, treatment of chronic disease accounts for an estimated three quarters of U.S. health care spending (Centers for Disease Control and Prevention [CDC] 2012). Chronic diseases directly affect overall health care budgets, employee productivity, and economies. Globally, noncommunicable diseases account for two-thirds of the overall disease burden in middle-income countries and are expected to rise to three-quarters by 2030, typically in parallel to economic development (World Bank 2011). Of particular concern to many low- and middle-income countries is that threats to population health occur on two fronts simultaneously: "In the slums of today's megacities, we are seeing noncommunicable diseases caused by unhealthy diets and habits, side by side with undernutrition" (WHO 2002).

Four modifiable risk factors are principal contributors to chronic disease, associated disability, and premature death: lack of physical activity, poor nutrition, tobacco use, and excessive alcohol consumption (CDC 2012). One in three adult Americans is overweight, another third is obese, and almost one-fifth of young people between

---

The opinions, findings, and conclusions of the author do not necessarily reflect the official position, views, or policies of the editors, the editors' host institutions, or the author's host institution.

H. Schmidt, MA, PhD (✉)
Department of Medical Ethics & Health Policy, Center for Health Incentives and Behavioral Economics, University of Pennsylvania, Philadelphia, PA, USA
e-mail: schmidth@mail.med.upenn.edu

D.H. Barrett et al. (eds.), *Public Health Ethics: Cases Spanning the Globe*, Public Health Ethics Analysis 3, DOI 10.1007/978-3-319-23847-0_5

6 and 19 years of age is obese, even though rates are not increasing at previous levels (Katz 2013). Although smoking has declined considerably over recent decades, about 20 % of Americans still smoke. Rates of smoking are markedly different across socioeconomic groups, and much higher among economically disadvantaged people (Garrett et al. 2011). Globally, deaths from smoking are expected to increase dramatically in low-income countries. In the twentieth century, tobacco-use killed around 100 million people worldwide. In the twenty-first century, an estimated one billion will die prematurely—a tenfold increase. By 2030, more than 80 % of deaths attributable to tobacco will be in low-income countries (WHO 2012).

In principle, if a risk factor can be modified, then much illness and suffering (morbidity) and early death (mortality) can be avoided or prevented. Therefore, prevention and health promotion policies seek ways in which the impact of modifiable risk factors can be reduced. How one analyzes the causal pathways that lead to the development of risk factors may encourage one to explore a range of different interventions. An obvious starting point is to focus on individual behavior or lifestyle, because what an individual does (or fails to do) typically plays a central role in chronic disease. Consider the following line of thought by John H. Knowles, an outspoken critic of the American health care system in the 1970s:

> Prevention of disease means forsaking the bad habits which many people enjoy—[but the] cost of sloth, gluttony, alcoholic intemperance, reckless driving, sexual frenzy, and smoking is now a national, and not an individual, responsibility. This is justified as individual freedom—but one man's freedom is another man's shackle in taxes and insurance premiums. I believe the idea of a 'right' to health should be replaced by the idea of an individual moral obligation to preserve one's own health—a public duty if you will. The individual then has the 'right' to expect help with information, accessible services of good quality, and minimal financial barriers (Knowles 1977).

Knowles comment is interesting on several counts. First, it underscores that even though population health usually features centrally in health promotion, cost considerations are never far removed and are equally prominent in current debates, especially in political fora.[1]

Second, in invoking three of the deadly sins (gluttony, sloth, and lust), Knowles illustrates in a frank way that discussions about health promotion are not confined to medical or public health concepts. Implicitly or explicitly, these discussions almost always entail moral concepts (such as personal responsibility or deservingness) that are embedded in deeply held normative frameworks.

---

[1]For an example of such a political debate, see the 2012 platform of the U.S.'s Republican Party: "... approximately 80 % of health care costs are related to lifestyle—smoking, obesity, substance abuse—far greater emphasis has to be put upon personal responsibility for health maintenance ..." (GOP 2012). Reforming Government to Serve the People is available at https://www.gop.com/platform/. This quote also illustrates the inaccurate use of statistics. Although the burden of chronic diseases is indeed roughly 80 %, it is an exaggeration to claim that personal responsibility alone accounts for the total burden. Exact estimates may not be straightforward due to complex interactions of different factors. Consequently, a more realistic estimate attributes 40 % to personal behavior, 30 % to genetic predispositions, 15 % to social circumstance, 10 % to inadequate health care, and 5 % to environmental causes (Schroeder 2007).

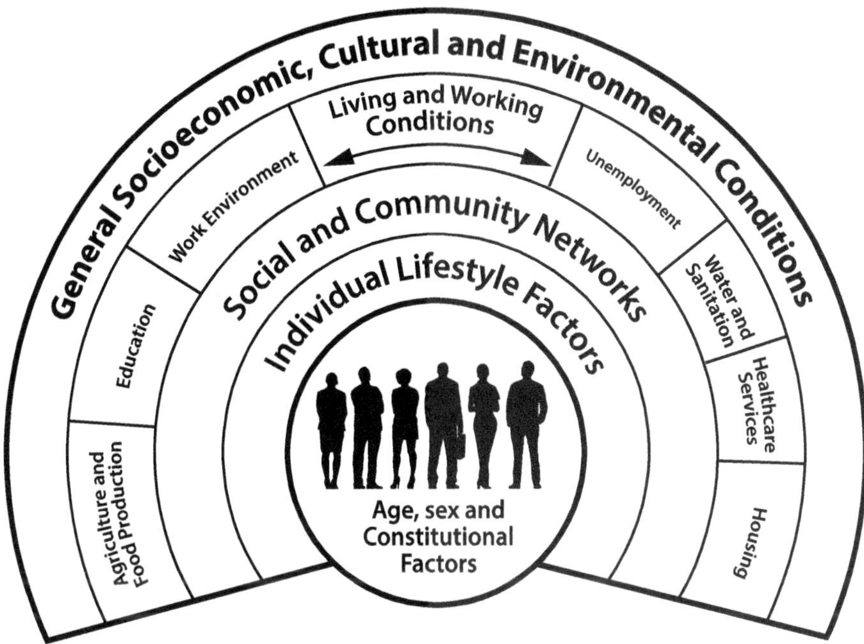

Fig. 5.1 Factors determining health and chronic diseases (Originally published in Dahlgren and Whitehead (1991). Reproduced from Acheson (1998). Reproduced with permission)

And finally—although Knowles acknowledges elsewhere in his essay the role of taxes and other measures to improve health and eradicate poverty—he concludes by stating "the costs of individual irresponsibility in health have now become prohibitive. The choice is individual responsibility or social failure" (Knowles 1977). The policy interventions he mentions aim for broader recognition of personal responsibility and therefore focus on education and information campaigns to empower people to behave responsibly. But this analysis is shortsighted. It fails to consider the responsibility of those who produce, market, and sell products (e.g., unhealthy foods, drinks, or tobacco) and of those who regulate markets or set business standards (e.g., trade groups or national or regional policy makers). His point could best be made if all people lived in similar environments and conditions, had sufficient disposable income, had ready access to healthy and affordable food, had equal opportunity to exercise, and experienced other health-conducive conditions. But this is not the case. People live in vastly different contexts, and many different factors determine health (Fig. 5.1).

Although Fig. 5.1 provides a useful overview of many factors that affect health, the concept of "lifestyle," commonly encountered in the broader debate around chronic diseases is problematic. It can suggest that people choose, for example, smoking or heavy drinking as others might decide between taking up golf or tennis as a hobby. The point is that "lifestyle" implies degrees of freedom and the possibility of genuine opportunity and choice. But assume that you grew up in an inner-city borough as a child of low-income obese and smoking parents. Many in your family and social environment smoke and are obese. Compared to the national average, you are among the most overweight, and you fail to lose weight as an adolescent. You remain obese. Calling your obesity a matter of lifestyle makes little sense. Now assume you started smoking as a minor (<18 years of age) just as 88 % of U.S. adults who smoke daily (U.S. Department of Health and Human Services 2012). It can be cynical to treat this "lifestyle" as voluntary and freely chosen if, for example, many of your role models smoke and if smoking in your social setting and challenging environment functions as a coping mechanism to relieve stress. The different spheres in the diagram therefore need to be understood as highly interdependent. Regarding terminology, the concept of lifestyle factors should be replaced with that of *personal behavior*. Doing so acknowledges that powerful constraints can severely infringe on the development of healthy habits and behavior. In the worst case, these constraints may thwart development of healthy habits and behaviors altogether, even when individuals have the best of intentions.

Focusing on just the individual is therefore overly narrow when identifying policies to prevent chronic diseases. Yet, removing the individual from the equation is also unhelpful (Schmidt 2009). The central ethical issues surrounding health promotion and prevention of chronic diseases concern the relative responsibilities of all agents whose actions influence the health of others. These agents include, in addition to individuals, health workers, governments (at different levels), and corporate entities.

5.2 Individuals

Except for some genetic conditions and extremely toxic environments (i.e., chemical exposure), individual behavior typically plays a causal role in bringing about bad—as well as good—health. People may or may not eat healthily; they may or may not use tobacco or illegal drugs; they may consume alcohol excessively or in moderation; they may exercise too little or too much; and they may regularly brush their teeth, go for medically recommended checkups, and take their medications—or fail to do so. However, it is important to recognize that implementation of measures such as praise or blame, or financial rewards, or penalties—although they presuppose a certain degree of causal responsibility—do not mean that individuals also automatically need to be held fully responsible in a moral (or legal) sense. Causal responsibility in the present context simply means that a person has behaved in ways that contributed to, say, poor health. Therefore, a smoker with lung disease arguably has some causal responsibility for the condition. But if it turns out that the smoker started becoming addicted as a child, it is clear that the outcome cannot simply be treated as the result of an entirely voluntary choice. Where there is no, or limited, opportunity of choice, there is the risk of "victim blaming" (Crawford 1977) and holding people responsible for factors that are, in fact, beyond their control. Conversely, ignoring the scope of possible behavior change can lead to fatalism and resignation (Schmidt 2009).

For individuals to take causal and other responsibility for their health, they require, among other things, information that they can understand, affordable access to health care, and, oftentimes far more important, environments conducive to health in which capabilities may be developed so that one can flourish in life (e.g., residential, work, and play settings) (Venkatapuram 2011; Ruger 2006). According to the adage "ought implies can," we can only hold people responsible for their actions if they could have acted otherwise. Of course, it is true in some sense that people who smoke, or overconsume unhealthy food, or fail to exercise, could oftentimes have acted otherwise, in principle: it was not literally impossible for them to act otherwise. However, the relevant question is not whether it is literally possible to engage in healthy behavior, but whether it reasonably feasible for people to engage in healthy behavior. Talk of personal responsibility therefore requires a clear focus on the settings in which people live and on their behaviors when presented with different choices. Consideration should also be given to the possibility that policies implementing personal responsibility through, for example, rewards and penalties, may impact core values underlying a health system, such as a sound doctor-patient relationship, equity, or risk sharing, which may affect their overall acceptability in positive or negative ways (Schmidt 2008).

5.3 Formal and Informal Health Workers

Health professionals play a central role in chronic disease prevention and health promotion (Dawson and Verweij 2007). In primary prevention, they focus on averting poor health in the first place and on promoting good health. In secondary prevention, they offer information, tests, and screenings aimed at early detection and treatment of diseases. Diabetes, blood pressure, and some cancer screenings can have utility, especially when targeting at-risk populations in a nonstigmatizing way. Primary care physicians are often in a good position to decide on the appropriateness of screenings. Their knowledge of patient background and overall situation can help them tailor tests on the supply side to the actual needs on the demand side, bearing in mind patient preferences and individual risks.

Cost effectiveness aside, a physician would be wrong to offer every available test to every patient because the clinical benefit is not always clear. A recent systematic review and meta-analysis of randomized controlled trials concerning general health checkups (i.e., comprising health risk assessments and biometric screening for high blood pressure, body mass index, cholesterol, and blood sugar) found no association with lower overall mortality or morbidity (Krogsbøll et al. 2012). On the basis of these findings, the researchers caution that checkups may needlessly increase diagnoses and use of drugs. They recommend clinically motivated testing of individuals to initiate preventive efforts but discourage screening at the population-level for lack of evidence. The authors acknowledge limitations in their research, including that most of the trials were relatively old and that changes in interventions and care pathways reduce applicability to current practice. All studies entailed voluntary invitations to get checkups, so selection bias may have overrepresented privileged people (in typically better health to start with) and not reached those needing attention the most (Krogsbøll et al. 2012). The focus on all-cause mortality has also been criticized as setting too high a threshold (Sox 2013). Yet despite the somewhat intuitive appeal of using general health checkups in secondary prevention, there is little robust evidence from randomized controlled trials to show any major impact on overall mortality.

An ethical problem arises when offering preventive screenings that do not follow evidence-based guidelines (U.K. National Screening Committee 2013). Such screenings may increase the number of "worried well" who oftentimes are confused by complex probabilities of detecting and preventing diseases. Clinicians must therefore do their utmost to understand risks and benefits of screening tests and communicate these to patients in ways that are easily comprehensible and not misleading (Wegwarth and Gigerenzer 2011). For example, a physician might tell his 50-year-old patient that she should undergo breast cancer screening because it reduces risk by 14 %. But this information is incomplete, as relative risk rates alone obscure the basic reference point against which the comparison is made. Another way of providing the same information would be to use absolute risk rates and to say that if one screens 1000 women for 20 years, four breast cancer deaths can be averted, even though eight among all screened women still die from breast cancer. In addition, over the 20 years, the 1000 women taking part in screening experience 412 false positives, and of 73 women who are diagnosed with breast cancer, 19 experience overdetection and are treated for a cancer that would not have developed into a lethal tumor, with treatment typically consisting of hormone- radio- or chemo-therapy, and partial or full surgical breast-removal (Hersch et al. 2015). This way of presenting data (Fig. 5.2), especially when combined with other relevant information about screening accuracy and rates of overdiagnoses, provides more adequate context for considering benefits and risks—yet, this presentation method is far from being universally adopted (Gigerenzer et al. 2010).

Adequate risk information in secondary prevention matters not only from a patient-empowerment perspective but also because it can mitigate real or perceived conflicts of interests of physicians. Physicians, anyone who markets or manufactures screening equipment, and those who analyze data typically experience financial gain when more patients undergo screening. Therefore, a central ethical issue of secondary prevention is not only how to avoid premature mortality in the most efficient and cost effective way but also how to eliminate potential conflicts of interests. Patients can become entangled in competing interests, as illustrated by the controversy surrounding prostate-specific antigen, or PSA, testing to detect prostate cancer. Although physicians and others experienced financial gain, patients experienced no reduced mortality and instead higher morbidity and loss of quality of life

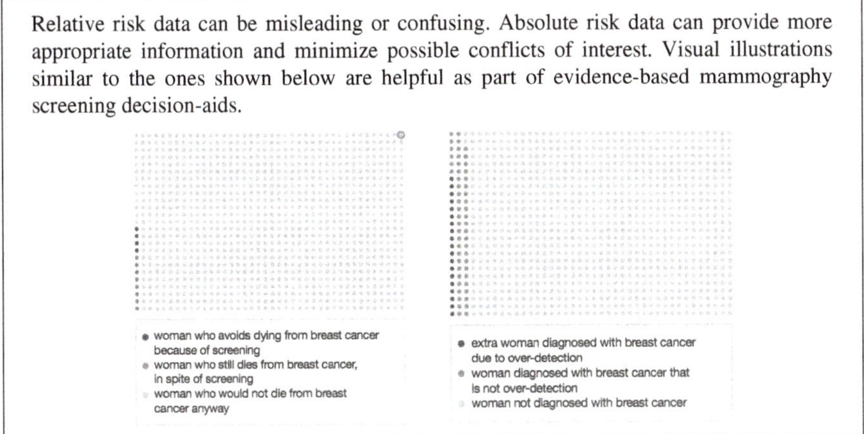

Fig. 5.2 Communicating benefits and harms of breast screening (Originally published in Hersch et al. (2015). Used with permission)

due to the entailed procedures (Ablin 2010). The question of "what is the magnitude of benefits and risks, and to whom?" is therefore an important one to ask in all secondary prevention, especially because the net gain for patients is not always obvious.

For these and other reasons, many in the public health community are skeptical about the relative utility of secondary prevention in a clinical context. Often this is paired with a call for shifting political and financial support to primary prevention and the broader sphere of public health (Sackett 2002; Mühlhauser 2007). Here, the objective is to avoid poor health in the first place by empowering people with different ways to lead healthy lives. Too often, only the privileged few in certain populations have this capability (WHO 2008).

Of course, this way of thinking immediately broadens the concept of health professional. Clearly, it is outside the scope of, say, a hospital-based general internist to reduce junk-food outlets or to increase exercise opportunities in a low-income part of town, even if the internist has good reasons to believe these structural features are key contributors toward rising levels of obesity among patients. But once we recognize how differences among settings in which people live can affect the incidence and prevention of chronic diseases, it becomes apparent that public health professionals outside the clinical context have as much, if not more, of a role to play compared to physicians when it comes to chronic disease prevention and health promotion.

A range of corresponding interventions are relevant to this discussion, including literacy, safe sex, hygiene and health awareness campaigns, financial subsidies for healthy food or gyms, exercise stations in parks, breastfeeding rooms in workplaces, and fluoridation of water. The public health field is heterogeneous and comprises numerous different actors both in and outside a clinical context. Public health, despite its many contexts and support from government and private sectors, is typically underfunded. This is especially true for informal grassroots campaigns, which often have a considerable competitive advantage over formal program structures. Grassroots campaigns evolve from the communities they seek to help. Because nearly every intervention that addresses chronic diseases has to do with how one lives one's life, top-down interventions are often experienced as intrusive forms of external meddling (Morain and Mello 2013). Conversely, initiatives led by a community member can be perceived more sympathetically than instructions from men in white coats who speak in formal and technical terms (unless, of course, that happens to be the target population, which, typically, it is not).

Health professionals working on chronic disease prevention and health promotion therefore span a wide field. In a looser sense, many professionals not generally seen as concerned with health could be included too, such as teachers, architects, town planners, or spiritual leaders. Each has perspectives that can be highly influential, but each is inherently limited in scope because chronic conditions result from complex interplay of different factors. This raises another key ethical issue involving how to determine the optimal mix of strategic approaches, bearing in mind the relative strengths and weaknesses.

Further, just as users and payers of health care should have a keen interest in having systematic studies and evaluations done to determine which of several drugs aimed at reducing, for example, severe headache, is most efficacious (and cost effective), we should be interested in the evidence base for possible benefits and harms of different interventions being implemented by health professionals concerned with chronic conditions. Yet, in an almost tautologic approach, health professionals often assume any preventive method will be good because its aim is prevention. But several strategies could be aimed at the same problem. Given that budgets are generally limited, it can be useful to determine which intervention is most effective and, for example, how its relative effectiveness and cost compare with its intrusion into peoples' lives. Such comparisons can help achieve value for money, even if the complex interplay of agents complicate this process.

5.4 Governments (At Different Levels)

Chronic disease prevention and health promotion policies often face criticism for promoting a "nanny state." This means that although government may legitimately use taxes and other measures to create health-conducive infrastructure that prevents chronic disease such as clean water supplies, sanitation services, or clean air acts, it should otherwise stay out of people's lives, and, in particular, refrain from telling citizens how to live their life (Childress et al. 2002; Gostin 2010; Dawson

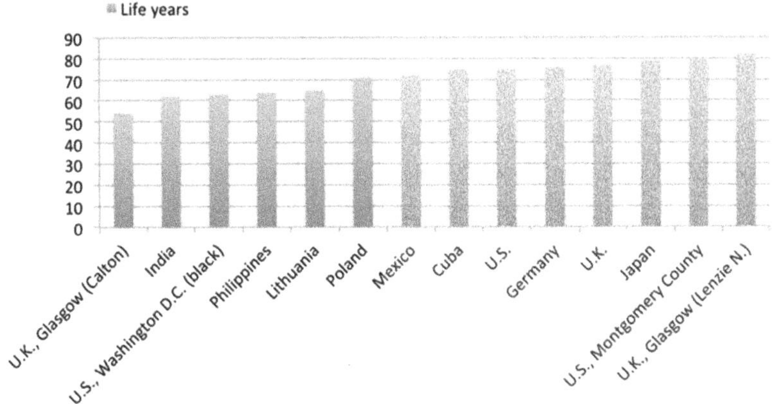

Fig. 5.3 Male life expectancy, between- and within-country inequities, selected countries (Figure is adapted from World Health Organization (2008))

and Verweij 2007). Many good reasons support this viewpoint. Still, many variables related to chronic diseases are linked to legitimizing governments in the first place.

For example, consider the U.S. Declaration of Independence. It declares that "all men are created equal; that they are endowed by their Creator with certain unalienable Rights; and that among these are Life, Liberty, and the pursuit of Happiness." Numerous countries express similar sentiments in legal frameworks and charge states with providing environments that enable conditions for a good life, and prevent harm. Moreover, building on the United Nations' (U.N.) *International Covenant on Economic, Social and Cultural Rights* of 1966 and clarifying *General Comment 14* by the U.N.'s Committee on Economic, Social and Cultural Rights, several countries have incorporated the right to health in their constitutions (WHO 2013). Yet, not all people live equally long, nor are they equally happy (in a nontrivial sense). For example, life expectancy differs widely, not just between countries at different levels of development, but also within countries, and sometimes with differences of almost 30 years across just 10 miles (see the data on two areas in Glasgow, Scotland, located near one another, Fig. 5.3). Chronic diseases are a major contributor to this variation.

Going back to the focus on personal responsibility, one might argue this variation in life expectancy is due to some people simply not wanting to be healthy or living long. But this is clearly myopic. Government planning at different levels has immense impact on both the prevalence and prevention of chronic diseases. It is sometimes argued that the best prevention is to instill in people the desire to live long and healthily (Rosenbrock 2013). For some, this might entail a state-guaranteed minimum income (irrespective of whether one works), since economic livelihood is of course a major factor in how one views one's own future. While a positive impact of such policies on the incidence of chronic disease and mortality would certainly be plausible, there is a wide range of less radical and politically more feasible options in the menu of different levels of government action. These include town planning, zoning laws, school and university meal plans, and, of paramount importance, regulation of industry where markets fail. These and other interventions can only be implemented by governments. An important part of chronic disease prevention and health promotion is to monitor where differences in morbidity and mortality are such that government action is warranted, and to impress on elected officials their responsibility in creating appropriate environments.

The monolithic notion of "the" government is, of course, an overly simplistic one. Key personnel in health departments may well wish to limit the size of, for example, soft drinks. Or they may wish to standardize ways in which nutritional content is shown on food packaging. Such measures would enable more informed consumer choice, and, more indirectly, incentivize producers to reconsider whether food composition can be optimized for health impact, given the secondary "showcasing" effect of labeling.[2] But their colleagues in trade or industry, as well as in the treasury, may point out the risk of tax shortfalls that could result from lower consumption. Or they may worry about pushback from lobbyists in the corporate sector who fear losing profits for their clients. Politicians may often be more concerned with their short-term re-election prospects than with making substantial (or even just incremental) longer-term progress on chronic disease prevention. These conflicting perspectives within government are inevitable. But only government can determine the playing field and ground rules for industries producing, selling and marketing food, drink, tobacco, and other products contributing to unhealthy behavior. In liberal economies that, typically, pursue a hands-off approach toward regulating markets, the central ethical challenge then is to decide at which points markets are considered to have failed, other options of market regulations are unfeasible, and government action is warranted, despite possible drawbacks.

A second closely related question is what intervention to pursue once the need for action has been identified. Figure 5.4 shows the Intervention Ladder published in a report by the Nuffield Council on Bioethics (2007) on public health ethics. The model suggests that governments have a range of different options at their disposal that become increasingly intrusive or paternalistic the higher one moves up the ladder. At the same time, each rung up the ladder requires more robust justification and evidence, although the report points out the bottom rung, "doing nothing or simply monitoring," also requires justification.

[2] For example, it has been shown that large U.S. chain restaurants changed menus in anticipation of a legal mandate requiring public calorie posting, resulting in a 12 % reduction in calories (or about 56 fewer calories per item, see Bleich et al. 2015).

In preventing chronic diseases and promoting health, governments have a range of policy options differing in justification, evidence requirements, and extent of intrusion.

- **Eliminate choice:** Prohibit substances such as transfats. Remove obese children from their home.
- **Restrict choice**: Ban unhealthy foods from shops or restaurants. Add fluoride to water.
- **Guide choice through disincentives:** Tax cigarettes. Discourage the use of cars in inner cities through charging schemes or by limiting parking spaces.
- **Guide choice through incentives:** Give tax breaks to commuters.
- **Guide choice by changing the default policy:** In restaurants, instead of providing fewer health options and including fries as a standard side dish (with healthier options available) make healthy options standard menu fare (with fries optional). Regulate salt levels of fast food meals because consumers can add salt afterwards.
- **Enable choice:** Create tax-funded smoking cessation programs, build cycle lanes, or provide free fruit in schools.
- **Provide information:** Implement campaigns to encourage people to walk more or to eat certain amounts of fruit and vegetables daily.
- **Do nothing or simply monitor the current situation.**

Fig. 5.4 The intervention ladder (Adapted from Nuffield Council on Bioethics (2007))

5.5 Corporate Entities

In the United States, the Institute of Medicine (1988) defines public health as "what we, as a society, do collectively to assure the conditions in which people can be healthy." In the United Kingdom, the Faculty of Public Health (2010) of the Royal Colleges of Physicians suggests that public health is the "science and art of preventing disease, prolonging life, and promoting health through organized efforts of society." These, and other conceptualizations, emphasize the collective nature of public health work (Verweij and Dawson 2007). Companies that facilitate consumer access to tobacco or to healthy and unhealthy food and drink are part of society and contribute via goods, services, and employment opportunities. In return, they often receive generous tax breaks. Company operations benefit further from diverse financial arrangements and infrastructures put in place by governments to ensure stability of civic and economic life, since both are essential to how markets function. It is therefore reasonable to ascribe some responsibilities for public health to companies. In many instances, this is achieved through voluntary corporate social commitments, such as charters or formal partnerships with charitable or community organizations. Increasingly, companies view their own ethical actions as an attractive side of their branding, especially in countries where consumers' awareness is high.

Although many companies generate profits through healthful products, many others benefit from bringing products to market that will likely cause harm. Product demand is rarely a function of basic human needs but, rather, is defined by social and cultural norms. These norms are often fueled—if not generated—by aggressive marketing to adults and children. The basic tension regarding the role of companies in relation to public health is their *prima facie* obligation to contribute to population health, while also maximizing owners or shareholders' profits. Public health would be promoted by measures such as providing honest nutritional information and other content of products; avoiding claims that are misleading (as is sometimes the case with vitamins, supplements, or some diagnostic tests); not denying or underplaying potential harm (as with so-called alcopops, which are high-alcohol drinks made to look like soft drinks); or not exploiting the "pester power" of children, particularly by marketing products to them and confusing the boundary between giving information and advertising. But realizing these aspirations typically curbs consumption and therefore reduces market shares and profits.

Companies therefore prefer as little regulation as possible and favor information-based over price-based interventions or more intrusive options (Fig. 5.4). In all high-income countries, company and government officials liaise to negotiate consumer protection policies, insofar as political and consumer pressure creates demand. These negotiations often reveal the limitations of corporate social responsibility, as perhaps illustrated most clearly by the tobacco industry. For decades, the industry pursued the strategy that there was no hard evidence that tobacco was harmful to health. When this strategy became too absurd to sustain, and, in particular, when the evidence of the harmful effects of secondary smoke became overwhelming, the industry caved in and agreed to implement a series of consumer protection measures in most developed countries (Brandt 2007). However, in many instances, this tug-of-war was repeated in other countries, despite a range of robust provisions in WHO's Framework Convention on Tobacco Control (2003), the only supranational hard law instrument on a major risk factor for chronic conditions that is legally binding in more than 170 countries. From a narrow business perspective, this behavior is entirely rational. But from an ethical viewpoint, it is extremely questionable. For example, it has been accepted in the United States and Europe that it is not appropriate to glorify tobacco on billboards, to give cigarettes away for free in promotions at rock concerts geared towards young people, or to sell them individually, then why should these and other practices be commonplace in many low-income countries, especially in Africa (Action on Smoking and Health 2007)? The obscene tenfold global increase in deaths attributable to tobacco in the twenty-first century has already been noted. What makes this prospect all the more appalling is the industry's refusal to take seriously the standards it agreed to uphold in high-income countries. For if these standards were upheld, history would not repeat itself with such horrific consequences.

5.6 Case Studies

In the following five cases, the reader is put in the position of a public health practitioner to illustrate how key ethical issues can arise in the prevention of chronic diseases and health promotion. The cases highlight several real-world, practical constraints: limited budgets; insufficient evidence for how interventions will work in structurally different settings; organizational constraints, particularly from specific formats for decision making; and clashes of perspectives and worldviews. Three cases concern children, an especially vulnerable population (Verweij and Dawson 2011). The cases ask whether the parents alone can make sound health decisions for their children, and if not, what interventions would be acceptable to reach the parents. The interventions range from chemical and behavioral to social ones, and central to each are ethical questions around their justification (because of competing interests) and oftentimes unclear evidence. Several cases touch on whether or not to engage the public in decision making—and if so, how? Public engagement is an increasingly popular approach being applied broadly to health policy. Yet, it is not always clear who should be involved in which decision-making processes and on what grounds (Kreis and Schmidt 2013).

Mah et al. provide an intriguing scenario in which a municipal public health department needs to decide whether to accept increased contributions to a youth after-school program from a local fast food-chain in exchange for mentioning the chain's name as part of the (renamed) program. The background section describes how food and beverages are marketed to children and notes that globally, self-regulation models are the most common approach. This case combines real and perceived conflicts of interests for the company and for notoriously cash-strapped public health workers. Woven into the case is the media's role. The discussion questions invite analyses from the vantage points of different stakeholders and address ways to modify the base scenario, adding layers of complexity.

Blacksher's case focuses on obesity prevention, media campaigns, and stigma. She describes the human and financial toll of obesity worldwide, focusing on children as an especially vulnerable group. She also presents a range of different policy options to address childhood obesity before charging the reader, acting as a state commissioner for health, to recommend a statewide obesity policy for a disproportionately poor and vulnerable population. The process for reaching consensus on this policy recommendation is common. A task force of a dozen members is appointed, half the seats are reserved for state legislator appointees, and half reserved for public health professionals and community representatives. Due partly to their different background and priorities, the task force disagrees about how intrusive the policy should be. Members settle, however, on a statewide media campaign aimed at changing social norms. Still, how hard-hitting should the campaign be? In the discussion questions, readers may consider, among other things, the evidence needed to justify different campaign types and if other stakeholders should (or need not) be included in the decision-making process to confer legitimacy.

The case by Goldberg and Novick focuses on an intervention program in which task force members grapple with whether the use of stigma might be acceptable under certain circumstances. The authors describe empirical research findings and conceptual arguments that suggest stigma is always correlated with negative health outcomes—especially in otherwise disadvantaged populations, and certainly in the case of obesity. They describe how stigmatizing approaches are based on certain conceptions of personal responsibility that fail to consider the broad underlying structural determinants of obesity. Then the case shifts focus to another situation often encountered in public health practice: applicability of evidence base in multiple settings. Here, a program intended to empower residents to take control of their weight through meal planning, physical activity, and behavioral modification proves effective in controlled studies. The director of the county health department, attracted to the program on grounds of potential cost effectiveness, readily embraces the program. Later, however, during a program meeting, one of the department's public health nurses expresses concern about an overly strong focus on personal responsibility, which she feels makes the program unfair. Based on her knowledge of the target population, she also feels the program will be rejected. Could the program nonetheless be effective? And how might risks of stigma be minimized? These and related issues form part of the questions section.

Whereas the first three cases are set in the United States, the case by Aspradaki et al. takes us to Greece and concerns issues raised by water fluoridation. The disease burden attributable to preventable tooth decay is laid out along with the risks of using fluoride. Oral disease is on the rise in low- and middle-income countries, with poorer populations disproportionately affected. The authors describe water fluoridation in different countries before suggesting that the primary ethical tension surrounding water fluoridation arises between the concepts of autonomy and paternalism. The case description puts the reader in the position of Greece's central oral health director providing a consult to the head of public health programs in the health ministry. Negotiations on a national strategy have been held up by political and organizational digressions and by public skepticism. Still, the health ministry wants to go ahead and put in place a countrywide fluoridation program. Your task is to identify which stakeholders should be involved, how the different elements of empirical data and ethical values should be considered, and what role economic pressures might play in the decision making.

The case by Aleksandrova-Yankulovsak is about banning smoking in public places in Bulgaria. Almost half of the men and a third of the women in Bulgaria are smokers. The case provides context to smoking in Europe and nearby regions before summarizing the regulatory framework that prompted Bulgaria to consider the ban. The political process, threatened by business interests and strife within government departments, is also addressed. The case then poses the question if you, as director of the regional health inspectorate, can guarantee implementation of the new law. Other questions invite discussion on whether the law is the right tool to achieve lower smoking rates, in principle, and how the public might view temporary legal provisions that could be repealed if political support dwindles. A further central point is how or whether economic costs can ever be set against cost in human welfare.

The cases illustrate but a fraction of the ethical issues that arise in chronic disease prevention and health promotion. Many cases will present differently depending on the country and its culture, infrastructure, health care system, and legal and political system. Similarly, this introduction is far from exhaustive. Yet, when combined, the cases and introduction introduce many central ethical issues that arise in global public health. Analyzing the ethical issues that featured centrally in justifying policies (or in the refusal of policy makers or other actors to change existing policies) will deepen the reader's engagement and reflection and, ideally, contribute to better policy and practice in the future.

Acknowledgements I am grateful to Anne Barnhill for helpful comments on an earlier version of this introduction.

References

Ablin, R.J. 2010. The great prostate mistake. *New York Times*, March 10, A27.

Acheson, D. 1998. *Independent inquiry into inequalities in health*. Department of Health: U.K. Government. http://www.archive.official-documents.co.uk/document/doh/ih/contents.htm. Accessed 20 Oct 2013.

Action on Smoking and Health. 2007. *Bat's African footprint*. http://www.ash.org.uk/files/documents/ASH_685.pdf. Accessed 20 Oct 2013.

Bleich, S.N., J.A. Wolfson, and M.P. Jarlenski. 2015. Calorie changes in chain restaurant menu items: Implications for obesity and evaluations of menu labeling. *American Journal of Preventative Medicine* 48(1): 70–75.

Brandt, A.M. 2007. *The cigarette century: The rise, fall, and deadly persistence of the product that defined America*. New York: Basic Books.

Centers for Disease Control and Prevention (CDC). 2012. *Chronic disease prevention and health promotion*. http://www.cdc.gov/chronicdisease/overview/index.htm#ref2. Accessed 21 Sept 2013.

Childress, J.F., R.R. Faden, R.D. Gaare, et al. 2002. Public health ethics: Mapping the terrain. *Journal of Law, Medicine & Ethics* 30(2): 170–178.

Crawford, R. 1977. You are dangerous to your health: The ideology and politics of victim blaming. *International Journal of Health Services* 7(4): 663–680.

Dahlgren, G., and M. Whitehead. 1991. *Policies and strategies to promote social equity in health*. Stockholm: Institute for Future Studies.

Dawson, A., and M.F. Verweij. 2007. Introduction: Ethics, prevention, and public health. In *Ethics, prevention and public health*, ed. A. Dawson and M. Verweij, 1–12. New York: Oxford University Press.

Faculty of Public Health, Royal Colleges of Physicians of the United Kingdom. 2010. *What is public health?* http://www.fph.org.uk/what_is_public_health. Accessed 20 Oct 2013.

Garrett, B.E., S.R. Dube, A. Trosclair, R.S. Caraballo, and T.F. Pechacek. 2011. Cigarette smoking United States, 1965 2008. *Morbidity and Mortality Weekly Report. Surveillance Summaries* 60(suppl): 109–113.

Gigerenzer, G., O. Wegwarth, and M. Feufel. 2010. Misleading communication of risk. *British Medical Journal* 341: c4830.

GOP. 2012. *Reforming government to serve the people*. Available at https://www.gop.com/platform/. Accessed 20 Oct 2013.

Gostin, L.O. (ed.). 2010. *Public health law and ethics: A reader*. Berkeley: University of California Press.

Hersch, J., A. Barratt, J. Jansen, L. Irwig, et al. 2015. Use of a decision aid including information on overdetection to support informed choice about breast cancer screening: A randomised controlled trial. *Lancet* 385(9978): 1642–1652.

Institute of Medicine. 1988. *The future of public health*. Washington, DC: National Academy Press.

Katz, D.L. 2013. Childhood obesity trends in 2013: Mind, matter, and message. *Childhood Obesity* 9(1): 1–2.

Knowles, J.H. 1977. The responsibility of the individual. *Daedalus* 106(1): 57–80.

Kreis, J., and H. Schmidt. 2013. Public engagement in health technology assessment and coverage decisions: A study of experiences in France, Germany, and the United Kingdom. *Journal of Health Politics, Policy and Law* 38(1): 89–122.

Krogsbøll, L.T., K.J. Jørgensen, C. Grønhøj Larsen, and P.C. Gøtzsche. 2012. General health checks in adults for reducing morbidity and mortality from disease. *Cochrane Database of Systematic Reviews* 10: CD009009. http://onlinelibrary.wiley.com/doi/10.1002/14651858.CD009009.pub2/abstract. Accessed 22 Oct 2013.

Morain, S., and M.M. Mello. 2013. Survey finds public support for legal interventions directed at health behavior to fight noncommunicable disease. *Health Affairs* 32(3): 486–496.

Mühlhauser, I. 2007. Ist Vorbeugen besser als Heilen? *Zeitschrift für ärztliche Fortbildung und Qualität im Gesundheitswesen* 101(5): 293–299. (Mühlhauser I. 2007. Is prevention better than healing? *German Journal for Evidence and Quality in Health Care* 101(5): 293–299.)

Nuffield Council on Bioethics. 2007. *Public health: Ethical issues*. London: Nuffield Council on Bioethics.

Rosenbrock, R. 2013. Die beste Prävention ist die Lust auf die eigene Zukunft. *Der Paritätische*, Ausgabe 3/2013, Soziales zählt, 16–18. (Rosenbrock R. 2013. The best prevention is the desire for their own future. *The Joint*, March edition, Social Matters, 16–18.)

Ruger, J.P. 2006. Health, capability, and justice: Toward a new paradigm of health ethics, policy and law. *Cornell Journal of Law and Public Policy* 15(2): 403–482.

Sackett, D.L. 2002. The arrogance of preventive medicine. *Canadian Medical Association Journal* 167(4): 363–364.

Schmidt, H. 2008. Bonuses as incentives and rewards for health responsibility: A good thing? *Journal of Medicine and Philosophy* 33(3): 198–220.

Schmidt, H. 2009. Personal responsibility in the NHS Constitution and the social determinants of health approach: Competitive or complementary? *Health Economics, Policy, and Law* 4(2): 129–138.

Schroeder, S.A. 2007. Shattuck lecture. We can do better—Improving the health of the American people. *New England Journal of Medicine* 357(12): 1221–1228.

Sox, H.C. 2013. The health checkup: Was it ever effective? Could it be effective? *Journal of the American Medical Association* 309(23): 2496–2497. doi:10.1001/jama.2013.5040.

U.K. National Screening Committee. 2013. *Criteria for appraising the viability, effectiveness and appropriateness of a screening programme*. http://www.screening.nhs.uk/criteria. Accessed 22 Oct 2013.

U.S. Department of Health and Human Services. 2012. *Preventing tobacco use among youth and young adults: A report of the surgeon general*. Atlanta: U.S. Department of Health and Human Services, Centers for Disease Control and Prevention, National Center for Chronic Disease Prevention and Health Promotion, Office on Smoking and Health.

Venkatapuram, S. 2011. *Health justice: An argument from the capabilities approach*. Cambridge: Polity Press.

Verweij, M., and A. Dawson. 2007. The meaning of 'public' in 'public health'. In *Ethics, prevention, and public health*, ed. A. Dawson and M. Verweij, 13–29. New York: Oxford University Press.

Verweij, M., and A. Dawson. 2011. Children's health, public health. *Public Health Ethics* 4(2): 107–108.

Wegwarth, O., and G. Gigerenzer. 2011. Statistical illiteracy in doctors. In *Better doctors, better patients, better decisions: Envisioning health care 2020*, ed. G. Gigerenzer and J.A.M. Gray, 137–151. Cambridge, MA: MIT Press.

World Bank. 2011. *The growing danger of non-communicable diseases: Acting now to reverse course*. Washington, DC: World Bank Human Development Network.

World Health Organization (WHO). 2002. *The World Health Report 2002: Reducing risks, promoting healthy life*. Geneva: World Health Organization.

World Health Organization (WHO). 2003. *WHO framework convention on tobacco control*. Geneva: World Health Organization.

World Health Organization (WHO). 2008. Commission on social determinants of health—final report. *Closing the gap in a generation: Health equity through action on the social determinants of health*. Geneva: World Health Organization. Online at http://www.who.int/social_determinants/thecommission/finalreport/en/index.html.

World Health Organization (WHO). 2011. *Noncommunicable diseases country profiles 2011*. Geneva: World Health Organization.

World Health Organization (WHO). 2012. *WHO report on the global tobacco epidemic, 2008: The MPOWER package*. Geneva: World Health Organization.

World Health Organization (WHO). 2013. *The right to health, fact sheet no. 323*. http://www.who.int/mediacentre/factsheets/fs323/en/. Accessed 8 Dec 2013.

Wu, S.Y., and A. Green. 2000. *Projection of chronic illness prevalence and cost inflation*. Santa Monica: RAND Health.

5.7 Case 1: Municipal Action on Food and Beverage Marketing to Youth

Catherine L. Mah
Faculty of Medicine
Memorial University
St. John's, NL, Canada
e-mail: catherine.mah@mun.ca

Brian Cook
Toronto Food Strategy, Toronto Public Health
Toronto, ON, Canada

Sylvia Hoang
Social and Epidemiological Research Department
Centre for Addiction and Mental Health
Toronto, ON, Canada

Emily Taylor
Dalla Lana School of Public Health
University of Toronto
Toronto, ON, Canada

This case is presented for instructional purposes only. The ideas and opinions expressed are the authors' own. The case is not meant to reflect the official position, views, or policies of the editors, the editors' host institutions, or the authors' host institutions.

5.7.1 Background

Children are exposed to a greater intensity and frequency of marketing than ever before. Evidence has demonstrated that marketing of food and beverages to children contributes adversely to health, affecting food knowledge, attitudes, dietary habits, consumption practices, and health status. Marketing to children has always raised concerns. But recently, numerous nongovernmental and international organizations and all levels of government have expressed their concern about food and beverage marketing and advertising to children as a public health issue.

Often used interchangeably with "advertising," the term "marketing," actually encompasses a broader range of issues. The World Health Organization (WHO) (2010) defines marketing as "any form of commercial communication or message that is designed to, or has the effect of, increasing the recognition, appeal and/or consumption of particular products and services. It comprises anything that acts to advertise or otherwise promote a product or service."

Two large-scale global systematic reviews of evidence in the last decade have concluded that food and beverage marketing substantially affects young people and is associated with adverse health outcomes. In 2003, the U.K. Food Standards Agency commissioned a systematic review of the influence of food promotion on children's food-related knowledge, preferences, and behaviors (Hastings et al. 2003). WHO updated the report in 2007 and 2009 (Hastings et al. 2007; Cairns et al. 2009). In 2006, the U.S. Institute of Medicine conducted a systematic review of the influences of food and beverage marketing on the diet and diet-related health of children and youth (McGinnis et al. 2006). Key findings from these reports follow:

- Food and beverages developed for and advertised to young people are predominantly calorie dense and nutrient poor;
- Marketing influences children's food and beverage preferences, purchase requests, and short-term consumption, even among young children (ages 2–5 years); and
- There is strong evidence that child and youth exposure to television advertising is significantly correlated with poor health status, although sufficient evidence of a causal link with obesity is not yet available.

The authors of the 2009 WHO report suggest that existing research "almost certainly underestimates the influence of food promotion" and that more research is needed, especially for newer forms of media (Cairns et al. 2009).

As part of its global strategy for the prevention and control of noncommunicable diseases (WHO 2004), WHO subsequently endorsed policy recommendations for governments to take action on food and beverage marketing to children (2010,

2012). The recommendations emphasize governments' key role in developing policies to protect the public interest, including leadership roles in managing intersectoral processes and negotiating stakeholder rights and responsibilities.

The scope of existing policy interventions that address food advertising to children includes statutory regulation (i.e., general restrictions or outright prohibitions) and industry self-regulatory codes. Globally, industry self-regulatory approaches tend to be the most common approach.

Many organizations promote the adoption of comprehensive public policy interventions, with the scope of these interventions ranging from total ad bans (all commercial advertising) to food ad bans or junk food ad bans (WHO 2012).

Other organizations suggest stepwise approaches that target particular exposures, products, ages, or specific forms of marketing or media. For example, such approaches could include limiting marketing in venues such as schools, restricting junk food, protecting children younger than a certain age, defining certain television broadcasts as children's programs, or restricting promotions in television broadcasts before 10 pm, respectively (WHO 2012).

In recent years, many food and beverage companies, working with industry associations, have issued voluntary pledges to alter marketing practices toward children. For example, such pledges typically include criteria for the nutritional quality of foods advertised to children, limitations on the use of licensed characters, and marketing in schools. However, critics argue that these types of voluntary changes are not sufficient to reduce the risks of food marketing to children in a substantive way.

Despite this array of interventions, the absence of widespread agreement on the most appropriate form of collective action has led many policy makers to default to inaction.

5.7.2 *Case Description*

You direct the Healthy Public Policy program for a large municipal public health department that recently has come under fire in a newspaper exposé about contributions from fast food companies to after-school programs for youth that the city government runs. The exposé highlighted the contributions of Big Boss Burger, a local fast food hamburger chain with 12 locations across the city. Big Boss Burger donates cooking equipment to the city's high-priority, after-school cooking program for 9- to 11-year-olds. Although the program is well-liked by youth, it is regularly threatened by funding cuts. The chain has recently offered to scale-up its annual cash donation to cover all food and equipment costs in exchange for renaming the program "The Big Boss Burger Community Kitchen" and for placing the chain's logo on all signage and promotional materials.

The highly successful Big Boss Burger chain is owned by a beloved, self-made restaurateur who has spent his entire career in the local food industry. Considered a colorful local personality, he frequently sends Twitter updates that reflect his over-the-top advertising style. One tweet, for example, offered a free sample of the chain's "quadruple bypass" burger to anyone who visited one of the chain's locations within the hour.

Media spokespersons for the mayor, meanwhile, have reiterated the community benefits of cultivating positive partnerships with local businesses. They note that only registered public health nutrition staff run the city's cooking programs, while insisting that Big Boss Burger has no influence whatsoever on city policies or youth curricula.

The media furor nevertheless has prompted city officials to explore developing a sponsorship policy for municipal child and youth programs. The Medical Health Officer has asked you to prepare a briefing note outlining the key public health considerations that such a sponsorship policy needs to address.

You face a dilemma. On the one hand, several years ago your Healthy Public Policy team launched a study of the impact of food and beverage advertising on children. Last year's update on the study to the Board of Health included a recommendation that city-operated venues and programs avoid commercial advertising of food and beverages targeting children younger than 13 years of age. Thus far, the recommendation has not led to any formal policy changes. Municipal employees partly attribute this inaction to the reluctance of local authorities to act when there are no state or national policies that govern sponsorship or marketing restrictions.

On the other hand, the financially strapped city relies on engagement with the local business community to fund many city-run programs, including health education activities. It is also well-known that the owner of Big Boss Burger grew up in a local low-income community and frequently volunteers his time at events in his former neighborhood.

5.7.3 Discussion Questions

1. What key points will you emphasize in your briefing note? How will scientific information from past public health reports and decisions influence your response? How should ethical considerations influence your briefing note?
2. What population groups are you most concerned about with regard to the sponsorship policy? What if the cooking program sponsored by Big Boss Burger was for 14- to 16-year-olds instead of 9- to 11-year-olds? For adults? For children in a high-income neighborhood?
3. Does corporate sponsorship constitute food promotion? What benefits to the municipality might be derived from Big Boss Burger's contributions (for example, local economic benefits or having increased public attention and private-sector support of priority neighborhoods)? How should the public health department weigh these benefits against population health benefits and harms? Consider your response if Big Boss Burger

   (a) Had offered its support without the naming rights request;
   (b) Had instead offered a cash donation to a parents' association supporting the program;

(c) Was an organic, vegan comfort food restaurant; or
(d) Was a large, multinational fast food corporation.

4. How will public opinion inform your briefing note? How will you handle the situation given that Big Boss Burger is a highly popular fast food chain and that the owner is a local public personality?
5. What are (and should be) the roles and responsibilities for various city departments in defining the sponsorship policy? Consider, for example, city departments responsible for public health, parks and recreation, municipal licensing, social services, and economic development.
6. Let's imagine that you are a parent of two girls, ages 6 and 9 years. In an ideal world, how much food and beverage marketing do you think they should be exposed to? How does your perspective as a parent enter into your professional decisions as director of the Healthy Public Policy program? How about your perspective as a voting citizen or city resident?

References

Cairns, G., K. Angus, and G. Hastings. 2009. *The extent, nature and effects of food promotion to children: A review of the evidence to December 2008*. Geneva: World Health Organization. http://whqlibdoc.who.int/publications/2009/9789241598835_eng.pdf. Accessed 29 May 2013.

Hastings, G., M. Stead, L. McDermott, et al. 2003. *Review of research on the effects of food promotion to children: Final report prepared for the food standards agency*. Glasgow: Centre for Social Marketing. http://tna.europarchive.org/20110116113217/http:/www.food.gov.uk/multimedia/pdfs/foodpromotiontochildren1.pdf.Accessed 29 May 2013.

Hastings, G., L. McDermott, K. Angus, M. Stead, and S. Thomson. 2007. *The extent, nature and effects of food promotion to children: A review of the evidence. Technical paper prepared for the World Health Organization*. Geneva: World Health Organization. http://whqlibdoc.who.int/publications/2007/9789241595247_eng.pdf. Accessed 29 May 2013.

McGinnis, J.M., J.A. Gootman, and V.I. Kraak (eds.). 2006. *Food marketing to children and youth: Threat or opportunity?* Committee on Food Marketing and the Diets of Children and Youth, Institute of Medicine of the National Academies. Washington, DC: National Academies Press.

World Health Organization (WHO). 2004. *Global strategy on diet, physical activity and health*. Geneva: World Health Organization. http://www.who.int/dietphysicalactivity/strategy/eb11344/strategy_english_web.pdf. Accessed 29 May 2013.

World Health Organization (WHO). 2010. *Set of recommendations on the marketing of foods and nonalcoholic beverages to children*. Geneva: World Health Organization. http://whqlibdoc.who.int/publications/2010/9789241500210_eng.pdf. Accessed 29 May 2013.

World Health Organization (WHO). 2012. *A framework for implementing the set of recommendations on the marketing of foods and non-alcoholic beverages to children*. Geneva: World Health Organization. http://www.who.int/entity/dietphysicalactivity/MarketingFramework2012.pdf. Accessed 29 May 2013.

5.8 Case 2: Obesity Prevention in Children: Media Campaigns, Stigma, and Ethics

Erika Blacksher
Department of Bioethics and Humanities
University of Washington
Seattle, WA, USA
e-mail: eb2010@u.washington.edu

This case is presented for instructional purposes only. The ideas and opinions expressed are the author's own. The case is not meant to reflect the official position, views, or policies of the editors, the editors' host institutions, or the author's host institution.

5.8.1 Background

Worldwide obesity has doubled since 1980 and kills some 2.8 million adults each year (World Health Organization [WHO] 2012). Childhood obesity also has increased at alarming rates with some 42 million children estimated to be overweight (WHO 2013). Among Organisation for Economic Cooperation and Development (OECD) countries, the United States has the highest rate of obesity (OECD 2012). More than 35 % of adults and almost 17 % of children are obese (Ogden et al. 2012), with especially high rates among poor and minority children (Centers for Disease Control and Prevention [CDC] 2012).

Childhood obesity has serious short- and long-term health consequences. Obese children are more likely to have risk factors for cardiovascular disease, including high cholesterol and blood pressure; type 2 diabetes; skeletal problems; sleep apnea; and mental health issues, such as low self-esteem and depression (CDC 2012; Reilly et al. 2003). Children now account for half of all new cases of type 2 diabetes. Obese children are also subject to systematic discrimination (Strauss 2002). More than 50 % of overweight children become obese adults who experience elevated health risks for heart disease, stroke, diabetes, osteoporosis, lower-body disability, some types of cancer, and premature mortality (Freedman 2011; CDC 2012).

The burdens of obesity are also economic. Rising health care costs are mostly driven by obesity-related costs. Estimates indicate that in 2008 some 10 % of medical spending in the United States was related to obesity, amounting to as much as $147 billion (Finkelstein et al. 2009). Experts estimate obesity-related costs will account for 21 % of medical spending by 2018 if obesity rates continue to rise (United Health Foundation 2009).

As the human and financial costs of obesity have become better recognized, government officials and public health leaders increasingly have called for strong action. Comprehensive approaches that act on environmental and social determinants of food choice and activity level are widely recommended (OECD 2012). The complexity of such an approach is reflected in the following recommended policies and strategies: taxing unhealthy foods and beverages, such as soda and snack food, to make them cost prohibitive; providing agricultural subsidies to lower the cost of healthy foods, such as fresh produce and whole grains; setting standards to lower sodium levels and prohibit the use of trans fatty acids in food products; banning unhealthy foods from public schools and child care facilities; restricting or banning the advertising of unhealthy foods to children; posting calorie counts on restaurant and take-out menus; using "counter-advertising" to show the harmful effects of unhealthy foods; redesigning communities and streets to incorporate parks, sidewalks, and bike paths; and reducing sedentary behavior by limiting time viewing television and playing computer games (Frieden et al. 2010; Butland et al. 2007).

Children's status as developing agents further complicates childhood obesity prevention. Parents have primary responsibility for rearing children and considerable discretion over cultural and lifestyle matters, including many daily decisions that directly affect a child's food and activity-related environments and behaviors (Blacksher 2008). Some measures would likely confer benefit regardless of parental behavior (e.g., banning food advertising to children or removing trans fats from packaged foods). But others will have their intended effect only if parents make certain choices, some of which will require that they change their health-related habits.

Many preventive measures will be controversial because they involve government action and seek to shape personal choice. Perhaps the least controversial of the measures enable healthier choices by providing people with information and making healthy options more available and affordable; however, many are more coercive, ranging from those that eliminate and restrict choice to those that guide choice through disincentives and default policies (Nuffield Council on Bioethics 2007). Intervening in voluntary choices where effects impose no harm to others constitutes strong paternalism and is difficult though not impossible to justify (Childress et al. 2002). However, society may justifiably intervene to prohibit behaviors that expose others to serious harms, and this "harm principle" has been appealed to as the basis for removing children from homes where parental practices are judged to contribute to severe childhood obesity and attendant comorbidities (Murtagh and Ludwig 2011). Removing a child from the home poses other potential harms, further complicating the ethical dilemma (Black and Elliott 2011). These ethical considerations in combination with the difficulty of changing health habits makes obesity prevention one of the more challenging public health priorities of the twenty-first century.

5.8.2 Case Description

Your state is the poorest in the nation with high rates of childhood poverty, obesity, and diabetes. Located in the southeastern part of the United States in what is known as the "stroke belt," adults disproportionately suffer from stroke and its risk factors—hypertension, high cholesterol, diabetes, and obesity. As the state's new commissioner of health, the governor has tasked you with making obesity prevention a public health priority. The governor is concerned about public health and rising health care costs. More than 50 % of the state's children and some 20 % of adults are enrolled in Medicaid (a federal-state program that provides health care services for low-income Americans), making it the largest item in the state budget.

The governor has requested that you convene and chair a 12-member task force to make recommendations for a statewide obesity prevention strategy. Six seats are reserved for state legislator appointees because the recommendations will need political support to be implemented. The other seats are reserved for public health, health care, and community representatives. For several months, task force members debated measures that eliminate or restrict adult choice through government action, such as taxes and bans on unhealthy foods and drinks. Those who favored such measures argued they would be the most effective, citing the success of tobacco taxes and smoking bans in reducing smoking, and could be justified on grounds that obesity-related costs constitute an economic harm to others (Pearson and Lieber 2009). Yet, many task force members, particularly elected representatives, found such measures objectionable forms of government intrusion into adult choices.

Task force members did, however, agree to tackle obesity prevention in children on grounds that the state has a role in protecting them. To that end, they endorsed measures to improve school lunches and to remove vending machines that sell soda and other sugary beverages from public school grounds. Task force members also wanted to invest in a statewide media campaign about the causes and harms of childhood obesity because they believed it would raise awareness and promote informed choices. They also thought a media campaign would help to change social norms, which they deemed essential to long-term change in their state, where fried and fatty foods are part of the cultural heritage.

Task force members cannot, however, agree on the orientation of such a campaign. Some favor an approach used by a nearby state that has attracted attention for its graphic depiction of obese and unhappy children accompanied by hard-hitting messages, such as "It's hard to be a little girl if you're not." Opponents believe the campaign blames the victims and further stigmatizes obese children. They propose instead an approach that highlights environmental barriers to healthy choices and depicts unhealthy food as the culprit, not those who consume it. But proponents of the more hard-hitting approach say it is honest about the facts and highlights the essential role of parents in regulating children's behavior. To support their case, they cite the use of similarly graphic media campaigns in tobacco cessation efforts and note that public health efforts have often relied on stigma as a tool of disease prevention, despite the controversy (Bayer 2008; Burris 2008). The task force has formulated a series of questions to take up at the next meeting.

5.8.3 Discussion Questions

1. What harms are associated with childhood obesity?
2. Are the harms of obesity and tobacco use analogous? Is the economic cost of obesity a harm to others in the same way that secondhand smoke is a harm to others?
3. Do public media campaigns that depict images of obese children stigmatize them? What is stigma?
4. Is it ever ethically permissible to use stigmatization as a tool of disease prevention and health promotion? If so, in what sort of cases? Should children ever be the targets of stigmatization?
5. Do public media campaigns that highlight the role of parents in regulating children's food and activity-related environments and choices blame the victims?
6. Should the task force consider gathering community input, particularly from people who are overweight or obese, about the sorts of messages they would find effective in changing their health habits and also find ethically acceptable? If so, should children be included in these focus groups? If so, at what age?

References

Bayer, R. 2008. Stigma and the ethics of public health: Not can we but should we. *Social Science & Medicine* 67(3): 463–472. doi:10.1016/j.socscimed.2008.03.017.

Blacksher, E. 2008. Children's health inequalities: Ethical and political challenges to seeking social justice. *Hastings Center Report* 38(4): 28–35.

Black, W., and R.L. Elliott. 2011. Childhood obesity and child neglect. *Journal of the Medical Association of Georgia* 100(4): 24–25.

Burris, S. 2008. Stigma, ethics, and policy: A commentary on Bayer's "Stigma and the ethics of public health: Not can we but should we". *Social Science & Medicine* 67(3): 473–475.

Butland, B., S. Jebb, P. Kopelman, et al. 2007. *Foresight. Tackling obesities: Future choices.* London: Government Office for Science.

Centers for Disease Control and Prevention (CDC). 2012. *Adolescent and school health: Childhood obesity facts.* http://www.cdc.gov/healthyyouth/obesity/facts.htm. Accessed 11 June 2013.

Childress, J.F., R.R. Faden, R.D. Gaare, et al. 2002. Public health ethics: Mapping the terrain. *Journal of Law Medicine & Ethics* 30(2): 170–178.

Freedman, D.S. 2011. Obesity—United States, 1988–2008. *Morbidity and Mortality Weekly Report. Surveillance Summaries* 60(01): 73–77.

Finkelstein, E.A., J.G. Trogdon, J.W. Cohen, and W. Dietz. 2009. Annual medical spending attributable to obesity: Payer- and service-specific estimates. *Health Affairs* 28(5): w822–w831.

Frieden, T.R., W. Dietz, and J. Collins. 2010. Reducing childhood obesity through policy change: Acting now to prevent obesity. *Health Affairs* 29(3): 357–363.

Murtagh, L., and D.S. Ludwig. 2011. State intervention in life-threatening childhood obesity. *Journal of the Medical Association* 306(2): 206–207.

Nuffield Council on Bioethics. 2007. *Public health: Ethical issues.* http://www.nuffieldbioethics.org/public-health. Accessed 11 June 2013.

Organisation for Economic Cooperation and Development (OECD). 2012. *Obesity update 2012.* http://www.oecd.org/health/49716427.pdf. Accessed 11 June 2013.

Ogden, C.L., M.D. Carroll, B.K. Kit, and K.M. Flegal. 2012. *Prevalence of obesity in the United States, 2009–2010*. National Center for Health Statistics Data Brief, no. 82. http://www.cdc.gov/nchs/data/databriefs/db82.pdf. Accessed 11 June 2013.

Pearson, S.D., and S.R. Lieber. 2009. Financial penalties for the unhealthy? Ethical guidelines for holding employees responsible for their health. *Health Affairs* 28(3): 845–852.

Reilly, J.J., E. Methven, Z.C. McDowell, et al. 2003. Health consequences of obesity. *Archives of Disease in Childhood* 88(9): 748–752.

Strauss, R.S. 2002. Childhood obesity and self-esteem. *Pediatrics* 105(1): 152–155.

United Health Foundation. 2009. *The future costs of obesity: National and state estimates of the impact of obesity on direct health care expenses*. United Health Foundation in collaboration with the American Public Health Association and Partnership for Prevention. http://www.nccor.org/downloads/CostofObesityReport-FINAL.pdf. Accessed 11 June 2013.

World Health Organization (WHO). 2012. *Obesity and overweight* (Fact Sheet no. 311), updated March 2013. http://who.int/mediacentre/factsheets/fs311/en/. Accessed 11 June 2013.

World Health Organization (WHO). 2013. *Global strategy on diet, physical activity and health. Childhood overweight and obesity*. http://who.int/dietphysicalactivity/childhood/en/. Accessed 11 June 2013.

5.9 Case 3: Obesity Stigma in Vulnerable and Marginalized Groups

Daniel S. Goldberg
Department of Bioethics and Interdisciplinary Studies, Brody School of Medicine
East Carolina University
Greenville, NC, USA
e-mail: goldbergd@ecu.edu

Lloyd Novick
Brody School of Medicine
East Carolina University
Greenville, NC, USA

This case is presented for instructional purposes only. The ideas and opinions expressed are the authors' own. The case is not meant to reflect the official position, views, or policies of the editors, the editors' host institutions, or the authors' host institutions.

5.9.1 *Background*

For empirical and normative reasons, stigma is an enormous public health problem that can have devastating psychosocial impact (Vanable et al. 2006; Chapple et al. 2004). Moreover, there is evidence that even after controlling for confounders, stigma is robustly correlated with adverse health outcomes (Vardy et al. 2002; Puhl and Brownell 2003). Stigma increases human suffering and diminishes health, both of which anchor ethical concerns. However, its ethical deficiencies are not solely a function of its health effects; as Burris notes, "even if [stigma] had no adverse effects on health … it may readily be seen as repugnant in a humane society" (Burris 2002; Courtwright 2013).

According to Hatzenbuehler et al. (2013), stigma in a public health context consists of two central components: (1) an in-group marks an out-group as different on the basis of some common demographic characteristic, and (2) the in-group assigns a negative evaluation to the characteristic. Stigma is therefore intimately connected to entrenched social power structures (Link and Phelan 2006; Scambler 2006). Unsurprisingly, while precise estimates are lacking, evidence suggests that the burden of such stigma is unequally distributed along the social gradient, and that already disadvantaged groups are more likely to experience more intense levels of stigma (Scambler 2006; Shayne and Kaplan 1991). The prospect of compound disadvantage and inequalities renders stigma a critical issue for public health ethics, one that strongly implicates concerns of distributive and social justice (Powers and Faden 2006; Courtwright 2009).

Recent data shows that the prevalence of obesity is 35.7 % in the United States (Ogden et al. 2012) and 12.0 % globally (Stevens et al. 2012). Tracking these high estimates, obesity stigma is one of the common and ethically alarming health stigmas (Puhl and Heuer 2009; Puhl and Brownell 2003). Puhl and Heuer (2010) expressly link the commonality of obesity stigma to the emphasis on personal responsibility in the United States, which is the subject of an active debate (Wikler 2002). This debate has nineteenth century roots but is ongoing (Leichter 2003) and influences public perceptions on whether collective action in the name of public health is warranted. Moreover, such perceptions vary with particular public health problems. For example, although many advocate for greater individual responsibility in wearing seat belts, few contend that such responsibility eliminates the need for guardrails and speed limits. The perceived linkages between obesity and personal responsibility suggest that approaches to health promotion emphasizing the latter run a significant risk of intensifying obesity stigma (Puhl and Heuer 2010). Goldberg (2012) argues that such risk renders these approaches ethically suboptimal.

In addition, it is well recognized that background socioeconomic conditions are primary components of obesity-creating environments (McLaren 2007; Pickett et al. 2005). The fact that socioeconomic conditions have an immense impact in determining patterns of obesity among and within populations suggests reasons for doubting that public health interventions targeted at individual lifestyle change will be particularly effective in countering obesity (MacLean et al. 2009). Indeed, the evidence obtained from analysis of other major risk factors, such as smoking, strongly suggests a lack of longitudinal efficacy for such interventions (Jarvis and Wardle 2006; Ebrahim and Smith 2001; Rose 1985).

There exists significant debate over the effectiveness of stigmatization in changing risky health behaviors. Some commentators argue that the denormalization and stigmatization of smoking has produced positive public health consequences given the overall decline in incidence in the United States (Bayer 2008; Bell et al. 2010) and in parts of Europe (Ritchie et al. 2010). One leading bioethicist even recently endorsed a kind of "stigmatization lite" as a tool to reduce obesity (Callahan 2013). Although the evidence for efficacy of stigma as a means to enhancing public health in general remains in dispute, the evidence as to obesity overwhelmingly suggests that stigma is more likely to exacerbate obesity than to reduce it (Puhl et al. 2013; Puhl and Heuer 2010).

Finally, there is excellent evidence that interventions that target individual behavior change have the unfortunate tendency to expand health inequalities. Capewell and Graham (2010) term such interventions "agentic" because the extent of their benefits depends on the resources the individual agent can bring to bear. Thus, for example, even when the least well-off are targeted, smoking cessation programs disproportionately benefit the affluent. The result is that effective programs targeting lifestyle change can unintentionally expand health inequalities, a fact that raises significant concerns of justice.

Ultimately, though efforts to counter obesity are critically needed, it is all too easy to implement public health interventions that intensify obesity stigma, expand health inequalities, and take little account of the role background social conditions play in structuring patterns of obesity and limiting health choices. Efforts to address obesity must therefore grapple with significant ethical issues centering primarily on justice and on health equity.

5.9.2 Case Description

The Brennan County Health Department (BCHD) is considering a new health promotion program to ameliorate the high and growing rates of adult obesity in the county (prevalence and incidence of 38 and 3.5 %). The program emphasizes the need to "Take Control" by (1) assessing weight; (2) losing weight; and (3) preventing weight gain (Centers for Disease Control and Prevention 2012). It highlights the significance of personal responsibility in countering obesity and aims to empower individuals to implement lifestyle change. The program consists of twice-weekly meetings facilitated by a nutritionist held over 8 weeks, with screening performed by a family nurse practitioner. The regimen consists of modules on meal planning, physical activity, behavioral modification, and cooking instruction. The meetings would occur at 6:30 pm at Brennan County Memorial Hospital.

The hospital is located in the town of Bernsville, which sits in the northwestern corner of the county. Brennan County is rural and geographically large, with a small population spread across large distances. Multiple bodies of water traverse the county. Road quality is uneven. Educational attainment is low, with only 43 % of residents having completed some college. Thirty-eight percent of children in Brennan County live in poverty, and the violent crime rate per 100,000 people is 605 (the national benchmark is 73). Unemployment is 14.2 %. Farming is a chief economic activity, with several migrant labor camps existing in the southeastern part of the county. In terms of demographics, 40 % of Brennan County residents are Caucasian, 35 % are African-American, 14 % are Hispanic/Latino, 10 % are Native American, and 1 % is Asian/Asian-American.

The BCHD obesity program is based on reasonably good evidence. Several controlled studies of model programs have demonstrated both reduction in body weight and prevention of weight gain. Such effects decreased over time, but statistically significant improvements were maintained at 8-month follow-up. Ongoing studies are intended to assess effect endurance at 18 and 24 months postintervention.

At a recent BCHD meeting, Pauline, a public health nurse employed by the health department, expressed concern about the implementation of the program. Surprised, several attendees ask Pauline why she is hesitant, and she replies that she is concerned that the obesity program's emphasis on personal responsibility and lifestyle change might not be received well in a resource-poor county that serves multiple vulnerable populations, many of whom have documented levels of medical and institutional mistrust. The BCHD director, James, admits that Pauline's concerns are legitimate, but he also notes the evidence suggesting the intervention's efficacy. He argues that such results are so important that they justify immediate implementation. James also notes that several county commissioners have publicly declared an obesity crisis in Brennan County and have privately indicated to him that BCHD is expected to lead a transparent and vigorous response. In addition, James points out that the county does not have the funds to devote to more upstream interventions and they have several staff already trained in lifestyle change methods, so that the costs could be low.

Pauline shakes her head and says that while it is critical to address obesity in Brennan County, the program ignores the environmental and background conditions in which the most at-risk communities in Brennan County live, work, and play. She reiterates her concern that the program as it currently stands is unfair.

5.9.3 *Discussion Questions*

1. To what extent does the program risk creating or intensifying obesity stigma against marginalized and vulnerable groups in Brennan County? Why does this matter ethically?
2. Why are the social and economic conditions residents of Brennan County experience relevant to an ethical assessment of the obesity program?
3. How does the rural nature of Brennan County influence the ethical analysis of the program?
4. What concerns related to justice and/or health equity does the program raise?
5. How should obesity interventions be structured to minimize risks of stigma?
6. To what extent should public health interventions intended to counter obesity target upstream social determinants of obesity and obesity-related diseases?

References

Bayer, R. 2008. Stigma and the ethics of public health: Not can we but should we. *Social Science & Medicine* 67(3): 463–472. doi:10.1016/j.socscimed.2008.03.017.

Bell, K., A. Salmon, M. Bowers, J. Bell, and L. McCullough. 2010. Smoking, stigma and tobacco 'denormalization': Further reflections on the use of stigma as a public health tool. *Social Science & Medicine* 70(6): 795–799.

Burris, S. 2002. Disease stigma in U.S. public health law. *Journal of Law, Medicine & Ethics* 30(2): 179–190.

Callahan, D. 2013. Obesity: Chasing an elusive epidemic. *Hastings Center Report* 43(1): 34–40.

Capewell, S., and H. Graham. 2010. Will cardiovascular disease prevention widen health inequalities? *PLoS Medicine* 7(8): e1000320.

Centers for Disease Control and Prevention. 2012. *Healthy weight.* http://www.cdc.gov/healthyweight. Accessed 20 Dec 2012.

Chapple, A., S. Ziebland, and A. McPherson. 2004. Stigma, shame, and blame experienced by patients with lung cancer: Qualitative study. *British Medical Journal* 328(7454): 1470.

Courtwright, A.M. 2009. Justice, stigma, and the new epidemiology of health disparities. *Bioethics* 23(2): 90–96.

Courtwright, A. 2013. Stigmatization and public health ethics. *Bioethics* 27(2): 74–80.

Ebrahim, S., and G.D. Smith. 2001. Exporting failure? Coronary heart disease and stroke in developing countries. *International Journal of Epidemiology* 30(2): 201–205.

Goldberg, D.S. 2012. Social justice, health inequalities and methodological individualism in U.S. health promotion. *Public Health Ethics* 5(2): 104–115.

Hatzenbuehler, M.L., J.C. Phelan, and B.G. Link. 2013. Stigma as a fundamental cause of population health inequalities. *American Journal of Public Health* 103(5): 813–821.

Jarvis, M.J., and J. Wardle. 2006. Social patterning of individual behaviors: The case of cigarette smoking. In *Social determinants of health*, 2nd ed, ed. M.G. Marmot and R.G. Wilkinson, 224–237. Oxford/New York: Oxford University Press.

Leichter, H.M. 2003. "Evil habits" and "personal choices": Assigning responsibility for health in the 20th century. *Milbank Quarterly* 81(4): 603–626.

Link, B.G., and J.C. Phelan. 2006. Stigma and its public health implications. *Lancet* 367(9509): 528–529.

MacLean, L., N. Edwards, M. Garrard, N. Sims-Jones, K. Clinton, and L. Ashley. 2009. Obesity, stigma and public health planning. *Health Promotion International* 24(1): 88–93.

McLaren, L. 2007. Socioeconomic status and obesity. *Epidemiologic Reviews* 29: 29–48.

Ogden, C.L., M.D. Carroll, B.K. Kit, and K.M. Flegal. 2012. *NCHS Data Brief No. 82: Prevalence of obesity in the United States, 2009–2010.* http://www.cdc.gov/nchs/data/databriefs/db82.pdf. Accessed 10 Apr 2013.

Pickett, K.E., S. Kelly, E. Brunner, T. Lobstein, and R.G. Wilkinson. 2005. Wider income gaps, wider waistbands? An ecological study of obesity and income inequality. *Journal of Epidemiology and Community Health* 59(8): 670–674.

Powers, M., and R. Faden. 2006. *Social justice: The moral foundations of public health and health policy.* New York: Oxford University Press.

Puhl, R.M., and K.D. Brownell. 2003. Psychosocial origins of obesity stigma: Toward changing a powerful and pervasive bias. *Obesity Reviews* 4(4): 213–227.

Puhl, R.M., and C.A. Heuer. 2009. The stigma of obesity: A review and update. *Obesity* 17(5): 941–964.

Puhl, R.M., and C.A. Heuer. 2010. Obesity stigma: Important considerations for public health. *American Journal of Public Health* 100(6): 1019–1028.

Puhl, R., J.L. Peterson, and J. Luedicke. 2013. Motivating or stigmatizing? Public perceptions of weight-related language used by health providers. *International Journal of Obesity* 37(4): 612–629.

Ritchie, D., A. Amos, and C. Martin. 2010. "But it just has that sort of feel about it, a leper"—Stigma, smoke-free legislation and public health. *Nicotine & Tobacco Research* 12(6): 622–629.
Rose, G. 1985. Sick individuals and sick populations. *International Journal of Epidemiology* 14(1): 32–38.
Scambler, G. 2006. Sociology, social structure and health-related stigma. *Psychology, Health & Medicine* 11(3): 288–295.
Shayne, V.T., and B.J. Kaplan. 1991. Double victims: Poor women and AIDS. *Women & Health* 17(1): 21–37.
Stevens, G.A., G.M. Singh, Y. Lu, et al. 2012. National, regional, and global trends in adult overweight and obesity prevalences. *Population Health Metrics* 10(1): 22.
Vanable, P.A., M.P. Carey, D.C. Blair, and R.A. Littlewood. 2006. Impact of HIV-related stigma on health behaviors and psychological adjustment among HIV-positive men and women. *AIDS and Behavior* 10(5): 473–482.
Vardy, D., A. Besser, M. Amir, B. Gesthalter, A. Biton, and D. Buskila. 2002. Experiences of stigmatization play a role in mediating the impact of disease severity on quality of life in psoriasis patients. *British Journal of Dermatology* 147(4): 736–742.
Wikler, D. 2002. Personal and social responsibility for health. *Ethics & International Affairs* 16(2): 47–55.

5.10 Case 4: Water Fluoridation: The Example of Greece

Aikaterini A. Aspradaki
Joint Graduate Programme in Bioethics
University of Crete
Crete, Greece
e-mail: kasprad@yahoo.gr

Ioannis Tzoutzas
School of Dentistry
National and Kapodistrian University of Athens
Athens, Greece

Maria Kousis
Center for Research and Studies in Humanities, Social Sciences and Pedagogics
University of Crete
Crete, Greece

Anastas Philalithis
Department of Social Medicine, Faculty of Medicine
University of Crete
Crete, Greece

This case is presented for instructional purposes only. The ideas and opinions expressed are the authors' own. The case is not meant to reflect the official position, views, or policies of the editors, the editors' host institutions, or the authors' host institutions.

5.10.1 Background

Dental caries is a condition with major public health impact worldwide. In most industrialized countries, it affects 60–90 % of school children and most adults, whereas in several Asian and Latin American countries, it is the most prevalent oral disease (Petersen and Lennon 2004). Dental caries significantly affects individuals and communities, leading to pain and discomfort, impairment of oral and general health, and reduced quality of life. It also highly correlates with health systems, living conditions, behavioral and environmental factors, and implementation of preventive measures (World Health Organization [WHO] 2005, 2007; Shariati et al. 2013). In low- and middle-income countries, the prevalence of oral diseases is on the rise; and in all countries, the greatest burden of oral diseases falls on disadvantaged and poor populations (Petersen 2008). Although oral disease ranks as the fourth most expensive disease to treat (WHO 2007), effective prevention and health promotion measures can greatly reduce the cost of dental treatment. As a result, the WHO has emphasized the importance of developing global oral health policies, especially the implementation of fluoride programs to prevent dental caries (WHO 2012).

For the past 60 years, fluoride use has consistently proven to be one of public health's most successful interventions (Clarkson et al. 2000). Used in tablets, mouthwash, toothpaste, gels or varnishes, fluoride also may be added to salt or drinking water to protect against dental caries (WHO 2011). High fluoride levels in drinking water (>10 mg l^{-1}), are associated with dental fluorosis, a discoloring or mottling of tooth enamel, while levels below 0.1 mg l^{-1} are associated with higher levels of dental decay (Edmunds and Smedley 1996). A level of about 1 mg l^{-1} is associated with lower incidence of dental caries, particularly in children (Fawell et al. 2006). Water fluoridation adjusts the fluoride concentration of a public water supply to an optimal level to prevent dental caries (WHO 2002). Countries such as Australia, Malaysia, Ireland, Spain, the United Kingdom, and the United States use water fluoridation, delivering fluoride to about 300 million persons worldwide (Clarkson et al. 2000).

Despite the demonstrated effectiveness of fluorides in preventing dental carries, public discussions about the effectiveness of water fluoridation continue (Awofeso 2012; Rugg-Gunn and Do 2012). Several publications discuss the benefits and harms of water fluoridation (McDonagh et al. 2000; European Commission, Directorate General for Health and Consumers, Scientific Committee on Health and Environmental Risks 2011; Phillips et al. 2011; Community Preventive Services Task Force 2013). However, a lack of good-quality evidence on the potential benefits and harms has been reported (Nuffield Council on Bioethics 2007). Moreover, with the advent of genomic techniques in studying oral diseases, susceptibility to dental caries has been shown in part to be due to genetic variations (Eng et al. 2012), increasing in this way the complexity and the multicausality of dental caries.

Implementing water fluoridation programs can be controversial and generate tension between competing ethical principles and values—primarily conflicts between the principles of paternalism and autonomy. While water fluoridation is considered to be a "test case" in the discussion about the paternalism of "collective decisions" (Dworkin 1988), appeals to paternalism point to water fluoridation's benefits for entire communities (e.g., health needs of children, reduction in health risks and health inequalities). However, those who prioritize autonomy point out that water fluoridation intervenes in an important area of personal life without the consent of those affected, essentially coercing adults to lead healthy lives (Nuffield Council on Bioethics 2007). Despite the controversy, water fluoridation is "the most celebrated example" of "collective action/efficiency" to justify public health programs and policies (Faden and Shebaya 2010). In deliberative democracies, governments tend to address the conflict between paternalism and autonomy by focusing on elements of procedural justice—rational explanations, transparency of the decision-making process, and involvement of individuals and stakeholder groups in decision making (Nuffield Council on Bioethics 2007).

Greece, a coastal Mediterranean country in southeastern Europe, has nearly 11 million people. Among 12-year-olds, the average number of dental caries—measured as the number of decayed, missing, or filled teeth—is 2.07 per child (Kravitz and Treasure 2009). Public institutions such as universities, hospitals, and health centers of the National Health System provide limited oral health care. Most oral health care takes place in private clinics, where dental patients pay the entire cost of care. Oral health care constitutes an estimated one-third of the total expenditure on private health care in Greece (Kravitz and Treasure 2009). Since 2009, Greece has faced a severe fiscal crisis. In providing health care, public health authorities have to deal with severe budget limitations. The financial crisis is also straining the ability of individuals to pay for private sector dental treatment.

The Greek central government regulates many public health programs, including oral disease prevention and oral health promotion policies, but implementation is local. Although the government mandated water fluoridation in 1974, as of 2013 the program had not been implemented because of diffuse public resistance to such interventions. In 2008, a special commission proposed to the Ministry of Health and Social Solidarity to include water fluoridation in the national strategy for public health (Ministry of Health and Social Solidarity 2008). Given the long hiatus in implementing the program, reasonable questions could be raised about its justification, political legitimization, and social acceptance. A two-part study on these questions was carried out (Aspradaki 2012). It included interviews with key figures in the dental community from academia, the professions, and trade unions. It also included a systematic content analysis of all mentions of water fluoridation by the involved actors (e.g., dental professionals, policy makers) reported in the *Journal of the Hellenic Dental Association* for 1983 through 2011. The results showed strong skepticism among professionals about the program's feasibility—reflecting the public's concerns over this issue. Significant concerns were about a lack of technical infrastructure and organizational problems in the institutions that would implement water fluoridation. The vigorousness of the opposing arguments in the autonomy/paternalism debate in terms of justice, procedural justice, and public interest added to the skepticism. Concerns were also raised about the overall importance of oral health for human life, the significance of prevention in dental care, and the concept of dental caries as an epidemic.

5.10.2 Case Description

You serve as the central oral health policy director. One morning you receive a call from Dr. Papadakis, head of the Public Health Programs and Policies Division at the Ministry of Health and Social Solidarity. Dr. Papadakis is considering implementing mandatory water fluoridation but is concerned about the many difficulties he may confront (i.e., ethical, legal, political and social challenges). Dr. Papadakis asks you to provide input about what to consider before mandatory water fluoridation is implemented in Greece.

5.10.3 Discussion Questions

1. Who are the stakeholders to consider in deciding if this program should be implemented? What are their values, perspectives, and primary interests?
2. How should the relevant values be considered, in particular, scientific evidence, ethical concerns, and economic factors?
3. Do public health institutions have special obligations to protect oral health?
4. When public health interventions are environmental, should public participation and democratic deliberation be considered in the decision-making processes?
5. How important is transparency about the benefits and risks of these interventions, in the light of the rapid progress and the tremendous achievements in life sciences and biotechnologies?
6. How would the rationale for such public health interventions change if the government and individuals were not facing a severe financial crisis?

Acknowledgements We thank the peer reviewers and editors for their comments. We also thank Professor Stavroula Tsinorema, Director of Studies of the Joint Graduate Programme in Bioethics, University of Crete, Crete, Greece, for her valuable support.

References

Aspradaki, A.A. 2012. *Autonomy and paternalism in medical care, with special emphasis on dental care.* Doctoral dissertation, University of Crete, Crete, Greece. http://elocus.lib.uoc.gr/search/?search_type=simple&search_help=&display_mode=overview&wf_step=init&show_hidden=0&number=10&. Accessed 30 Mar 2013.

Awofeso, N. 2012. Ethics of artificial water fluoridation in Australia. *Public Health Ethics* 5(2): 161–172.

Clarkson, J.J., K. Hardwick, D. Barmes, and L.M. Richardson. 2000. International collaborative research on fluoride. *Journal of Dental Research* 79(4): 893–904.

Community Preventive Services Task Force. 2013. Preventing dental caries: Community water fluoridation. In *The guide to community preventive services: The community guide: What works to promote health.* http://www.thecommunityguide.org/oral/fluoridation.html. Accessed 13 Aug 2013.

Dworkin, G. 1988. Paternalism: Some second thoughts. In *The theory and practice of autonomy*, 121–129. Cambridge: Cambridge University Press.

Edmunds, W.M., and P.L. Smedley. 1996. Groundwater geochemistry and health: An overview. *Geological Society, London, Special Publications* 113(1): 91–105. doi:10.1144/GSL.SP.1996.113.01.08.

Eng, G., A. Chen, T. Vess, and G.S. Ginsburg. 2012. Genome technologies and personalized dental medicine. *Oral Diseases* 18(3): 223–235.

European Commission, Directorate General for Health & Consumers, Scientific Committee on Health and Environmental Risks. 2011. *Critical review of any new evidence on the hazard profile, health effects, and human exposure to fluoride and the fluoridating agents of drinking water.* Brussels: European Union. http://ec.europa.eu/health/scientific_committees/environmental_risks/docs/scher_o_139.pdf. Accessed 10 Nov 2012.

Faden, R., and S. Shebaya. 2010. Public health ethics. In *Stanford encyclopedia of philosophy*, ed. E. N. Zalta. http://plato.stanford.edu/archives/sum2010/entries/publichealth-ethics/. Accessed 10 Mar 2011.

Fawell, J., K. Bailey, J. Chilton, E. Dahi, L. Fewtrell, and Y. Magara. 2006. *Fluoride in drinking–water*. London: World Health Organization, IWA Publishing.

Kravitz, A.S., and E.T. Treasure. 2009. *Manual of dental practice (version 4.1).* See esp. pp. 171–178 part 11: "Individual Country Sections -Greece" Council of European Dentists: Cardiff. http://abdentist.com/en/assets/files/man_dent_prac.pdf. Accessed 15 Nov 2012.

McDonagh, M.S., P.F. Whiting, P.M. Wilson, et al. 2000. Systematic review of water fluoridation. *British Medical Journal* 321(7265): 855–859.

Ministry of Health and Social Solidarity. 2008. *National plan of action on public health. National plan of action on oral health 2008–2012.* http://www.moh.gov.gr/articles/health/domes-kaidra-seis-gia-thn-ygeia ethnika-sxedia-drashs/95-ethika-sxedia-drashs?fdl=222. Accessed 3 June 2015.

Nuffield Council on Bioethics. 2007. *Public health: Ethical issues.* http://nuffieldbioethics.org/project/public-health/. Accessed 20 Dec 2011.

Petersen, P.E. 2008. World Health Organization global policy for improvement of oral health—World Health Assembly 2007. *International Dental Journal* 58(3): 115–121.

Petersen, P.E., and M.A. Lennon. 2004. Effective use of fluorides for the prevention of dental caries in the 21st century: The WHO approach. *Community Dentistry and Oral Epidemiology* 32(5): 319–321.

Phillips, C., B. Amphlett, and I.J. Robbé. 2011. The long-term effects of water fluoridation on the human skeleton. *Journal of Dental Research* 90(5): 683.

Rugg-Gunn, A.J., and L. Do. 2012. Effectiveness of water fluoridation in caries prevention. *Community Dentistry and Oral Epidemiology* 40(suppl 2): 55–64.

Shariati, B., M.I. MacEntee, and M. Yazdizadeh. 2013. The economics of dentistry: A neglected concern. *Community Dentistry and Oral Epidemiology* 41(5): 385–394.

World Health Organization (WHO). 2002. *World water day 2001: Oral health* by R. S. Smith. http://who.int/water_sanitation_health/oralhealth/en/. Accessed 10 Dec 2012.

World Health Organization (WHO). 2005. *The Liverpool declaration: Promoting oral health in the 21st century. A call for action.* http://www.who.int/oral_health/events/liverpool_declaration/en/. Accessed 10 Dec 2012.

World Health Organization (WHO). 2007. WHA60.17 Oral health: Action plan for promotion and integrated disease prevention. In *Sixtieth world health assembly: Resolutions and decisions,*

annexes. Geneva: WHO. http://apps.who.int/gb/ebwha/pdf_files/WHASSA_WHA60-Rec1/E/cover-intro-60-en.pdf. Accessed 10 Dec 2012.
World Health Organization (WHO). 2011. *Guidelines for drinking-water quality*, 4th ed. Geneva: World Health Organization. http://www.who.int/water_sanitation_health/publications/2011/dwq_guidelines/en/. Accessed 10 Dec 2012.
World Health Organization (WHO). 2012. *Oral health*, Fact Sheet No. 318. Geneva: World Health Organization. http://www.who.int/mediacentre/factsheets/fs318/en/. Accessed 30 Mar 2013.

5.11 Case 5: The Prohibition of Smoking in Public Places in Bulgaria

Silviya Aleksandrova-Yankulovska
Faculty of Public Health, Department of Public Health Sciences
Medical University of Pleven
Pleven, Bulgaria
e-mail: silviya_aleksandrova@hotmail.com

This case is presented for instructional purposes only. The ideas and opinions expressed are the author's own. The case is not meant to reflect the official position, views, or policies of the editors, the editors' host institutions, or the author's host institution.

5.11.1 Background

Chronic noncommunicable diseases, including cardiovascular diseases, malignant neoplasms, and noninfectious pulmonary diseases, are a major cause of the global burden of disease in the European Region[3] (86 % of the 9.6 million deaths and 77 % of the 150.3 million disability-adjusted life years (DALYs) (Vassilevsky et al. 2009). Commonly associated risk factors include smoking, alcohol consumption, unhealthy diet, and low physical activity.

Tobacco smoking alone produces 12 % of the global disease burden in the European Region (ranges from 3 to 27 % for the individual countries) and it causes 2–21 % of all deaths. For Bulgaria, these rates are 13.5 % and 12.4 %, respectively (Vassilevsky et al. 2009). Annually, more than four billion people die worldwide from diseases related to tobacco products. By 2030, this number is expected to reach ten million, which will turn tobacco smoking into the biggest single cause of death (World Bank 1999).

Bulgaria is among the countries with the highest level of morbidity and mortality from cardiovascular diseases, especially cerebrovascular disease. Standardized death rates of all smoking-related causes of death for 2011 were estimated to be 318

[3]As of 2015, the European Region includes 51 countries (see http://www.who.int/choice/demography/euro_region/en/).

per 100,000 people, whereas the average for the European Union (EU)[4] was 195 per 100,000 people. Standardized death rates of stroke in Bulgaria were about three times higher than the average level for the EU. Only Ukraine, Moldova, Kyrgyzstan, and Russia had higher rates (World Health Organization [WHO] 2012).

At the same time, Bulgaria is a leading country in cigarette use among Central and Eastern European countries (Ministry of Health, Bulgaria 2008). About 40 % of the population are smokers: 47 % of men and 33 % of women (Vassilevsky et al. 2010). Cigarettes smoked per person per year in Bulgaria (2793 cigarettes) is significantly higher than the average for the European Region (1681 cigarettes) (WHO 2012). Smoking among teenagers in Bulgaria is also among the highest in Europe—40 % of teenagers smoke (36 % of boys and 44 % of girls) (Tsolova et al. 2010). A 2011 survey found that Bulgaria was fourth out of 36 countries in teenage smokers (Hibell et al. 2012).

These data are alarming. But additional concern for public health is the effect of secondhand smoking. The risk of death from coronary heart disease increases 30 % from exposure to secondhand smoke (American Heart Association 2013). Secondhand smoke—"passive" smoking—increases a child's risk of developing pneumonia, asthma, and other allergic conditions (Naydenov et al. 2007). A survey of countrywide integrated noncommunicable disease intervention (CINDI) programme-Bulgaria found more than 80 % of teenagers were exposed to passive smoking daily (20 % of teenagers were exposed for 1–2 h per day; 50 % were exposed for more than 2 h per day). Exposure was higher among girls than boys (43.1 % of boys and 56.7 % of girls were exposed to secondhand smoke for more than 2 h per day) (Tsolova et al. 2010).

As a member of the EU, Bulgaria has had to harmonize its legislation with European legislation. The first smoke free legislation in Europe was adopted in March 2004 in Ireland (Howell 2004). Currently, all EU member countries have some form of regulation aimed at limiting exposure to secondhand smoke. However, the scope of these regulations differs widely within the EU (European Public Health Alliance 2012). First attempts to prohibit smoking in public places in Bulgaria date back to January 2005. Restaurants and other food and drink places were separated into zones for smokers and nonsmokers. The Bulgarian society also split into groups of supporters of the changes and opponents of smoking restrictions.

On November 7, 2005, Bulgaria ratified the World Health Organization Framework Convention on Tobacco Control. Article 8 of the Convention stipulates that "effective legislative, executive, administrative and other measures, providing for protection from exposure to tobacco smoke in indoor workplaces, public transport, indoor public places and, as appropriate, other public places should be taken" (WHO 2003).

On May 17, 2012, the parliament voted to amend the Bulgarian Health Act prohibiting smoking in public places (Republic of Bulgaria Council of Ministers 2012). According to the new regulation, which took effect June 1, 2012, smoking was

[4]As of 2013, the European Union consisted of 28 member countries (see http://europa.eu/about-eu/countries/member-countries/).

prohibited in all indoor public places and workplaces including stadiums, children playgrounds, kindergartens, and other schools. Still, Bulgarian society remained conflicted about the issue.

In November 2012, two independent members of the Bulgarian parliament raised the issue of business losses from the smoking ban. They claimed that 10,000 people lost jobs due to fewer patrons of food and drink establishments and pleaded for revision of the law (Todorova 2012). Official data about business losses were not provided, and such surveys have not been done. Nevertheless, these claims increased public debate about the smoking bans. On December 10, 2012, the Bulgarian Hotel and Restaurant Association officially protested the law and insisted it be revised. The prime minister initially agreed that some revision could be possible but later supported the minister of health, who opposed changing the law. The minister of health pointed out that pitting business against health was unacceptable and, instead of discussing business losses, the government should be discussing the cost of treating oncological and cardiovascular diseases (Dimitrova 2012). The minister of economy, energy, and tourism favored a more flexible application of the law. Eventually, decision making was transferred to parliament's Economic Committee with the idea that the ban on smoking could be abolished through the Law of Tourism, particularly if certain amendments were adopted to allow smoking in specific areas of bars and restaurants. On December 18, 2012, the Economic Committee rejected any amendment to the law. Thus, despite the controversy and public debates, the law prohibiting smoking in public places has survived without change as of May 2013.

5.11.2 Case Description

The law prohibiting smoking in public places has been enacted. You are aware of the public debate and tension surrounding the issue. What would you, as a director of the regional health inspectorate, do to guarantee the implementation of the law in the region?

5.11.3 Discussion Questions

1. When is it acceptable to limit personal autonomy to benefit of the health of others?
2. How should economic interests be weighed in public health decision making? Specifically, how should health care expenditures due to smoking-related diseases be weighed against economic losses incurred by the ban on smoking?
3. Law is usually regarded as the strongest measure of public control. Is law the best approach for influencing health behavior in a society where citizens traditionally feel no responsibility for their own health or the health of others?

4. What long-term effects could repealing or revising the smoking ban have on the public's trust and support?
5. In future years, if a new government decides to revisit the law, what would you, as an expert in public health, advise the new minster of health? Who are the relevant stakeholders, and which of their values should the minister of health consider?

References

American Heart Association. 2013. *Heart disease and stroke statistics—2013 update.* http://circ.ahajournals.org/content/127/1/e6.full.pdf+html. Accessed 7 June 2013.

Dimitrova, D. 2012. *Smoking prohibition confronted two ministers—The Minister of Economics Dobrev and the Minister of Health Atanasova.* http://dnes.dir.bg/news/zabrana-deljan-dobrevmerki-srestu-pusheneto-12592161. Accessed 10 Dec 2012.

European Public Health Alliance. 2012. *Updated European smoking bans: Evolution of the legislation.* http://www.epha.org/a/1941. Accessed 10 Dec 2012.

Hibell, B., U. Guttormsson, S. Ahlström, et al. 2012. *The European school survey project on alcohol and other drugs: The 2011 ESPAD report, substance use among students in 36 European countries.* http://www.espad.org/Uploads/ESPAD_reports/2011/The_2011_ESPAD_Report_FULL_2012_10_29.pdf. Accessed 10 Dec 2012.

Howell, F. 2004. Ireland's workplaces, going smoke free. *British Medical Journal* 328(7444): 847–848.

Ministry of Health, Bulgaria. 2008. National health strategy: 2008–2013. *State Gazette* 107/16.12.2008.

Naydenov, K., T. Popov, D. Markov, and A. Melikov. 2007. The influence of smoking on allergy morbidity among children in Sofia and Burgas at age 2–7 years. *Modern Medicine* 58(4): 13–20.

Republic of Bulgaria Council of Ministers. 2012. Bulgarian health act. *State Gazette* 70/10.08.2004 (effective 01.01.2005). Amended 17th May 2012. *State Gazette* 40/29.05.2012 (effective 01.06.2012 г.). http://lex.bg/laws/ldoc2135489147. Accessed 1 Dec 2012.

Todorova, T. 2012. *Parliamentarians require changing the prohibition of smoking.* http://dnes.dir.bg/news/tutunopushene-merki-srestu-pusheneto-kiril-gumnerov-12413757. Accessed 10 Dec 2012.

Tsolova, G., N. Vassilevsky, P. Dimitrov, and A. Manolova. 2010. Surveillance of risk factors for non communicable diseases among children aged 14–18 years within the zones of CINDI programme-Bulgaria 2008. *Bulgarian Journal of Public Health* 2(3): 35–60.

Vassilevsky, N., L. Ivanov, G. Tsolova, and P. Dimitrov. 2009. National behavior risk factors survey among population aged 25–64, 2007. *Bulgarian Journal of Public Health Supplement* 1(3): 3–42.

Vassilevsky, N., G. Tsolova, P. Dimitrov, and A. Manolova. 2010. Surveillance of risk factors for non-communicable diseases among population aged 25–64 within the zones of CINDI programme- Bulgaria 2007. *Bulgarian Journal of Public Health* 2(3): 3–32.

World Bank. 1999. *Curbing the epidemic: Governments and the economics of tobacco control. Development in practice.* Washington, DC: World Bank. http://documents.worldbank.org/curated/en/1999/05/437174/curbing-epidemic-governments-economics-tobacco-control. Accessed 7 June 2013.

World Health Organization (WHO). 2003. *WHO framework convention on tobacco control.* Geneva: World Health Organization. http://www.who.int/fctc/text_download/en/index.html. Accessed 7 June 2013.

World Health Organization (WHO). 2012. *European health for all database.* http://data.euro.who.int/hfadb. Accessed 15 Dec 2012.

Chapter 6
Environmental and Occupational Public Health

Bruce Jennings

6.1 Environment and Workplace: Key Venues for Public Health

Environmental health and occupational health and safety have long been established subfields of public health research, policy, and practice (Frumkin 2010). More so perhaps than areas such as infectious disease or health promotion, environmental and occupational health remind us that the health of a society is profoundly affected by its economic system and economic development. Today, the environmental health field is largely concerned with a human-made (anthropogenic) environment brought about by urbanization, the extraction of natural resources, industrial manufacture, the physical separation of home and workplace, and the transportation systems needed to support this mode of economy and pattern of living. Economic development alters the natural environment and sometimes harms ecosystems in terms of the humanly useful services they provide, their diversity, and their resilience. We are coming to understand that all of this has significant consequences for human health.

Environmental health has been understood as a public health issue in relation to air quality, water quality, and exposure to environmental pollutants that are toxic, carcinogenic, or teratogenic or are chemically bioactive in other ways. The rise of fossil fuels as the energy base for economic production and transportation, the industrial-scale advances in mining and metallurgy, and the creation and widespread presence of synthetic chemical substances have contributed to environmental health risks throughout the past two centuries. Indeed, these changes have redefined the meaning of environmental health. For the most part, environmental health involves

---

The opinions, findings, and conclusions of the author do not necessarily reflect the official position, views, or policies of the editors, the editors' host institutions, or the author's host institution.

B. Jennings, MA (✉)
Center for Biomedical Ethics and Society, Vanderbilt University, Nashville, TN, USA
e-mail: brucejennings@humansandnature.org

D.H. Barrett et al. (eds.), *Public Health Ethics: Cases Spanning the Globe*,
Public Health Ethics Analysis 3, DOI 10.1007/978-3-319-23847-0_6

the domain of chronic illness and disease, and it investigates factors that increase population risk and susceptibility to patterns of physical and mental illness in various forms. Epidemiological investigation is key to public health response to environmental health hazards.

If the public health of entire populations is affected in the background by modernization and industrialization in the form of environmental hazards, the personal health of a large number of individuals—especially people who work in industrial settings or are otherwise exposed to workplace hazards—is also affected directly in often injurious ways (Bayer 1988). Despite struggles to protect people in the workplace, the literature on occupational health is replete with examples of work-related cancers and pulmonary disease. Moreover, issues of safety and health go hand in hand in the occupational arena. Occupational accidents and injuries are a substantial factor in the overall health profile of society. Some occupational sectors remain particularly dangerous due to inherent features of the work environment, the necessary technology and equipment, or the absence of adequate policies and protections for workers. The recent emphasis in public health research and policy on personal injury and trauma may lead to renewed interest in occupational health as a public health issue.

More effective public health policy in regard to environmental and occupational health is made difficult by the fact that they tend to have distinct regulatory structures. Each is governed by different authorizing statutes and accumulated bodies of administrative rules and is overseen by different agencies of varying government levels (particularly in countries with federal systems). Nonetheless, occupational health and environmental health should be viewed in relation to each other, since both ultimately spring from a common root in the recent history of the impact of science and technology on society. Moreover, the public health responses to these two areas has varied with different understandings of the appropriate role of the state and public authority. This is to be expected, given that health matters overall, though biologically and biochemically connected, raise political, economic, and social issues. Major disparities in environmental and occupational risk, for example, stem from race and socioeconomic status (Shrader-Frechette 2005), and thus raise ethical questions about political and social rights, economic entitlements and welfare safety nets, and the just distribution of risk, wealth, and power.

One additional feature of a contemporary perspective on environmental and occupational public health should be noted: Our paradigm for understanding the interrelationships of health, the natural environment, and the workplace environment is broadening. Lang and Rayner (2012) distinguish among five models for public health, each with its own historical origins and core ideas. These models are (1) the sanitary-environmental model; (2) the biomedical model, both individual and population focused; (3) the social-behavioral model; (4) the techno-economic model; and (5) the ecological model.

The first four models take an essentially human-centered approach. In these models, the term "environment" is understood as a mere backdrop or aggregation of conditions and risks for states of human health and illness. By contrast, model five, the ecological model, understands the natural environment to be comprised of complex *systems*, not as an array of separate factors. The environment is the functional and relational context in which human health and behavior emerge, not just a set of background conditions. The growing influence of the ecological model of public health is reorienting the study and regulation of both environmental health and occupational health, and this model has the potential to bring them into closer alignment.

There are several reasons for this. First, research on the social determinants of health indicates that distinguishing the social from the natural aspects of an environment's health effects is not straightforward. Even in remote wilderness areas, the natural environment is shaped by human activity. Moreover, the social features of everyday life include not only psychological effects (happiness and well-being) but also physiological effects (cardiovascular, hormonal) on the internal biological environment of the human body.

Second, the growing discussion around the health effects of global climate change contributes to this reorientation of environmental health by reminding us that ecosystems are holistic and complex networks of interrelationships and interdependencies. Therefore, hazards to human health take the form of both discrete threats and general factors that undermine the integrity or functioning of ecosystems upon which the health and functioning of all life ultimately depend. For example, a recent literature review on the public health effects of climate change summarizes the situation as follows:

> Impacts of climate change cause widespread harm to human health, with children often suffering the most. Food shortages, polluted air, contaminated or scarce supplies of water, an expanding area of vectors causing infectious diseases, and more intensely allergenic plants are among the harmful impacts. More extreme weather events cause physical and psychological harm. World health experts have concluded with "very high confidence" that climate change already contributes to the global burden of disease and premature death. IPCC [Intergovernmental Panel on Climate Change] projects the following trends, if global warming continues to increase, where only trends assigned very high confidence or high confidence are included: (*1*) increased malnutrition and consequent disorders, including those related to child growth and development, (*2*) increased death, disease and injuries from heat waves, floods, storms, fires and droughts, (*3*) increased cardiorespiratory morbidity and mortality associated with ground-level ozone. While IPCC also projects fewer deaths from cold, this positive effect is far outweighed by the negative ones (Hansen et al. 2013, 8).

Third, the way the built environment is developed can affect not only greenhouse gas emissions but also lifestyle factors that impinge on human health–for example, land use and zoning patterns that lead to suburban housing sprawl and automobile dependency (Frumkin and McMichael 2008).

Environmental health hazards can no longer be thought of simply as discrete entities (e.g., pathogens, toxic chemicals, carcinogenic substances) within an otherwise health-neutral field (Kassel and Stephens 2011). Previously environmental health hazards (even air and water pollution) were viewed on rather narrow local or regional scales and in close proximity to effected human populations. Now we must view the health hazards emerging from systemic disruptions or dysfunctions as operating on far broader scales and far more remotely than previously suspected. Deforestation in tropical areas involves a chain of factors that ultimately affects the quality of life of people with asthma in Central Asia; changes in the salinity and temperature of the oceans will affect heat emergency events in Europe. A contaminated well is a *localized* health risk.

Conversely, environmental changes on the Himalayan plateau that alter the hydrology of a river spanning miles upon which hundreds of millions depend for fresh water, represents a different challenge for public health analysis and response. The problem is *global* and *institutional*, which is to say, fundamentally political and economic. The public health response needs to involve not only specific protections and rules or laws aimed at individual decisions and behaviors, such as toxic dumping in a particular site, or the point source pollution of a river, but also the institutional and systemic governance that alters the structure of power and wealth, and the process by which decisions and policies are made. The perennial debate between an approach aimed at individual behavior and one aimed at structural change is endemic to both environmental health and occupational health and safety.

Because both environmental and occupational public health raise public issues that involve public perception, a couple of the thorniest ethical problems concern the concept of acceptable risk and criteria for risk management and risk reduction. Environmental risks to the public's health can be managed (or prevented) in multiple ways. The same can be said of workplace risks, especially when conditions put workers in contact with dangerous machinery or industrial processes; expose workers to harmful substances; and, in the case of health care professionals and biomedical researchers, expose them to infectious diseases. The debate always concerns how risk management should be done and at what cost.

6.2 Population Benefits, Individual Rights, and Ethically Acceptable Risk

The four intriguing cases in this chapter provide examples of policy, decision making, and public health practice under specific circumstances. Looming in the background of each case are fundamental questions about power, equality, and social justice. The cases indicate the need for a more systemic understanding of environmental and occupational health factors, from the small-scale ecosystem of potentially contagious organisms within the human body to the large-scale natural ecosystem's reaction to the effects of mining technology and operations.

Here are the main themes and issues that the cases in this chapter pose for environmental and occupational health, especially from the perspective of an ecological model of public health ethics:

- How should a society democratically set priorities and manage its economic sectors to ensure productivity in the global economy and at the same time protect its limited natural resources, its core values, and cultural diversity of regional and ethnic ways of life? Snyder and colleagues address this theme in their case on mining and health equity.
- How should vulnerable populations, such as hospitalized patients, be protected from serious infection, and to what extent should those measures impinge on individual rights and careers of health professionals who are subject to screening and possible exclusion from clinical practice? This theme is addressed by Rump

and colleagues in their case involving the exclusion of physicians who test positive for Methicillin-resistant *Staphylococcus aureus* (MRSA) from performing patient related interventions.

- How should nongovernmental organizations (NGOs) working on development projects in resource poor and underserved areas allocate limited resources effectively and equitably? What responsibility does the NGO have when its programs inadvertently pose health risks to the community that also may threaten its future capacity to provide services? This theme is addressed in Hayward's case about well construction in areas without access to safe drinking water. Hayward compares the health risks and benefits to the cost of different construction methods.
- What are the ethical responsibilities of organizations whose staff and volunteers do public health work in areas lacking public safety and security resources? What balance should be struck between outreach to those who need services and the personal health and safety of the organization's employees? This case, also by Hayward, describes how Peace Corps volunteers use motorcycles to reach otherwise inaccessible areas, which increases their risk of traffic accidents.

As mentioned previously, the forces of economic, scientific, and technological development brought environmental health and occupational health and safety issues to the forefront of contemporary public health. Indeed, public health as we know it today is an outgrowth of the industrial revolution, which has brought about both great advances and significant disparities of wealth and power. Worldwide, public health operates amid highly urbanized social systems stratified by class, race, and ethnicity. In its quest for optimal health outcomes on a population basis, public health is ethically constrained by individual rights and liberties that may conflict with that goal, just as it is politically constrained by powerful vested interests. Nonetheless, social inequality is an obstacle against which public health pushes. For the most part, certainly in the post-World War II era, the direction of public health has been toward greater access to the resources and conditions necessary for widespread health and well-being, greater social and economic equality, and fairness for the most vulnerable and marginalized.

Operating within that trend, decision making about environmental and occupational health draws primarily on two ethical concepts of public health: One is a utilitarian ethic of population well-being, and the other is an ethic of human rights, dignity, and justice.

Utilitarianism defines the ethical rightness of human acts toward maximizing aggregate net social benefit (happiness, utility, preference satisfaction). Not surprisingly, utilitarianism is a significant aspect of public health ethics. Its orientation toward aggregative outcomes befits its concern for populations rather than individual health—weighing and balancing options rather than delimiting intrinsic value or ethical absolutes.

Rights- and justice-based ethics focus on intrinsic rightness or wrongness of specific acts and general actions—*not* on the consequences of those acts. Actions embody fundamental values such as respect, dignity, equality, autonomy, and inclusiveness and therefore have intrinsic rightness. This ethical orientation appeals to cultures with a heritage of humanitarian concern and to political and legal systems that are simultaneously democratically egalitarian and protective of individual liberty.

Utilitarian ethics and rights-based ethics may conflict when situations pit aggregate net population benefits (i.e., health and welfare) against equity and fairness perspectives that reject discrimination and are unwilling to violate the rights of one, or a few, to achieve well-being among many. Such dilemmas and trade-offs often arise in public health practice.

For example, one conflict involving individual rights arises in the case from Rump and colleagues. In this case, a precautionary policy of exclusion provides safety for hospitalized patients who have contact with a medical student who is a carrier of MRSA. But at the same time, the exclusion policy burdens the medical student who faces personal and professional risk to her livelihood. An individual's rights may be violated when health status becomes the basis for discriminatory treatment or for the loss of liberty or opportunity. A physician or other health care professional with a condition that poses undue risk to patients illustrates the conflict between individual rights or freedom and protection of patients health collectively, or indeed, protection of patient health individually. To resolve such conflict, one must strike a balance among competing values, informed by factual (biomedical) knowledge. No individual has the right to intentionally harm an innocent person, and no physician has a right to deliberately harm a patient. These conflicts typically arise when facts are uncertain and knowledge is imperfect or probabilistic. Thus, the question turns not on *absolute* right and wrong, but on *reasonably acceptable* risk. Is a policy that provides a blanket exclusion of health workers who are MRSA positive appropriate? Or is this policy overly inclusive and cautious? Moreover, how do we ethically factor in the costs or harms done by exclusion of risk? Perhaps a gifted physician who poses a low risk of infecting patients may greatly benefit them. If so, then considerations of nondiscrimination for the individual (physician) and aggregate net benefit for the population (patients) could coincide.

Hayward presents a mirror image in her case on threats to personal safety. This case involves transportation safety in the developing world, a significant public health problem to everyone living and working there. Under discussion is a policy that prohibits staff and volunteers from using dangerous forms of travel, such as motorcycles, even when alternative means of accessing remote areas do not exist. This would affect many field staff and volunteer health workers who strive to maximize client services by minimizing transportation time, even at the risk of a traffic accident. The rights-based question in this case has to do with individual freedom of choice versus paternalistic protection by institutional authorities, again within the context of ethically acceptable risk. The utilitarian question may be framed as a cost–benefit comparison of population harm done by the death or injury of health workers (to themselves, their families, and their clients) and the harm done by suboptimal service delivery (slower, but safer modes of transportation). A far-reaching consequence may be the loss of public health and economic development programs that benefit the community.

Risk and harm appear in yet another guise in Hayward's case on safe water standards and well construction in rural Africa. An ethical dilemma arises because a less expensive drilling technique (shallow rather than deep-drilled wells) can produce more water for more people; however, the risk of contamination and harm to users will increase. How can decision makers resolve the trade-off between water quantity and quality to benefit the aggregate net population's health and welfare? In this instance, an organizational and programmatic risk is also involved. The dilemma decision makers face has broad implications for future public health initiatives in the region. If too few wells with a high per unit cost are produced, the community might perceive that the needs of many are not being considered. Similarly, they might perceive their health and safety are being neglected if the wells are inexpensive. Decision makers should strive to preserve community trust if they are to gain cooperation in future public health initiatives.

These three cases illustrate how almost every conceivable approach to risk management can pose one or more ethical problems. Risk management interventions may protect some while shifting the exposure and burden of risk to others, raising serious questions of distributional equity or fairness. Or, interventions to mitigate risk and protection efforts may supplant or inhibit other programs or public health activities since intervention is expensive and may lay claim to scarce resources.

Moreover, the concept of risk is seemingly impossible to define in value-neutral terms and is inherently controversial. Even more ethically charged are the questions of what level or degree of risk is socially acceptable, who should decide, and how exposure to risk should be distributed across the affected population. Routine public health practice in environmental and occupational risk management involves interventions and policies designed to prevent harm to individuals and to lower health risks within the population. Interventions include various forms of public health surveillance—screening and testing—of different groups, with the attendant untoward effect of discrimination or social stigma. Policies may involve regulations with substantial financial consequences in the form of job loss in regulated industries and hence higher unemployment rates in the overall economy or higher production costs and hence higher prices for consumers.

The question of ethically justifiable public health paternalism versus individual autonomy arises when individuals want to continue engaging in activities that put themselves, third parties, or the general public at risk. Among the difficult issues raised about situational ethics are (*1*) identifying the genuine interests and agendas of public health authorities who follow seemingly paternalistic programs to reduce risks and harms; (*2*) identifying when individuals knowingly (and willingly) expose themselves to environmental or occupational risks, given the context of inequalities of power and wealth involved and the lack of employment or residential options available to these individuals and their families; (*3*) determining a reasonable level of acceptable risk in the face of scientific uncertainty; and (*4*) gauging how a policy to reduce public health risk will affect public perception and trust.

6.3 Systems and Power: The Ethical Importance of Ecological and Social Context

We generally know that human health is undermined when the diversity, services, and functioning of ecosystems are compromised. We also know that various economic activities that extract raw materials, manufacture commodities, and provide jobs often secure these benefits at the expense of the environment. On a local or regional scale, the health burdens are often felt by people in the immediate area, whereas the benefits and wealth often accrue to people far removed from the local environmental disturbances and health risks. When viewed as a manifestation of economic systems, environmental health and occupational health are inseparable from questions of global health justice, and these are very difficult theoretical and practical questions indeed. Moreover, these dimensions of the ethics of environmental public health are evolving. Today, given what is known about climate change, we can reasonably say that economic activity virtually anywhere can be environmentally damaging—from oil drilling in the Artic to land clearing in tropical rain forests—and that such damage affects the health and well-being of people everywhere, not just of those in the local or regional areas where the environmental damage takes place.

If environmental public health cannot be divorced from economics, neither can it be understood apart from conditions of governance at international, national, and local levels. International policies and interventions, including the Millennium Development Goals and climate change response defined by international protocols beginning with the Kyoto treaty, are forms of global governance in which environmental public health and public health ethics play indispensable roles.

Questions are no less complex for public health and for ethics at the national level. In the developing world, particularly countries still experiencing widespread poverty and lacking fundamental infrastructure and services, economic growth remains a priority and benefit. Nonetheless, there is a trade-off between short-term economic gains and long-term national (and global) interest in health, economic sustainability, and environmental conservation. For example, ecosystems like rainforests perform a vital function in absorbing atmospheric CO_2. This global function can be undermined by economically driven decisions about land use and other commercial activities that lead to deforestation. Climate change is only one, albeit dramatic, illustration. The collective carbon footprint of developing countries is growing, often placing the preservation of their ecosystems, biodiversity, and fresh water at risk. Putting the economic growth of developing nations on a more sustainable path is not only critical to global control of greenhouse gas emissions, it is also key to each nation's economic future and to global public health.

Economic development is no longer simply an issue for each national government to acknowledge in its internal affairs and domestic policy. In our global market, external forces impinge on options and resources of individual countries, even wealthy and powerful ones. Yet in the absence of international governance, it is the government of each country that remains ethically responsible for the health and welfare of its citizens and should legislate and regulate its social and economic affairs accordingly. In a democracy, public participation, debate, and consensus in viewpoint and among plural groups are valued and essential components of governance.

The case from Snyder and colleagues provides an opportunity to examine the global and systemic dimensions of environmental public health ethics and governance. In Mongolia's economy, which is heavily dependent on the mining industry and mining operations, the trade-off between economic growth and environmental protection is acute. The country clearly needs investment and job opportunities to combat poverty. But issues of social justice, including health equity, are made complex by the stratification of wealth and income and by the uneven development of different regions and sectors of the society. Mining operations can threaten a complex and fragile ecosystem and adversely affect health (e.g., toxic waste, air and water pollution). Mining operations can also create social dislocations (work migration) and change patterns in land use, especially in areas with a long cultural and economic tradition of pastoralism.

The case by Hayward questions whether to drill expensive deep wells or less expensive shallow water wells in sub-Saharan Africa. Part of the health risk posed by the shallow wells requires a change in cultural behavior by preventing livestock from contaminating the wells and by controlling surface run-off. Thus, any successful public health effort cannot be assessed apart from the capacity of the local society to manage and behave toward both its natural and constructed environment in prudent and sustainable ways. Similarly, but on a larger scale, Mongolia's regulation of economic growth and its mining industry raise questions of cultural rights and cultural capacity as well as questions of social equity and institutional capacity to govern in an effective and socially legitimate fashion.

In summary, environmental and occupational health policy and practice is an ethical minefield. Overly cautious approaches when predicted outcomes fail to materialize may reduce the general public's attentiveness and compliance with public health warnings, recommendations, and directives in the future. Insufficient, cautious responses leading to health consequences that could have been avoided can carry a heavy political price for officials involved.

As you read and examine the cases in this chapter, pay particular attention to how public opinion is formed, ethical decisions are justified, and inclusive and participatory deliberation and consensus are achieved. We need effective and meaningful approaches for engaging the public in health decisions. In particular, we need to find ways to make a participatory and deliberative form of democracy practical and effective, especially in the context of environmental and occupational health. Civic education about environmental health and ethical literacy will prepare not only stakeholders but all citizens to make wise decisions about economic interests and the use of technology. What would motivate genuine deliberation and not simply special interest advocacy? And civic deliberation is not free-standing; it requires special organizational forums and needs to move from spontaneity to institutionalized practice if it is to make a lasting difference. Proper access to information and the cooperation of experts with specialized technical knowledge are examples of the organizational side of effective grassroots participation and discussion of key environmental and occupational health issues. How can public health professionals facilitate and contribute to the formation of civic practice and democratic public judgment in this sense?

References

Bayer, R. (ed.). 1988. *The health and safety of workers: Case studies in the politics of professional responsibility*. New York: Oxford University Press.

Frumkin, H. (ed.). 2010. *Environmental health: From global to local*, 2nd ed. San Francisco: Jossey-Bass.

Frumkin, H., and A.J. McMichael. 2008. Climate change and public health: Thinking, communicating, acting. *American Journal of Preventive Medicine* 35(5): 403–410. doi:10.1016/j.amepre.2008.08.019.
Hansen, J., P. Kharecha, M. Sato, et al. 2013. Assessing "dangerous climate change": Required reduction of carbon emissions to protect young people, future generations and nature. *PLoS ONE* 8(12): e81648. doi:10.1371/journal.pone.0081648.
Kessel, A., and C. Stephens. 2011. Environment, ethics, and public health. In *Public health ethics: Key concepts and issues in policy and practice*, ed. A. Dawson, 154–173. Cambridge: Cambridge University Press.
Lang, T., and G. Rayner. 2012. Ecological public health: The 21st century's big idea? *British Medical Journal* 345: e5466. doi:10.1136/bmj.e5466.
Shrader-Frechette, K. 2005. *Environmental justice: Creating equality, reclaiming democracy*. New York: Oxford University Press.

6.4 Case 1: Assessing Mining's Impact on Health Equity in Mongolia

Jeremy Snyder
Faculty of Health Sciences
Simon Fraser University
Burnaby, BC, Canada
e-mail: jcs12@sfu.ca

Craig Janes
School of Public Health and Health Systems
University of Waterloo
Waterloo, ON, Canada

Colleen Davison
Clinical Research Centre and Department of Emergency Medicine
Kingston General Hospital
Kingston, ON, Canada

Department of Public Health Sciences
Queen's University
Kingston, ON, Canada

Oyunaa Lkhagvasuren
Leading Researchers
Ulaanbaatar, Mongolia

Lory Laing
School of Public Health
University of Alberta
Edmonton, AB, Canada

Meghan Wagler
Faculty of Health Sciences
Simon Fraser University
Burnaby, BC, Canada

This case is presented for instructional purposes only. The ideas and opinions expressed are the authors' own. The case is not meant to reflect the official position, views, or policies of the editors, the editors' host institutions, or the authors' host institutions.

6.4.1 Background

Mongolia is a landlocked country bordered by Russia to the north and China to the south. Although one of the largest countries in Asia in land area (1.56 km^2), it has a small population (2.74 million in 2010). Nearly two-thirds of the population is urban and reside in provincial capitals and cities. Nomadic pastoralists who tend mixed herds of animals across the desert and steppe grasslands primarily make up the remaining third of the population (Central Intelligence Agency 2010).

Beginning in 1990, Mongolia transitioned from a single-party socialist state to a multiparty democracy, which led to withdrawal of Soviet aid and termination of trade relations with Soviet bloc countries. The loss of state subsidies and price controls and implementation of trade liberalization caused the economy to falter during the transition (Stiglitz 2002). Not until 2004 did the gross domestic product (GDP) return to pre-transition levels (Rossabi 2005). Since then, macroeconomic growth has been strong, driven by a rapidly expanding mineral sector.

Although resource extraction had been a major economic activity in Mongolia for some time, the scale of exploration and investment increased markedly in the early 2000s (Central Intelligence Agency 2010). As of 2008, general mining exploration licenses covered a quarter of the country. Copper, gold, and coal dominate mining activities, with much of the product exported to neighboring China (The Economist 2012). The mining industry's proportion of the total GDP tripled from 11 to 33 % during 2003 through 2007, the sector contributing about one-third of government tax revenues (World Bank 2013). Propelled by mining and related construction and transportation sectors, in 2011 Mongolia became the world's fastest growing economy, reporting annual economic growth of 17 % (World Bank 2011).

Mining in Mongolia occurs in a context of a lower middle-income country with a GDP of $8.8 billion, rural underdevelopment, and social and economic inequality (World Bank 2013). Mongolia exhibits significant wealth disparities: more than one-third of the population lives in poverty, a proportion that has persisted despite rapid economic growth. Although income poverty levels in rural areas exceed those in urban areas, both settings have large numbers of vulnerable poor. In rural settings, those lacking sufficient herd animals to sustain livelihoods, especially female-headed households, rank among the poorest of the poor. Urban areas are inundated with rural migrants forced into cities by weather disasters and lack of employment. There they labor in the informal economy, typically living in squatter or "ger" settlements without access to running water, sewerage, or electricity.[1]

[1] A ger settlement, or "yurt," is a rural parcel of land in Mongolia comprising several detached and portable dwellings (gers) or shanties. Traditional ger settlements were occupied by pastoralists (nomadic Mongolian people). Gers typically lack modern conveniences such as water, sewage, and electricity. Occupants, although mostly self-sufficient, rely on some communal services such as wells.

Although mining potentially can provide employment, improve infrastructure, and support government services, it also poses substantial social, environmental, and health risks. Adverse environmental impacts noted in Mongolia include dust pollution, diminution and degradation of ground and surface water, and loss of traditional grazing lands by erosion and pollution. Especially concerning is the influx of thousands of mine and construction workers, their families, entrepreneurs, job seekers, and artisanal miners into rural mining areas (World Bank 2006). This influx, which greatly strains infrastructure in some areas, can potentially increase the risk of local epidemics of infectious disease, including HIV. As a result, resource development in Mongolia has become a hotly contested political issue, which has subjected the mining sector to increased public and regulatory scrutiny (Reeves 2011). Mongolians retain a strong identity with their pastoralist history and culture, which has manifested itself in strong pressure to develop resources that benefit the nation while protecting vulnerable herder populations. Recently, and with international donor support, the government of Mongolia began addressing some of these concerns. In May 2012, the efforts culminated in landmark environmental legislation that took into its purview the broad social and health impacts of mining (Mongolian Mining Journal 2012). This legislation demonstrates Mongolian interest in mitigating the negative health impacts of mining, though administering this legislation will be challenging.

Expansion of the Mongolian mining sector raises ethical challenges in three areas. First, the Mongolian government must assess a proposed mining project's impact on Mongolian stakeholders, taking into account the economic, environmental, social, and health impacts. Because projects will affect stakeholders differently, the assessment should adopt an equity lens, with differential impacts noted. A wide-ranging assessment of this kind requires that the government determine how equity will be assessed and how competing negative and positive impacts will be measured and compared. Second, the Mongolian government must use the assessment to help mitigate potential negative social and health impacts. Third, however, the government must consider how regulations could deter mining investments and reduce potential economic benefits of this industry. In a country with a growing population and limited economic development, the loss of these benefits could impact the country's welfare significantly, limiting modernization and expansion of the health care system.

Before the equity impacts of mining activities can be assessed, stakeholders must first agree to a *standard of equity* to prevent misunderstandings. These include equality, priority to the least advantaged, and sufficiency accounts where the aim is to achieve a threshold level of well-being for all people. Second, officials must determine whether any local populations who are particularly vulnerable to mining's impact merit special consideration. Third, to meet the diverse needs of the Mongolian people, an impact assessment must be locally appropriate and assume various forms. For example, different remediation requirements may apply to different mine developers, depending on circumstances. Fourth, one needs to be clear about when differential impacts of mining become problems of equity. Finally, officials should investigate what requirements for mitigating equity impacts should be included in any policy (Snyder et al. 2012).

6.4.2 Case Description

The rapid urbanization and social upheaval brought on by the mining industry and economic liberalization in Mongolia threaten to destabilize the country and squander its resources. To avert these threats, Mongolia has already developed robust legislation to assess the environmental and health impacts of mining. Some government officials believe that an equity-focused health impact assessment policy represents the logical next step in the country's management of its rapid economic development. Implementation of an equity-focused health impact assessment for new mining projects could ensure that economic benefits are distributed equitably. Doing so could improve health and social cohesion without disproportionately burdening some populations with mining's adverse consequences (Douglas and Scott-Samuel 2001). A policy of this kind, while difficult to develop and implement, is crucial to Mongolia's future.

A panel that includes public health professionals is being organized to make recommendations to the Mongolian government on its equity-focused health impact assessment policy for new mining projects. The agenda for discussion includes the following three areas:

- How to best include stakeholders in the development of the policy?
- How should health equity be conceptualized?
- How can an equity-focused health impact assessment be applied broadly?

6.4.3 Discussion Questions

1. Giving a fair hearing to stakeholders in deliberations about issues that affect them is central to democratic deliberation.
   (a) How important or practical is it in Mongolia to give a meaningful voice to all stakeholders in the deliberations about whether and how a mining project should be allowed to develop?
   (b) What level of consultation constitutes meaningful participation?
   (c) Should stakeholders be given veto power over decisions and an equal voice in a democratic process?
   (d) Is consultation by the government without a vote in the final decision adequate?
2. Equity can be conceptualized differently, leading to various interpretations and attendant misunderstandings.
   (a) Are stakeholders unfamiliar with theories of health equity sufficiently qualified to discuss health equity impacts?
   (b) If not, how can they prepare for discussions of this kind?

   (c) Should stakeholders undertaking an equity-focused health impact assessment be asked to reach a consensus on a concept of equity?
   (d) Is it preferable to supply a single conception of equity?
   (e) How can cultural and linguistic differences in understanding concepts such as equity and fairness be resolved?

3. Some countries are incorporating a health equity assessment component in all policies.

   (a) Is there any unique feature of mining development that sets it apart from other developments (e.g. road or housing construction)?
   (b) Could equity-focused health impact assessment be used more generally to assess the health equity impacts of projects and policies?
   (c) What are the challenges of doing so, especially in a fledgling democracy?

4. Should the panel recommend to the Mongolian government that it apply an equity-focused health impact assessment policy to new mining projects?

Acknowledgements We thank everyone who participated in a workshop on equity-focused health impact assessments in Mongolia in October 2010. This workshop was funded through a Health Equity Catalyst Grant from the Canadian Institutes of Health Research.

References

Central Intelligence Agency. 2010. *The world factbook: Mongolia.* https://www.cia.gov/library/publications/the-world-factbook/geos/mg.html. Accessed 21 May 2013.

Douglas, M., and A. Scott-Samuel. 2001. Addressing health inequalities in health impact assessment. *Journal of Epidemiology and Community Health* 55(7): 450–451.

Mongolian Mining Journal. 2012. The amended law on environmental impact assessment. September 25. http://en.mongolianminingjournal.com/content/34726.shtml. Accessed 23 Jan 2014.

Reeves, J. 2011. Resources, sovereignty, and governance: Can Mongolia avoid the 'resource curse'? *Asian Journal of Political Science* 19(2): 170–185.

Rossabi, M. 2005. *Modern Mongolia: From Khans to Commissars to Capitalists.* Berkeley: University of California Press.

Snyder, J., M. Wagler, O. Lkhagvasuren, L. Laing, C.M. Davison, and C. Janes. 2012. An equity tool for health impact assessments: Reflections from Mongolia. *Environmental Impact Assessment Review* 34: 83–91.

Stiglitz, J.E. 2002. *Globalization and its discontents.* New York: W. W. Norton.

The Economist. 2012. *Booming Mongolia: Mine, all mine.* January 21. www.economist.com/node/21543113. Accessed 23 Jan 2014.

World Bank. 2006. *Mongolia: A review of environmental and social impacts in the mining sector.* Washington, DC: World Bank. http://siteresources.worldbank.org/INTMONGOLIA/Resources/Mongolia-Mining.pdf. Accessed 23 Jan 2014.

World Bank. 2011. *Mongolia quarterly economic update—August 2011.* www.worldbank.org/en/news/2011/08/24/mongolia-quarterly-economic-update-august-2011. Accessed 15 May 2013.

World Bank. 2013. *Data: Mongolia.* http://data.worldbank.org/country/mongolia. Accessed 15 May 2013.

6.5 Case 2: Exceptions to National MRSA Prevention Policy for a Medical Resident with Untreatable MRSA Colonization

Babette Rump
Department of Infectious Disease Control
Municipal Health Service Utrecht
Zeist, The Netherlands
e-mail: brump@ggdmn.nl

Carla Kessler
Ethics Institute
Utrecht University
Utrecht, The Netherlands

Ewout Fanoy
Department of Infectious Disease Control
Municipal Health Service Utrecht
Zeist, The Netherlands

National Institute for Public Health and the Environment
Centre for Infectious Disease Control
Bilthoven, The Netherlands

Marjan Wassenberg
Department of Medical Microbiology
Utrecht University Medical Centre
Utrecht, The Netherlands

André Krom
Technology Assessment
Rathenau Institute
The Hague, The Netherlands

Marcel Verweij
Department of Social Sciences, Communication, Philosophy and Technology: Centre for Integrated Development
Wageningen University
Wageningen, The Netherlands

Jim van Steenbergen
National Institute for Public Health and the Environment
Centre of Infectious Disease Control
Bilthoven, The Netherlands

Leiden University Medical Centre
Centre for Infectious Diseases
Leiden, The Netherlands

This case is presented for instructional purposes only. The ideas and opinions expressed are the authors' own. The case is not meant to reflect the official position, views, or policies of the editors, the editors' host institutions, or the authors' host institutions.

6.5.1 Background

Antimicrobial resistance (AMR) is an increasingly serious threat to global public health. First described in 1961, methicillin-resistant *Staphylococcus aureus* (MRSA) is one of the best known antimicrobial resistant (AMR) pathogens. It has become an increasingly serious cause of health care associated infections worldwide (Boyce et al. 2005). People infected with MRSA, which resists standard beta-lactam antibiotics, can present symptoms or be asymptomatic carriers.

In a community setting, most MRSA carriers have few or relatively minor symptoms. In hospitals, however, open wounds, invasive devices, and weakened immune systems pose a greater risk of infection, making MRSA a serious health problem. The presence of Panton-Valentine leukocidin (PVL) cytotoxin in a *Staphylococcus aureus* has the potential to cause more severe infections, such as pneumonia and skin infections, although these are rare events considering the number of asymptomatic carriers (Gorwitz 2008).

Worldwide, prevalence of MRSA among the general public and in hospitals varies widely, as do the strategies used to control hospital-acquired MRSA (Boyce et al. 2005). In the Netherlands and Scandinavia, for example, MRSA causes less than 1 % of all cases of *Staphylococcus aureus* bacteraemia. This percentage contrasts with percentages of up to 50 % in other European countries (Wertheim et al. 2004). To maintain this low incidence, hospitals in the Netherlands and Scandinavia follow a strict AMR related search and destroy policy. This policy consists of active screening of patients and staff for MRSA, strict enforcement of contact precautions, and judicious use of broad-spectrum antibiotics (Boyce et al. 2005).

In the Netherlands, the Working Party on Infection Prevention (WIP) has incorporated this search and destroy policy into national MRSA guidelines. The WIP, funded by the Dutch Ministry of Health, was founded 25 years ago by respective professional societies of physicians, hygienists, and microbiologists. WIP-issued guidelines are professional standards most health professionals and institutes follow (Boyce et al. 2005).

The 2012 WIP guidelines for MRSA prevention in hospital settings involve three principal procedures, which address both symptomatic and asymptomatic patients, since carriers can also transmit the infection. First, patients with MRSA are isolated in single rooms and treated to eradicate MRSA. Isolation procedures require those entering the patient's room to wear a gown and mask. Second, hospital patients at increased risk of being carriers are also placed in isolation until proven MRSA free. Patients considered potential carriers include all patients (a) transferred from hospitals abroad to Dutch hospitals, (b) transferred from Dutch hospitals with an existing MRSA condition, and (c) placed in the same room as a patient subsequently detected unexpectedly with MRSA. Third, hospital staff who care for MRSA patients are screened for MRSA and treated with antibiotics and mupirocin nasal ointment if found positive (Boyce et al. 2005).[2]

Nationally, this search and destroy policy has proved highly successful and effective at maintaining a low prevalence of MRSA in Dutch hospitals (van der Zee et al. 2013). However, MRSA screening and treatment of health care staff can seriously affect their lives because they cannot return to work unless testing confirms MRSA-negative status. Fortunately, MRSA colonization (antibiotic-resistant strain of bacteria that lives on skin) is usually temporary, but when persistent, eradication requires longer-term efforts. Although untreatable colonization is rare, it can necessitate job change (Boyce et al. 2005).

6.5.2 Case Description

A Dutch medical student has the potentially more virulent Panton-Valentine leukocidin (PVL) form of MRSA colonization yet shows no signs or symptoms of infection. More than a year ago, a routine MRSA screening of health care personnel providing care for MRSA-positive patients detected the colonization. Since then, the student has been treated intensively but unsuccessfully in an attempt to decolonize her. During this decolonization period, the medical student was barred from performing patient-related interventions, temporarily interrupting her medical residency. After initial treatment with mupirocin nasal ointment and antibiotics proved ineffective, a more stringent hygiene regime was added that included hand, nose, hair, and body scrubbing with disinfecting soap. Additional precautions included simultaneous treatment of household members and disinfection of the family home. Despite these efforts, her MRSA status has remained positive. WIP guidelines bar any health care worker diagnosed with MRSA from performing patient-related interventions. Unable to complete the residency requirement of at least 1 year of patient care, the medical student was advised to pursue a career in another profession.

Refusing to accept this verdict, she united with other similarly excluded medical students to launch a protest that gained media attention. In a press interview, she acknowledged that potential iatrogenic spreading of MRSA could risk institutional or community safety. However, she questioned the seriousness of this risk and argued that the protesting students were being unfairly targeted. She pointed out that medical staff are not routinely screened for MRSA unless they have cared for a MRSA-positive patient or have worked in a country with high MRSA prevalence. Because MRSA can be acquired in the community, potentially many undiagnosed MRSA-colonized medical staff or residents currently work in hospitals. She also pointed out that other European countries, despite a higher MRSA prevalence, allow MRSA carriers to work in health care settings. Despite being persistently MRSA positive, these professionals can safely work in medical specialties that do *not* involve direct patient contact.

[2] An English version of the WIP guidelines is available at http://www.wip.nl

As a result of this press coverage, the public has pressured the WIP to reconsider its guidelines. Because iatrogenic spreading of disease has public health implications, you, as a public health professional, have been asked to serve on a WIP committee charged with considering whether the guidelines need to be changed to address these and future cases. The chair of the committee wants to discuss the following questions.

6.5.3 Discussion Questions

1. Who are the main stakeholders in this case, and what are their primary interests?
2. What is the ethical rationale for allowing or not allowing medical students who are MRSA carriers to continue their medical education?
3. What would be your ethical justification for either recommending or not recommending universal screening for all medical students and doctors?
4. How would it change your recommendation if
   (a) The MRSA of this student was not PVL positive?
   (b) The overall prevalence of MRSA in the Netherlands was high or rapidly increasing?
   (c) There was little or no evidence that excluding colonized health care workers decreases risks to patients?
   (d) The students agreed to pursue medical specialties that do not involve patient care?
5. Although the European Union (EU) is increasingly standardizing its AMR policy, some EU countries have less stringent regulations than others. Would it be ethical to advise the medical students in question to finish their education in a European country with a less stringent MRSA policy?

References

Boyce, J.M., B. Cookson, K. Christiansen, et al. 2005. Meticillin-resistant *Staphylococcus aureus*. *Lancet Infectious Diseases* 5(10): 653–663.

Gorwitz, R. 2008. Understanding the success of methicillin-resistant *Staphylococcus aureus* strains causing epidemic disease in the community. *Journal of Infectious Diseases* 197(2): 179–182. doi:10.1086/523767.

van der Zee, A., W.D. Hendriks, L. Roorda, et al. 2013. Review of a major epidemic of methicillin resistant *Staphylococcus aureus* : The costs of screening and consequences of outbreak management. *American Journal of Infection Control* 41(3): 204–209.

Wertheim, H.F., M.C. Vos, H.A. Boelens, et al. 2004. Low prevalence of methicillin-resistant *Staphylococcus aureus* (MRSA) at hospital admission in the Netherlands: The value of search and destroy and restrictive antibiotic use. *Journal of Hospital Infection* 56(4): 321–325.

6.6 Case 3: Safe Water Standards and Monitoring of a Well Construction Program

Alison Hayward
Department of Emergency Medicine, Yale School of Medicine
Yale University
New Haven, CT, USA

Uganda Village Project
Iganga, Uganda
e-mail: ahs.hayward@gmail.com

This case is presented for instructional purposes only. The ideas and opinions expressed are the author's own. The case is not meant to reflect the official position, views, or policies of the editors, the editors' host institutions, or the author's host institution.

6.6.1 Background

The lack of access to safe drinking water is a serious public health problem affecting many developing countries. More than 780 million people, mostly located in sub-Saharan Africa, lack safe drinking water. Sub-Saharan Africa only has coverage with safe drinking water sources for 61 % of its population, a stark contrast with regions such as Latin America, northern Africa, and most of Asia, which have all achieved greater than 90 % coverage (World Health Organization/United Nations Children's Fund Joint Monitoring Programme for Water Supply and Sanitation 2012). The Millennium Development Goals (MDGs) have specified that by 2015, the proportion of people who lack access to safe water and sanitation should be halved (United Nations 2013). Significant progress has been made towards achieving this goal; however, vast inequities emerge when comparing populations of rural areas to urban ones, and of more impoverished communities to those with a higher socioeconomic status. As such, progress toward achieving access to safe water and sanitation facilities is not likely to be equitable. As an example, one estimate by the United Nations Development Program suggests that the world overall will attain the safe water and sanitation MDGs by 2016 and 2022 respectively, but sub-Saharan Africa is not projected to attain these goals until 2040 and 2076 (Jimenez and Pérez-Foguet 2010).

In sub-Saharan Africa, 19 % of the rural population resort to using surface water collected from streams, rivers, ponds, or other such sources. Unprotected water sources are particularly dangerous because those who fetch water contaminate the water source by reaching their hands into the water and wading into it as they fill their basins and jerrycans. Open defecation and lack of sanitation also contribute to contamination, as does fecal runoff from livestock wandering through unprotected water sources. Water that is not contaminated at the source runs a high risk of becoming contaminated on its way to the drinking cup due to inadequate home storage and dispensing methods that allow children or other household members to reach into the water while serving it. As a result of this rampant drinking water contamination, diarrheal disease is common in residents of areas without access to safe water. Diarrheal disease is deadliest for young children, the elderly, and immunocompromised community members, such as people living with HIV/AIDS. In children younger than 5 years of age, diarrheal disease is the second leading cause of death (World Health Organization 2009). With proper access to safe water and sanitation, most of these deaths would be prevented.

Access to safe water can prevent many other potentially lethal infectious diseases. These include schistosomiasis, intestinal worms, and malnutrition from repeated diarrheal and intestinal worm infections. Diarrheal disease, however, represents the bulk of the disease burden contributed by poor sanitation, hygiene, and drinking water quality (Prüss-Üstün et al. 2008).

The World Health Organization (WHO) publishes a simple set of recommendations to help small communities with limited water supplies maintain water safety. One key recommendation calls for the creation of, and adherence to, a Water Safety Plan (WSP), using illustrated pamphlets to convey the need for preventive maintenance of water supplies. Another recommendation calls for innovative monitoring strategies such as the use of mobile phones to send data from the field to public health inspectors (WHO 2010). Water treatment products like chlorine can be added either at the well, when the water is collected, or at the point of use in the home to reduce the risk of water contamination (WHO 2011).

The WHO also has detailed guidelines for drinking water quality. These guidelines promote the use of health-based targets, which take into account local variables such as public health status, contribution of drinking water to the transmission of infectious disease, and social and cultural factors. Some international organizations set inflexible water quality standards for pathogen concentrations used in analyzing data from water sources and drinking water. The WHO instead suggests that such targets be modified to realistic and attainable goals. In order to most appropriately allocate limited resources, the WHO additionally suggests "less stringent transitional targets supported by sound risk management systems" to achieve a "tolerable disease burden" for waterborne illness, with incremental improvement in a health-based transitional target eventually progressing towards tight water quality control, as resources allow. Such transitional targets can be developed with the aid of risk management theory. Data collection and advanced statistical modelling may be challenging in countries with limited resources. Estimations of organisms per liter in raw water can be combined with information on risk of diarrheal illness from a given infection, and health outcome targets, to calculate performance targets for reducing pathogens through water source control or treatment interventions. Modifiable targets should consider the relevant risks and benefits in a local area to attain the desired reduction in illness occurrence, and thus, health outcomes, as measured in disability-adjusted life years per person per year. These targets should be outlined in the Water Safety Plan (WHO 2011).

6.6.2 Case Description

You are a managing director for a small nongovernmental organization (NGO) in rural sub-Saharan Africa. Your organization partners with rural villages to construct protected shallow wells in areas where residents otherwise need to walk more than 2 km to reach the nearest safe source. This program was designed to be as cost effective as possible, with village residents volunteering their time and manual labor for well construction.

Organization members debated whether to use borehole drilling or cheaper, hand-dug protected shallow wells. Because boreholes draw water from deep underground, the likelihood of contamination from surface runoff is far less. In contrast, shallow wells risk contamination, particularly if steps are not taken to address the problem, such as constructing a fence around the site to keep grazing livestock away. The nonprofit board concluded that boreholes would be about ten times as expensive to drill, allowing construction of one-tenth the number of wells for the same funding. They therefore decided to focus on shallow well construction to reach the greatest number of communities in need. Still, questions remained about the relative health risks of an approach prone to contamination. Some members of the organization are concerned that the shallow well method was pushed, in part, because it was less expensive and the number of wells constructed would impress donors.

The program was designed in collaboration with the District Water Office for sustainability. Although the District Water Office agreed to assume responsibility for testing the water quality of wells being built, its ability to conduct the tests has been limited by a lack of financial resources. Your organization therefore has undertaken its own water quality testing of roughly 50 wells constructed in the district. Your well construction program manager has reported to you the discouraging results of the water quality tests. Of the wells tested, 20 % have coliform bacteria present in levels unacceptable to international standard drinking water guidelines, which the staff use as a target for water quality as part of the program's monitoring and evaluation plan. The program manager, who has been in discussions with the District Water Office and other nonprofits involved in well construction, has several ideas to improve the well construction process and strengthen protection against coliform contamination in the wells. He also wants to remediate the wells that failed the testing.

Before committing to any of these ideas, you hold an organizational meeting to help you decide whether or how to convey these results to the community members who use the wells, knowing they mistrust both governmental and nongovernmental programs. You particularly worry about the damage to your organization's reputation in trying to convey that the water from wells it has built is dangerous to drink. One staff member suggests holding community meetings to discuss the issue. Meanwhile, all heavily contaminated wells would be marked with signs and red tape to indicate the water is unsafe to drink. Another staffer argues that marking the wells in such a way might frighten community members and discourage them from drinking from the wells even after remediation. He notes that if told not to use these sources, community members might prefer using nearby but similarly (or worse) contaminated open water sources to walking a long distance to find another protected source.

Although the educational workshops the organization offers have always emphasized the need for boiling water or chemically treating it with a chlorination product to ensure its safety, you know that in practice, many community members consider water from a protected source to be "safe," regardless of whether it is boiled or treated. As you leave the meeting, you realize you have four key questions to resolve.

6.6.3 Discussion Questions

1. What ethical implications are raised by considering whether or not to publicize the water quality test results? Which option is more justified, and why?
2. What ethical concerns are raised by the use of shallow well construction, which allows more wells to be constructed at lower cost but at higher risk of water contamination?
3. If the water quality test results are publicized, what participatory approach might best address the problem with water quality?
4. Considering that lower water quality standards could result in more illnesses and deaths in the community, is the WHO's risk-benefit approach the most appropriate way to determine what is environmentally, economically, and socially possible? Would it be better to base one's strategy on an internationally recognized standard for acceptable water quality?

References

Jimenez, A., and A. Pérez-Foguet. 2010. Challenges for water governance in rural water supply: Lessons learned from Tanzania. *International Journal of Water Resources Development* 26(2): 235–248.

Prüss-Üstün, A., R. Bos, F. Gore, and J. Bartram. 2008. *Safer water, better health: Costs, benefits and sustainability of interventions to protect and promote health.* Geneva: World Health Organization. http://whqlibdoc.who.int/publications/2008/9789241596435_eng.pdf. Accessed 15 May 2013.

United Nations. 2013. *Millennium development goals.* http://www.un.org/millenniumgoals/. Accessed 27 May 2013.

World Health Organization (WHO). 2009. *Diarrhoeal disease fact sheet no. 330.* http://www.who.int/mediacentre/factsheets/fs330/en/index.html. Accessed 15 May 2013.

World Health Organization (WHO). 2010. *Small and safe: Investing in small community water supplies will reduce waterborne disease outbreaks and overall costs.* http://www.who.int/water_sanitation_health/WHS_WWD2010_small_systems_2010_4_en.pdf. Accessed 15 May 2013.

World Health Organization (WHO). 2011. *Guidelines for drinking water quality*, 4th ed. http://www.who.int/water_sanitation_health/publications/2011/dwq_guidelines/en/index.html. Accessed 15 May 2013.

World Health Organization/United Nations Children's Fund Joint Monitoring Programme for Water Supply and Sanitation. 2012. *Progress on drinking water and sanitation.* http://www.unicef.org/media/files/JMPreport2012.pdf. Accessed 15 May 2013.

6.7 Case 4: Implementation of Global Public Health Programs and Threats to Personal Safety

Alison Hayward
Department of Emergency Medicine, Yale School of Medicine
Yale University
New Haven, CT, USA

Uganda Village Project
Iganga, Uganda
e-mail: ahs.hayward@gmail.com

This case is presented for instructional purposes only. The ideas and opinions expressed are the author's own. The case is not meant to reflect the official position, views, or policies of the editors, the editors' host institutions, or the author's host institution.

6.7.1 Background

Many global public health agencies and organizations from high-income countries conduct programs in locations where the personal safety of workers and volunteers cannot be guaranteed. Staff and volunteers of nonprofit organizations and government aid agencies face a variety of threats. In 2012, aid workers were harmed in 100 discrete incidents involving 187 aid workers, 43 of whom were international aid workers (Humanitarian Outcomes 2013). These incidents included kidnappings, murder, and traumatic injury. The profile of deaths amongst aid workers and volunteers who serve in conflict zones significantly differs (Sheik et al. 2000). Contrary to popular belief, tropical infectious diseases rarely cause death in aid workers (Hargarten et al. 1991). A systematic review of unintentional injury in international travelers found that only 2 % of traveler deaths were secondary to infectious disease, whereas injury represented a major cause of death. Motor vehicle accidents were the leading cause of fatal injury to travelers (McInnes et al. 2002).

According to the World Health Organization's *Global Status Report on Road Safety*, more than 90 % of the world's road fatalities occur in low and middle-income countries. The report further notes that the majority of road fatalities in these countries occur among vulnerable road users—pedestrians, cyclists, and riders of motorized two-wheeled vehicles (World Health Organization 2009). Little research has been conducted on health and safety policies and procedures for international nongovernmental organizations (O'Sullivan 2010). One exception is the U.S. Peace Corps. A study done of fatalities in the Peace Corps between 1962 and 1983 revealed that unintentional injuries caused 70 % of deaths, with motor vehicle crashes the top cause of fatality, and motorcycle collisions responsible for 33 % of the deaths related to motor vehicles (Hargarten and Baker 1985).

After release of the report, the Peace Corps banned motorcycle use in many countries in which their volunteers serve and mandated a motorcycle safety course and helmet usage in countries where the use of motorcycles was still permitted. A follow-up study of fatalities through 2003 concluded that injury prevention measures instituted as a result of the prior study had significantly decreased the risks faced by Peace Corps volunteers (PCVs), although, once again, motor vehicle collisions topped the list of causes of death. In the 20 years prior to institution of the helmet rules, 22 of 105,539 PCVs died in motorcycle collisions. In the following 20 years, another 71,198 PCVs participated in the program, but only 2 died in motorcycle collisions (Nurthen and Jung 2008). These studies provide evidence that preventive measures can save the lives of aid workers and volunteers even in low-income countries with poor transportation safety and infrastructure.

6.7.2 Case Description

In rural sub-Saharan Africa, you oversee the operations of a nonprofit organization that provides public health programs to remote communities. Needs assessments have shown that these areas have the greatest poverty, as well as lack of access to safe water sources and health care facilities. But the roads leading to the villages, which become little more than footpaths at some points, pose challenges to travelers that include erosion, flooding, and large potholes as well as the physical obstacles of livestock, children, other pedestrians, and bicyclists. The optimal strategy for reaching the villages is to use a motorcycle.

While working on a grant proposal one afternoon at the office, you receive a cell phone call from Moses Izimba, a program manager for your nonprofit. Earlier in the day, several staff and volunteers had taken "boda-bodas" (motorcycle taxis) to a remote village to offer a sanitation outreach program. Despite passenger warnings to drive slowly due to the road conditions, the taxi drivers were speeding when a car that pulled suddenly into their path caused a collision.

One victim is a staff member who had left without his motorcycle helmet as the group rushed to depart. With a quivering voice, Moses reports that this staff member did not survive the collision. Another victim is a volunteer who had purchased a helmet at a local shop, which likely was not safety certified by the Ministry of Transportation. This helmet now lies shattered near the accident scene, while the volunteer, still bleeding from a large scalp laceration, is alive but comatose.

The only four-wheeled vehicle on hand for transportation is the car involved in the accident, which now has a broken windshield, but the driver has offered to transport the victims to a health care facility. You urge Moses to get the injured staff member to the district hospital quickly. As you end the phone call, shocked by the tragic news, several thoughts come immediately to mind. Could this accident have been prevented? How can the organization best deal with a serious trauma to one of its staff members during fieldwork?

You convene a committee to discuss the ramifications of the accident. The committee's pragmatic charge will be to examine staff insurance benefits, including evacuation coverage and repatriation of remains; organizational policy improvements to minimize the likelihood of riding without a helmet; appropriate standards for safety equipment; an alert system to warn of hazardous road or transportation conditions; and innovative strategies to optimize transportation safety under local conditions. But the committee has also been asked to consider three areas of ethical challenge the situation has presented.

6.7.3 Discussion Questions

1. Under what circumstances should you limit humanitarian aid based on the assessment of risk to workers or volunteers? What is an acceptable level of risk, and what harms—to the organization, its staff, and the communities being served—could potentially result from limiting or ending aid?
2. What are the obligations of nonprofits or humanitarian agencies to protect their workers from safety threats, given that they frequently operate in dangerous environments where infrastructure is lacking? Do the obligations of nonprofits differ from the private sector when it comes to protecting the health and safety of their staff, and if so, how?
3. How can a nonprofit or humanitarian agency best deal with a tragic accident resulting in the death or serious injury of a volunteer or worker? Consider the ethical pros and cons of the potential approaches that could be taken to prepare for risks to aid worker health and safety and address such a situation as it unfolds, including risk communication.

References

Hargarten, S.W., and S.P. Baker. 1985. Fatalities in the Peace Corps. A retrospective study: 1962 through 1983. *Journal of the American Medical Association* 254(10): 1326–1329.

Hargarten, S.W., T.D. Baker, and K. Guptill. 1991. Overseas fatalities of United States citizen travelers: An analysis of deaths related to international travel. *Annals of Emergency Medicine* 20(6): 622–626.

Humanitarian Outcomes. 2013. *Aid worker security database*. https://aidworkersecurity.org/incidents/report/summary. Accessed 4 June 2015.

McInnes, R.J., L.M. Williamson, and A. Morrison. 2002. Unintentional injury during foreign travel: A review. *Journal of Travel Medicine* 9(6): 297–307.

Nurthen, N.M., and P. Jung. 2008. Fatalities in the Peace Corps: A retrospective study, 1984 to 2003. *Journal of Travel Medicine* 15(2): 95–101.

O'Sullivan, S.L. 2010. International human resource management challenges in Canadian development INGOs. *European Management Journal* 28(6): 421–440.

Sheik, M., M.I. Gutierrez, P. Bolton, P. Spiegel, M. Thieren, and G. Burnham. 2000. Deaths among humanitarian workers. *British Medical Journal* 321(7254): 166.

World Health Organization (WHO). 2009. *Global status report on road safety: Time for action.* http://www.who.int/violence_injury_prevention/road_safety_status/2009/en/. Accessed 4 June 2015.

Chapter 7
Vulnerability and Marginalized Populations

Anthony Wrigley and Angus Dawson

7.1 Introduction

Public health practitioners attempt to identify and then remove, or at least reduce, threats of harm. However, harm does not affect everyone in the same way. Some people and communities are resilient, whereas others are more susceptible to potential harm. Much public health work is carried out by, or on behalf of, governments. Where people or communities are at great risk of harm, government has a clear and firm responsibility to protect its citizens. One way of describing a potential source of such a risk of harm is to focus on the idea of *vulnerability*. This introduction explores the concept of 'vulnerability' and the role that it may play in public health.

Vulnerability is a concept often used in public health ethics and more broadly in bioethics—but its exact meaning is unclear. Roughly, it indicates that an individual or group is thought to have a particular status that may adversely impact upon their well-being, and that this implies an ethical duty to safeguard that well-being because the person or group is unable to do so adequately themselves. This concept, although important, consistently eludes precise definition. The difficulty in defining the concept arises from disagreement as to how to characterize the idea of "special status" and to whom it applies. As a result, more and more categories of individuals and groups are being classified as vulnerable in an ever-increasing range of situations. This raises the concern that almost everyone can be classified as vulnerable in some

The opinions, findings, and conclusions of the authors do not necessarily reflect the official position, views, or policies of the editors, the editors' host institutions, or the authors' host institutions.

A. Wrigley, PhD
Centre for Professional Ethics, Keele University, Staffordshire, UK

A. Dawson, PhD (✉)
Center for Values, Ethics and the Law in Medicine, Sydney School of Public Health,
The University of Sydney, Sydney, Australia
e-mail: angus.dawson@sydney.edu.au

D.H. Barrett et al. (eds.), *Public Health Ethics: Cases Spanning the Globe*,
Public Health Ethics Analysis 3, DOI 10.1007/978-3-319-23847-0_7

way and, in turn, that almost every activity now requires this additional attention. If true, then the concept of 'vulnerability' ceases to be useful because if everyone is vulnerable, then no one is.

There is currently no clear, single, definitive account of this concept that is universally accepted, although numerous different approaches have been adopted by, for example, various international bodies in their guidelines. In this chapter, we shall critically examine some leading definitions of vulnerability and attempt to explain and classify them to make clear the differences in approach. Then we will offer an account of vulnerability that seeks to provide a universal basis for the everyday use of the concept while avoiding the pitfalls associated with the other definitions. Our approach aims to reduce the concept to a simple role, not as a basic moral concept in its own right, but as a marker, or signal, to public health practitioners that something in the situation before them requires ethical attention. The real ethical work is to be done by the practitioner, not by vague appeal to the idea of vulnerability, but via the application of other concepts and ethical concerns that are already familiar in public health and bioethics. We shall use case studies to illustrate how this approach works.

7.2 Different Approaches to the Concept of Vulnerability

Before looking at the approaches taken to define vulnerability, a worthwhile starting point is to examine the concept that can be derived from the term's everyday use. Vulnerability, in line with the etymological root of the word meaning "to wound," is widely interpreted as

(**V1**) Open to harm or under threat of harm.

This basic definition is perfectly adequate, for a range of uses, with context determining the nature and kind of harm at stake. However, such a definition only captures a broad background use as to how the concept should be employed. Though this definition will be sufficient for most purposes, further clarity and greater specificity of the concept is needed here. In attempting to refine this basic definition, several challenges arise. First, how we formulate any definition will change whether or not we see someone as vulnerable. Therefore, in providing a more substantial definition, one has to avoid the problem of inadvertently excluding those who should be considered genuinely vulnerable or including those who are not vulnerable. Second, if we want the concept of vulnerability to function as something that generates a duty or responsibility to prevent harms from befalling people, then we must move beyond a basic, factual description and include some normative ethical element, something along the lines of what Goodin characterizes as "the principle of protecting the vulnerable" (1985, 110).

Providing a sound definition of vulnerability that satisfies these elements is more difficult than might be expected. Hurst (2008) captured this difficulty well by likening it to the attempts of six blind men trying to describe an elephant. As each blind man touches a different part of the elephant—the trunk, ear, tusk, tail, etc.—they cannot agree on how to describe the animal. This analogy maps directly to the challenge of defining vulnerability. Because different perspectives abound on what constitutes the grounds of vulnerability, consensus on the definition is difficult to reach (Schroeder and Gefenas 2009).

Much of the focus on vulnerability in the bioethics literature has been in research ethics, where many international guidelines recommend or impose some duty to provide extra protection for those considered vulnerable. However, these guidelines generally fail to define the concept (although the Council for International Organizations of Medical Sciences [CIOMS] (2002) does provide a definition) and, instead, list groups commonly considered vulnerable (U.S. Department of Health, Education, and Welfare 1979; World Medical Association 2013; CIOMS 1993). Although this practice is slowly changing, strategies for analyzing and defining the concept are usually limited to simply adding or subtracting from a list of properties, conditions, or categories that typify what it is to be considered vulnerable.

The approaches taken to define vulnerability beyond everyday use (**V1**) can be categorized broadly into three basic types:

(**V2**) Vulnerability is a universal condition that humanity has in virtue of our physical or social nature (Fineman 2008; Hoffmaster 2006; Turner 2006; Rogers et al. 2012; MacIntyre 1999; International Bioethics Committee of UNESCO [IBC] 2013; and to some extent Hart 1961).

or

(**V3**) Vulnerability involves one or more specific attributes, contexts, or group types (Rendtorff 2002; and this is perhaps also the approach taken by the International Bioethics Committee of UNESCO when it considers what it calls special vulnerabilities, 2013, 5–6).

or

(**V4**) Vulnerability involves one (or more) familiar but overarching ethical concept(s) (Goodin 1985; Wrigley 2010).

Before we critically examine each approach, it is worth noting that all definitions are perfectly adequate depending on what we want the concept to do or what role we want it to play. One possible explanation for the failure to produce a single, universally agreed-upon definition of this concept is that, put simply, those who use the term have different aims and roles in mind.

7.3 Concerns Surrounding Approach (V2): Universal Condition

Approaches to the concept along the lines of (**V2**) use vulnerability to mark every human as somehow open to harm—including physical injury, dependency on others, loss of power, and so forth—just by virtue of being human (Fineman 2008). Hence, by that logic, everyone is vulnerable because we all have bodies that can be injured, disabled, and fail through illness and old age. On this view, we are also vulnerable because whilst we live in social units that require interdependence, high quality interaction does not always exist.

(**V2**) is a very particular way of thinking about the concept of vulnerability inasmuch as it motivates and drives discussion of the human condition in general. However, the major problem with such accounts is that the general truth that we, as humans, are open to harms of various kinds or that we live in social groups, fails to pick out a special category because it applies to absolutely everyone. It becomes difficult to talk of '*degrees*' or '*types*' *of* vulnerability on such accounts. This, in turn, has led to the criticism that such an approach results in the "naturalizing" of the concept, whereby it is held to be normal or natural to be vulnerable in one way or another (Luna 2009). Of course, if the idea behind using the term '*vulnerable*' is (*a*) to articulate a fundamental aspect of the human condition, (*b*), to say something substantive about the interdependence of humans, and, perhaps, (*c*) to thereby affirm a natural commitment to human solidarity, then much substantive (and controversial) content is built into the concept, and our discussion moves far from the everyday meaning of vulnerability. If we are all vulnerable, then appealing to this concept as a means to avoid a harm or seek special protection becomes problematic, as it is hard to see how particular priorities can be set.

This approach makes vulnerability far too broad to serve as anything other than an underlying presumption about all human beings, and so it is unable to generate ethical duties beyond what we owe to every human by virtue of being human. As a result, this approach does not provide an account of vulnerability that can identify cases where people or groups are potentially open to harm in any special way.

7.4 Concerns Surrounding Approach (V3): Specific Attributes, Contexts, or Groups

In direct contrast to the approach taken in (**V2**), (**V3**) characterizes vulnerability by identifying it with some specific attribute, context, or group membership. This approach focuses on vulnerability *in terms of something*, such as physical vulnerability, social vulnerability, vulnerability *in terms of* lacking capacity, vulnerability *in terms of* belonging to a certain identifiable group, or vulnerability because of belonging to a marginalized population, etc.

This approach to defining the concept is an excellent way of illustrating the sorts of conditions that we might want to pick out as requiring special consideration in terms of susceptibility to harm. As such, (**V3**) serves as a useful heuristic device because it gives examples of the sorts of things that are often considered vulnerabilities. However, this check-list approach is to borrow David Lewis's (1986) phrase, an attempt at explanation by "way of example," whereby we provide some key paradigmatic examples or illustrations of what constitutes vulnerability and state that vulnerabilities are "these sorts of things."

This approach does a poor job of defining vulnerability. Listing everything that falls under a concept, even if it were possible, does not give us a good definition of that concept. (**V3**) neither tells us whether the examples listed are appropriate nor guides our decision making on controversial cases where identifying someone as vulnerable is unclear. Further, by using the (**V3**) approach, attention is directed away from the underlying question of what vulnerability *is*; and instead, the focus is on whether or not to add a particular group to a continually expanding unstructured list of examples (Rogers et al. 2012). Of course, any such list might prove useful as an aide memoir during, for example, an emergency event. Such a pragmatic role may be useful, but it should not be mistaken for an ontological category or conceptual boundary.

The (**V3**) approach has therefore met with the criticism that it is both too broad and too narrow to satisfactorily define vulnerability (Levine et al. 2004; Schroeder and Gefenas 2009; Luna 2009). Concerns about being too broad stem from the list of vulnerabilities becoming inflated to the point where "virtually all potential human subjects are included" (Levine et al. 2004). As such, the same concern for (**V2**) applies to (**V3**), since both approaches fail to specify in sufficient detail those who need additional or special protection from harms.

(**V3**) is also, potentially, too narrow because it focuses all attention onto specific or group characteristics and therefore fails to address concerns outside the particular designated categories (Rogers et al. 2012). It will, therefore, potentially miscategorize certain individuals or groups as *not* being vulnerable if, for example, they are a group that has not been encountered previously or if some trait has not made it onto the list of specified characteristics. Moreover, by focusing on specific or group characteristics, (**V3**) can stereotype individuals who fall under category headings (Scully 2013). If, for example, we assign names to different categories of vulnerability (e.g., 'the elderly', 'the disabled,' or 'women,' or 'the poor' as categories of vulnerability), then many people could be classified as vulnerable without them necessarily being at any greater risk of harm.

7.5 Concerns Surrounding Approach (V4): Overarching Concepts

The (**V4**) approach explains vulnerability in terms of one or more overarching but more familiar ethical concept(s). Perhaps the best example of this kind is Goodin's (1985) account of vulnerability, which builds on the everyday use of the term (**V1**)— open to or under threat of harm— but goes a step further by exploring what the relevant harms might be. This leads Goodin to interpret "harm" in terms of a person's "welfare" or "interests" so giving us an initial definition of being vulnerable in terms of '*being susceptible to harms to one's interests*'(1985, 110–114).

However, as the concepts of 'welfare' and 'interests' can in turn be open to a great deal of interpretation, including the possibility of focusing on subjective explications involving the satisfaction of preferences or desires, further clarification is needed. To this end, Goodin suggests that a particular sub-group of interests, that is—people's "vital interests" or "needs"—are the universally important welfare considerations that we need to be concerned about. On this view, one is vulnerable if one's needs are threatened. And one is most vulnerable if one's most vital needs are threatened.

Goodin also adds an explicit normative role to the concept of vulnerability by imposing an ethical duty to safeguard the potentially vulnerable from harm. This role is imperative if the concept of vulnerability is to be anything more than a factual description of an individual's or a group's characteristics. Goodin does this by linking his account of vulnerability to the "principle of protecting the vulnerable," which is, essentially, an obligation to protect the vital interests of others. Hence there is a direct link between the classification of someone as being vulnerable, with a requirement on the part of others to protect them from any potential harms.

Despite being a highly influential account of vulnerability, this approach has been criticized. One concern is that it potentially promotes widespread paternalism in an attempt to meet others' needs (Rogers et al. 2012), thereby characterizing all vulnerable people as, in some way, being helpless. This criticism misses the mark, though, because being vulnerable by Goodin's account does not mean one is powerless. More telling, however, are the concerns that this account does nothing more than reduce the concept of vulnerability to the well-recognized concept of needs, together with a moral theory that demands we aid those in need. In essence, this implies that the concept of vulnerability is redundant and could be replaced with the concept of being in (serious) need.

7.6 Simplifying the Concept of Vulnerability (V5): The Moral-Marker Approach

Rather than continuing this attempt to define vulnerability along the lines of the approaches already mentioned (**V2**, **V3**, **and V4**), an account of vulnerability can be offered in much simpler terms. Instead of seeking a substantive definition that tries to establish conditions for vulnerability, another option is to interpret the word "vulnerability" as nothing more than an empty marker or signal for potential moral concern. This approach can be seen in Hurst's view of vulnerability as a sign of "increased likelihood of incurring additional or greater wrong" (2008). However, this view can be taken further. A formal moral-marker approach simplifies the account of vulnerability by avoiding any reliance on moral theory or preconceived wrongs as part of the definition. On this account, vulnerability will simply be

(**V5**) A marker that additional consideration needs to be given to whatever existing ethical issues there may be.

It can be seen that what is then in dispute between the different accounts presented is what sorts of considerations are the relevant ones. However, if we stop at the point where "vulnerability" is recognized as just a warning marker, we don't need to engage with the substantial task of trying to provide a catch-all definition that somehow incorporates all physical, mental, or emotional, etc. cases that might constitute vulnerability. Instead, we can focus on substantive ethical concepts such as harm, consent, exploitation, etc. and explore how each applies to the particular case before us. On the basis of this approach, "vulnerability" says nothing at all about what generates the need for any special scrutiny because the substantive ethical weight of the concern (and how to address it) requires us to engage with these substantive moral concepts. So, for example, it says little to talk about marginalized populations as being vulnerable, but if we recognize the 'moral marker' of vulnerability here, we might then explore how exploitation, inequity, and harm are relevant when deliberating about a particular case. One of the priorities for educating public health professionals about ethical issues is to seek to increase their sensitivity to the relevant features of each situation, rather than teach them the formulaic application of rules or vague concepts such as that of "vulnerability" (Coughlin et al. 2012).

The (**V5**) approach offers other advantages as well. For example, it avoids stereotyping based merely on belonging to a specified category; it avoids exclusion on the grounds of not already being on the list of vulnerable groups; and it avoids the vacuity of identifying "all" as vulnerable, while maintaining the crucial aspect that the concept marks out the need for special ethical scrutiny. Trying to provide more substantial components to the definition of vulnerability diverts scrutiny and energy from where it matters most—sensitive, rational thought about specific problems—and instead, promotes a formulaic approach to ethical safeguarding.

Although other writers on vulnerability, such as Levine et al. (2004) and Luna (2009), criticize this approach claiming generic guidance about paying "special attention" or giving "special consideration" to something is not useful, the same criticism could also apply to an account that identifies specific categories or relies on some overriding concept. For example, if we try the specific category or context route (**V3**) so that, say, we hold "the elderly" vulnerable, how would that guide our actions without reference to established concerns about, for example, physical harms or exploitation? The same holds true of (**V4**) accounts such as Goodin's focus on vulnerability as being open to harms to one's interests, which then requires further analysis of "vital" needs. The best that can be said for such accounts is that each provides something of a heuristic, teaching anyone who wants to learn ways in which harms or wrongs might arise.

The importance and implications of these issues become apparent as we consider the various cases in the rest of this chapter. The implications of (**V2**), the approach focused on vulnerability as arising from the human condition, is that all are vulnerable, including the police and immigration officials in Blight's and McDougall's cases, the public health officials with responsibility for launching national programs to reduce Sudden Infant Death Syndrome (SIDS) in the Jonas and Haretuku case, and the prison governor in Christopher et al.'s case. This outcome demonstrates the key problem with this view. The very concept of vulnerability ceases to have much meaning, although presumably there might be a retreat to the thought that some individuals and populations are 'more' vulnerable than others, although it is unclear how this is to be specified.

Many of the cases could more obviously be used to endorse (**V3**), the approach focused on specific groups, contexts, or categories. Many of these cases focus on marginalized groups within society, such as prison inmates (Christopher et al.), immigrants, asylum seekers, refugees (McDougall; Blight), substance abusers (Christopher et al.), minority communities of various kinds (Bernard et al.; Blight; Jonas and Haretuku), and the poor (Vergès et al.). This is a traditional, influential, and powerful way of thinking about vulnerability. However, as stated previously, this approach has its problems. Does it necessarily follow that if you belong to one of these groups that you are vulnerable? You may well be at increased risk of harm of various kinds if you belong to such groups. However, you might also be at increased risk of harm as a recreational drug user, skydiver, or American football player, although individuals belonging to such groups are not likely to be seen, intuitively, as being necessarily vulnerable.

The more specific focus on providing a normative explanation for vulnerability presented in the work of writers such as Goodin (**V4**), is more useful, in that we can begin to clearly identify subgroups that are at risk of harm to their vital interests (the girl fed through a tube and unable to feel pain involved in a forced deportation case: Blight), rather than just being routinely disadvantaged (the surrogate encouraged to take on that role because of poverty: Vergès et al.) or at increased risk of harm due to the cultural traditions or choices of their parents (Jonas and Haretuku). How should we think about risk factors and vulnerability? Some will think of smoking around children (increasing the risk of SIDS) as being an individual's choice. Others will argue that it is unfair to assume that it is always individuals that are responsible for such choices and the resultant outcomes, as people may be addicted to nicotine or they may have become smokers through the influence of norms within their social environment.

The advantage of the 'moral-marker' approach (**V5**) is that it allows us to dive beneath the surface offered by the label of 'vulnerability' and offer more sophisticated explanations for the situations described in the cases, as well as providing the opportunity to develop strong normative reasons to respond. For example, all of these cases are about various kinds of injustice, disadvantage, and inequities in society, and their impact on individual and community health. They are appropriate issues for those working in public health to be concerned about precisely because they provide reference to the identification of various harms at the population-level, and many of the solutions to these issues will have to come through collective and public action.

As the discussion of the different approaches to defining vulnerability considered above illustrate, most of the approaches to vulnerability do little more than encourage us to engage in additional ethical scrutiny using already well recognized and well understood moral concepts. The final 'moral-marker' approach (**V5**) suggests that this is exactly what the concept should be used for, and nothing more.

References

Coughlin, S.S., A. Barker, and A. Dawson. 2012. Ethics and scientific integrity in public health, epidemiological and clinical research. *Public Health Reviews* 34(1): 71–83. http://www.publichealthreviews.eu/upload/pdf_files/11/00_Coughlin.pdf. Accessed 20 June 2015.

Council for International Organizations of Medical Sciences (CIOMS). 1993. *International ethical guidelines for biomedical research involving human subjects*, 1st ed. Geneva: CIOMS.

Council for International Organizations of Medical Sciences. 2002. *International ethical guidelines for biomedical research involving human subjects*, 2nd ed. Geneva: CIOMS.

Fineman, M.A. 2008. The vulnerable subject: Anchoring equality in the human condition. *Yale Journal of Law and Feminism* 20(1): 1–23.

Goodin, R.E. 1985. *Protecting the vulnerable: A reanalysis of our social responsibilities*. Chicago: University of Chicago Press.

Hart, H.L.A. 1961. *The concept of law*. Oxford: Oxford University Press.

Hoffmaster, B. 2006. What does vulnerability mean? *Hastings Center Report* 36(2): 38–45.

Hurst, S.A. 2008. Vulnerability in research and health care, describing the elephant in the room? *Bioethics* 22(4): 191–202.
International Bioethics Committee (IBC) of UNESCO. 2013. *The principle of respect for human vulnerability and personal integrity*. http://unesdoc.unesco.org/images/0021/002194/219494e.pdf. Accessed 20 June 2105.
Levine, C., R. Faden, C. Grady, et al. 2004. The limitations of "vulnerability" as a protection for human research participants. *American Journal of Bioethics* 4(3): 44–49.
Lewis, D. 1986. *On the plurality of worlds*. Oxford: Blackwell.
Luna, F. 2009. Elucidating the concept of vulnerability: Layers not labels. *International Journal of Feminist Approaches to Bioethics* 2(1): 121–139.
MacIntyre, A. 1999. *Dependent rational animals: Why human beings need the virtues*. Chicago: Open Court.
Rendtorff, J.D. 2002. Basic ethical principles in European bioethics and biolaw: Autonomy, dignity, integrity and vulnerability—Towards a foundation of bioethics and biolaw. *Medicine, Health Care, and Philosophy* 5(3): 235–244.
Rogers, W., C. MacKenzie, and S. Dodds. 2012. Why bioethics needs a concept of vulnerability. *International Journal of Feminist Approaches to Bioethics* 5(2): 11–38.
Schroeder, D., and E. Gefenas. 2009. Vulnerability: Too vague and too broad? *Cambridge Quarterly of Healthcare Ethics* 18(2): 113–121.
Scully, J.L. 2013. Disability and vulnerability: On bodies, dependence, and power. In *Vulnerability: New essays in ethics and feminist philosophy*, ed. C. Mackenzie, W. Rogers, and S. Dodds. New York: Oxford University Press.
Turner, B. 2006. *Vulnerability and human rights*. University Park: Pennsylvania State University Press.
U.S. Department of Health, Education, and Welfare. 1979. *The Belmont report: Ethical principles and guidelines for the protection of human subjects of research*, vol. Publication No. (OS) 78-0012. Washington, DC: U.S. Government Printing Office.
Wrigley, A. 2010. Vulnerable and non-competent subjects. In *European textbook on ethics in research*, ed. J. Hughes, 49–74. Luxembourg: Publications Office of the European Union.
World Medical Association. 2013. *Declaration of Helsinki—Ethical principles for medical research involving human subjects*. http://www.wma.net/en/30publications/10policies/b3/. Accessed 6 June 2014.

7.7 Case 1: Reducing Sudden Infant Death Syndrome in a Culturally Diverse Society: The New Zealand Cot Death Study and National Cot Death Prevention Programme

Monique Jonas
School of Population Health, Faculty of Medical and Health Sciences
The University of Auckland
Auckland, New Zealand
e-mail: m.jonas@auckland.ac.nz

Riripeti Haretuku
Maori SIDS and Research
MauriOra Associates
Auckland, New Zealand

This case is presented for instructional purposes only. The ideas and opinions expressed are the authors' own. The case is not meant to reflect the official position, views, or policies of the editors, the editors' host institutions, or the authors' host institutions.

7.7.1 Background

Sudden Infant Death Syndrome (SIDS) involves the death of apparently healthy sleeping infants, usually within the first year of life. It is a diagnosis of exclusion, that is, it denotes an unknown cause of death (Willinger et al. 1991; American Academy of Pediatrics 2011). It is also known as cot or crib death and is classified as a form of Sudden Death in Infancy (SUDI).

Unlike many public health issues, SIDS unites clinical and forensic considerations, as this finding of cause of death can determine attribution of criminal (and moral) responsibility. Police collect evidence and coroners assess the circumstances of the death and release judgments. This is the method by which a SIDS death is determined. Context heightens the ethical significance of SIDS diagnosis, research, and prevention.

In 1991, when the New Zealand Cot Death Study (NZCDS) commenced, New Zealand's rate of SIDS was high by international standards at 4 deaths per 1,000 live births (Mitchell et al. 1997) compared, for example, to the Netherlands (1.3/1,000 in 1989) (de Jonge et al. 1989) and Hong Kong (0.3/1,000 in 1986–1987) (Lee et al. 1989). Within New Zealand, SIDS deaths occurred in the indigenous Māori population at twice the rate of the non-Māori population (Mitchell et al. 1994). The reason for this significant disparity was not well understood.

The NZCDS was the first national case-control study designed to identify risk factors for SIDS. By comparing infants whose deaths were attributed to SIDS with a representative sample of live births, within a year, the NZCDS had identified a number of risk factors. The study confirmed an association between increased risk of SIDS and lower socioeconomic status, along with a range of associated maternal factors, including fewer years of education, younger age at first pregnancy, greater number of previous pregnancies, and lower attendance at prenatal classes (Mitchell et al. 1991). The NZCDS selected three risk factors to address among this range of findings: lack of breast-feeding, maternal smoking, and placing infants to sleep in a prone position (Mitchell et al. 1991).

The ensuing national prevention campaign focused on publicizing these risks, which parents were seen as able to influence. These were categorized as 'modifiable risk factors.' Many parents changed their practices in response to the campaign (Cowan 2010). Abandonment of the prone sleeping position was the most readily and widely adopted measure and is credited with delivering the largest proportion of the national reduction in SIDS rates (Mitchell et al. 1997). Factors that were less susceptible to parental alteration were classified as 'nonmodifiable risk factors.' Nonmodifiable factors included the baby's sex, the mother's age, and the family's socioeconomic status.

Analysis of the second year's data revealed another risk factor: bed-sharing (Mitchell et al. 1992). Bed-sharing was categorized as a modifiable risk factor, and parents were advised to avoid sleeping on the same surface as their baby or allowing others (for instance, other children) to do so. The study's findings were immediately fed into the prevention campaign.

Communicating with parents about this particular risk factor became more problematic than initially anticipated. The difficulties partly reflected a developing understanding about the subtle nature of bed-sharing risk. While early messages counselled against all bed-sharing, subsequent findings prompted adjustments (Cowan 2010). Now bed-sharing is not viewed as a significant risk unless coupled with maternal smoking or with the baby's bedmate being intoxicated or excessively tired. Other factors such as the baby's age, the site, and duration of bed-sharing have also been identified as affecting the magnitude of risk. These considerations make it difficult to summarize the risk in a way that is scientifically sound and that parents can easily understand. Also, the prevention campaign took place against a backdrop of numerous changes in prevailing thought since the 1950s about the causes of SIDS. These changes were associated with changing advice about parental practices, which created uncertainty within families about which advice should be followed.

The cultural significance attributed to bed-sharing meant that there were different reactions among groups to advice not to bed-share. While bed-sharing is not traditional among New Zealand European (Pākehā) families, it is firmly rooted in Māori and Polynesian child-rearing practices (Tipene-Leach et al. 2000). In these communities, bed-sharing is seen as positive and beneficial, promoting bonding between mother and child and enabling mothers to comfort and care for their child (Abel et al. 2001; Tipene-Leach et al. 2000). The message that bed-sharing is risky had serious implications, then, for Māori and Polynesian child-rearing practices.

The early years of the SIDS prevention campaign succeeded in reducing the rate of SIDS, but the tenor of the anti-bed-sharing message alienated many, particularly indigenous Māori, consequently turning whānau (wider family networks) away from SIDS prevention messages altogether (Stewart et al. 1993; Tipene-Leach et al. 2000; Cowan 2010). Some interpreted the campaign as blaming Māori for infant deaths. After an infant death, the involvement of police, pathologists, and a coroner's court compounds overtones of culpability, intensifying the guilt and grief associated with the loss of a child (Clarke and McCreanor 2006).

Several years after the ongoing SIDS prevention campaign was launched, rates of SIDS among Māori remained disproportionately high. In 2009, the rate of SIDS for Māori was 1.5 per 1,000 live births, compared with 0.6/1,000 for Pacific Peoples, and 0.3/1,000 for Other, including Pākehā (Ministry of Health 2012).

Several modifiable risk factors for SIDS, including maternal smoking and bed-sharing, are more prevalent in the Māori community. Māori parents less frequently attend prenatal classes than non-Māori parents. Along with the modifiable factors, many nonmodifiable factors are more likely to apply to Māori families, including lower socioeconomic status, younger age of mother at first pregnancy, greater number of pregnancies, and fewer years of education (Mitchell et al. 1993). These contributors to rates of SIDS among Māori do not receive the same level of scrutiny in the media as modifiable parental practices, and prevention campaigns continue to focus upon altering parental practices.

A sense of injustice and a perception that the state lacks a true commitment to addressing the societal factors underpinning SIDS prevails in parts of the Māori community. The prevention campaign's focus upon discouraging bed-sharing contributes to the community's sense that the campaign undermines rather than supports traditional Māori practices. In particular, the coronial process—the investigations into the cause of death, the invasive process of autopsy, and the slow return of the body to whānau—cannot easily accommodate the deep-felt need of whānau to complete the traditional Tangihanga process, the spiritual rituals and burial proceedings following a death (Clarke and McCreanor 2006; McCreanor et al. 2004). Nor is the high profile of the bed-sharing risk matched by a commitment to tackle other risk factors, which may require more resources. Some have therefore called for examination of the process by which risk factors are categorized as modifiable or nonmodifiable (Tipene-Leach 2010; McManus et al. 2010).

The government has committed substantial resources to culturally appropriate SIDS prevention for Māori and Polynesian families and is conducting trials of appropriate supports for families to bed-share safely (Tipene-Leach 2010). Meanwhile, criminal proceedings against Māori parents relating to the deaths of their infants while co-sleeping continue to receive media attention (R v Tukiwaho 2012; APNZ 2013). No wonder, then, that the strong sense of parental responsibility for SIDS deaths, where bed-sharing is a factor, remains. Although inequities underwrite the high exposure of Māori families to both modifiable and nonmodifiable risk factors, both government-funded health promotion and media coverage of SIDS remain focused on parental practice.

7.7.2 Case Description

Following high-profile media coverage of the greater burden of SIDS among Māori, new funding is available for a SIDS prevention campaign to reduce SIDS in Māori and Polynesian families. Part of this funding is reserved for the generation of new guidelines acceptable to Māori. There is also an opportunity to brief the Minister of Health and the Minister of Social Development about measures that can reduce rates of SIDS deaths among Māori infants.

7.7.3 Discussion Questions

1. Evidence suggests that several factors affect the magnitude of risk and that bed-sharing in the absence of these factors does not significantly increase the risk of SIDS. But the interplay of risks can be complex and difficult to communicate effectively in a national campaign. Can a definitive "no bed-sharing" message be defended, on ethical grounds, if it causes less confusion but overstates the risk to some groups? What are the most important ethical considerations here?

2. What weight should be attributed to the cultural significance of bed-sharing when generating guidelines, and why? Should risks that relate to culturally significant parental practices, such as bed-sharing, be treated differently from risks relating to practices that are not held to be culturally significant?
3. Māori and Polynesian families value bed-sharing because of the health and social benefits they attribute to it. These benefits are not captured in studies investigating SIDS risk. Should the health and social benefits attributed to bed-sharing by families who practice it be accorded weight when formulating guidelines? If so, how much weight? If not, why not?
4. Colonization has imposed and continues to impose an assault upon Māori culture. Anti-bed-sharing advice might be seen to extend that assault, privileging a narrow range of health concerns. The inherent beliefs and practices that led Māori to value bed-sharing, such as bonding between mother and child that promotes strong social bonds, seems particularly worth preserving. How can respect for Māori social practices and ways of viewing the world inform SIDS-related health promotion? How much difference does the magnitude of the relevant health risk make? If the risk is less serious, would you favor a different approach?
5. Consider how risk factors might be categorized as modifiable or nonmodifiable. What role should fairness play in this process?
6. Consider the role guidelines might play in coroners' investigations to identify contributing factors to an infant death. Should this possibility be kept in mind when guidelines are being drafted? Why? Why not?
7. Does parental responsibility require compliance with child health guidance? How should parents evaluate conflicting or changing advice about risk?
8. Parents can control some risk factors for SIDS, but others involve broader societal issues, such as socioeconomic status. Does social justice require that prevention campaigns targeting parental practices be coupled with efforts to tackle social and economic disparities and inequities? Who should be responsible for ensuring that this is the case? What should researchers do when they identify a parental practice as risky if resourcing for broader action is not forthcoming?

Acknowledgements Many thanks to Carol Everard, Dr. Sally Abel, and Dr. David Tipene-Leach for their patient and generous reflections and sharing of knowledge about SIDS in New Zealand. Thanks also to Professor Ed Mitchell, Professor Robert Scragg, and Alistair Stewart for their major contributions.

References

Abel, S., J. Park, D. Tipene-Leach, S. Finau, and M. Lennan. 2001. Infant care practices in New Zealand: A cross-cultural qualitative stud. *Social Science & Medicine* 53(9): 1135–1148.

American Academy of Pediatrics, Taskforce On Sudden Infant Death Syndrome. 2011. SIDS and other sleep-related infant deaths: Expansion of recommendations for a safe infant sleeping environment. *Pediatrics* 128(5): 1030–1039. doi:10.1542/peds.2011-2284.

APNZ. 2013. Parents sentenced over babies death. *New Zealand Herald*, March 15. http://www.nzherald.co.nz/nz/news/article.cfm?c_id=1&objectid=10871515. Accessed 1 June 2015.

Clarke, E., and T. McCreanor. 2006. He wahine tangi tikapa …: Statutory investigative processes and the grieving of Maori families who have lost a baby to SIDS. *Kōtuitui: New Zealand Journal of Social Sciences Online* 1: 25–43.

Cowan, S. 2010. Creating change: How knowledge translates into action for protecting babies from sudden infant death? *Current Pediatric Reviews* 6: 86–94.

de Jonge, G.A., A.C. Engelberts, A.J.M. Koomen-Liefting, and P.J. Kostense. 1989. Cot death and prone sleeping position in The Netherlands. *British Medical Journal* 298(6675): 722.

Lee, N.N.Y., Y.F. Chan, D.P. Davies, E. Lau, and D.C.P. Yip. 1989. Sudden infant death syndrome in Hong Kong: Confirmation of low incidence. *British Medical Journal* 298: 721.

McCreanor, T., D. Tipene-Leach, and S. Abel. 2004. The SIDS care-workers study: Perceptions of the experiences of Maori SIDS families. *Social Policy Journal of New Zealand* 23: 154–166.

McManus, V., S. Abel, T. McCreanor, and D. Tipene-Leach. 2010. Narratives of deprivation: Women's life stories around Maori sudden infant death syndrome. *Social Science & Medicine* 71(3): 643–649.

Ministry of Health. 2012. *Fetal and infant deaths 2008 and 2009*. Wellington: Ministry of Health.

Mitchell, E., R. Scragg, A.W. Stewart, D.M. Becroft, B. Taylor, and R.P. Ford. 1991. Results from the first year of the New Zealand cot death study. *New Zealand Medical Journal* 104(906): 71–76.

Mitchell, E.A., B.J. Taylor, R.P. Ford, et al. 1992. Four modifiable and other major risk factors for cot death: The New Zealand study. *Journal of Paediatrics and Child Health* 28(suppl 1): S3–S8.

Mitchell, E.A., A.W. Stewart, R. Scragg, et al. 1993. Ethnic differences in mortality from sudden infant death syndrome in New Zealand. *British Medical Journal* 306(6869): 13–16.

Mitchell, E.A., J.M. Brunt, and C. Everard. 1994. Reduction in mortality from sudden infant death syndrome in New Zealand: 1986–92. *Archives of Disease in Childhood* 70(4): 291–294.

Mitchell, E.A., P.G. Tuohy, J.M. Brunt, et al. 1997. Risk factors for sudden infant death syndrome following the prevention campaign in New Zealand: A prospective study. *Pediatrics* 100(5): 835–840.

R v Tukiwaho, NZHC 1193 (2012).

Stewart, A., E.A. Mitchell, D. Tipene-Leach, and P. Fleming. 1993. Lessons from the New Zealand and UK cot death campaigns. *Acta Paediatrica Supplement* 82: 119–123.

Tipene-Leach, D. 2010. Sudden infant death and co-sleeping: A better message. *The New Zealand Medical Journal* 123(1309): 137–138.

Tipene-Leach, D., S. Abel, S.A. Finau, J. Park, and M. Lennan. 2000. Maori infant care practices: Implications for health messages, infant care services and SIDS prevention in Maori communities. *Pacific Health Dialog* 7(1): 29–37.

Willinger, M., L.S. James, and C. Catz. 1991. Defining the sudden infant death syndrome (SIDS): Deliberations of an expert panel convened by the National Institute of Child Health and Human Development. *Pediatric Pathology* 11(5): 677–684.

7.8 Case 2: Medical Tourism and Surrogate Pregnancy: A Case of Ethical Incoherence

Claude Vergès
Children's Hospital
University of Panama
Panama City, Panama
e-mail: vergeslopez@hotmail.com

Jorge Rodríguez
Sexual and Reproductive Health, Ministry of Health
Panama City, Panama

Panamanian Family Medicine Association
Panama City, Panama

Raquel de Mock
Adult Health Program, Ministry of Health, University of Panama
Panama City, Panama

This case is presented for instructional purposes only. The ideas and opinions expressed are the authors' own. The case is not meant to reflect the official position, views, or policies of the editors, the editors' host institutions, or the authors' host institutions.

7.8.1 Background

Advances in biotechnology regularly generate novel ethical challenges that fall between the cracks of safeguards designed for conventional cases. Innovations—especially in reproductive technologies—can even create new classes of vulnerable people. Such novel cases often force us to thoroughly reexamine ethical safeguards and reveal the legal and ethical gaps.

Panama, like most Latin American countries, divides its health care system into public and private systems. Public insurance covers roughly 81 % of the population (Contraloria de la Republica de Panamá 2012). Families lacking permanent work and unable to afford insurance can find public assistance for health services through the Ministry of Health (MoH). The MoH by law regulates most health research and health services, including regulation and supervision of hospitals and public and private clinics (Asamblea Nacional de Panamá 1947). The private system, although legally supervised by the Ministry of Commerce, exists mostly free of external control and relies heavily on self-regulation. Medical doctors, after initial MoH certification, are no longer monitored (Decreto de Gabinete 1970).

Like the certification process, the ethical guidance that applies to doctors is not overseen. Although a Panamanian Medical College code of ethics has applied to doctors since 2009, its ethics committee meets only to consider malpractice charges brought against doctors (Colegio Médico 2012). Independent associations for medical specialties exist, but they focus on academic and social matters, not on public health issues. Only recently have some associations begun to discuss the ethical, legal, and social implications of their specialty-related health topics such as transplantation, blood banks, storage of biological tissues, sale of organs for transplant, and rights and obligations of organ donors and recipients.

In response to a growing burden of maternal mortality, sexually transmitted diseases, and adolescent pregnancy, the World Health Organization in 2000 began a sexual and reproductive health program (World Health Organization 2000). This initiative prompted the Panamanian government to begin covering infertility problems and permitting the public health care system to treat married couples (Ministerio de Salud 2000). Although the MoH did not include in-vitro fertilization (IVF) and surrogate pregnancy in this program, a public institution, the Gorgas Institute for Health Research, announced in 2011 that it would launch an IVF program in 2013 for couples with limited resources (Soto 2012). The government, however, was silent about IVF, so the regulations governing IVF remain unclear. However, a law governing organ transplantation, which permits donation of living cells, comes closest to offering legal guidance for IVF. This law requires the donor and recipient to give written consent but does not permit the donor to receive compensation. Nor does it protect the health and confidentiality of the donor and recipient or offer treatment of medical complications (Asamblea Nacional de Panamá 2010). Nowhere, does this law or any other address surrogacy.

Medical tourism is a new and growing industry in Central America, where a quarter of the world's medical tourism occurs (Martinez 2011). At 16 %, Costa Rica commands the largest industry share in Central America; but according to estimates of its National Science and Technology secretary, Panama will achieve a 12 % share in 2015 through services offered by its four private hospitals. At these hospitals, medical tourism may represent nearly 20 % of the patients being treated. The patients, who come mainly from Canada and the United States, usually seek surgery for orthopedic problems, infertility, and cardiac disease. Although private advertisements for medical tourism have been appearing since 2007 (Sbwire 2013), lawmakers have not yet created a national legal framework to address the issue.

Couples from neighboring countries or the United States come to Panama seeking infertility treatment because it is inexpensive, is largely unregulated, and performed by Panamanian doctors noted for technical ability. Moreover, anyone who travels to Panama for treatment is entitled to receive it. IVF using fertilized eggs from anonymous donors has become standard practice, but surrogacy is not officially offered. No medical or legal problems with IVF surfaced until 2011 when the Panamanian MoH was asked to weigh in on a high-profile case of an abandoned child born with severe birth defects to a Panamanian woman acting as a surrogate for a foreign couple.

7.8.2 Case Description

A Panamanian woman, who was married with two children, had a primary school education. She worked in her own home but was experiencing economic difficulties because her husband could not find permanent employment. Why she agreed to surrogacy is unknown, but presumably economic considerations played a major role. Because her first two pregnancies had presented no problems, she signed a surrogacy contract to carry the fertilized egg of a married couple who had traveled to Panama seeking surrogacy services. Little is known about how the foreign couple and the Panamanian woman came to know each other, because no lawyer participated in this transaction. Nor did the surrogate's husband learn of the transaction until after she had signed the contract. Why no one thought to include the husband is a mystery. After signing the informed consent form, the surrogate was inseminated in a private clinic in Panama. Doctors involved in the case state that they followed medical recommendations and obtained the informed consent of the surrogate and the egg donor. Neither the procedure nor the pregnancy presented any problems, but the surrogate unexpectedly died after severe complications developed during delivery. These complications, which also caused hypoxia and convulsions in the newborn, left him with severe cerebral paralysis. As a result of his birth defects, he will never walk or speak and will require care for the remainder of his life.

The couple rejected the child, arguing that the contract specified "a healthy child." The husband of the Panamanian surrogate also rejected the child claiming it was neither his wife's, nor his, especially as he had not participated in the contract. He also pleaded that he now had to cope with his wife's death and raising two motherless children. Appealing to the MoH, the clinic sought state custody of the child. The MoH offered medical assistance, but it declined to accept long-term responsibility for the child. Instead, the MoH charged a ethics panel to examine the case and, pending its outcome, sent the child to a religious orphanage.

The ethics panel has been charged not only with making a ruling on this case, but in recommending measures to regulate surrogacy in the future, particularly cases involving medical tourism.

7.8.3 Discussion Questions

1. In the context of surrogacy and medical tourism, who is responsible for raising this child, and who should pay for his care and upbringing? What role should government and professional associations play in these cases? What is the responsibility of doctors involved in such practices?
2. What measures should the ethics panel recommend to protect vulnerable women in the future who have agreed to surrogacy?
3. What ethical basis could justify compensation for surrogates or their families in the case of death or injury to the surrogate?
4. What measures should the ethics panel recommend for protecting medically compromised and abandoned infants when surrogacy-involved pregnancy or delivery goes radically wrong? How should informed consent forms be modified to anticipate such outcomes?
5. Do cases of medical tourism require international regulation of medical technologies? If not, why not? If so, how should the panel's ethical arguments be incorporated into legal agreements between countries to guarantee the protection of vulnerable populations?

Acknowledgments To Sandra Lopez Vergès and Elizabeth King for their English edits.

References

Asamblea Nacional de Panamá. 1947. *Por la Cual se Aprueba el Código Sanitario.* Ley 66 de 10 de noviembre de 1947. Gaceta Oficial, 10467. https://www.panamaemprende.gob.pa/descargas/Ley%2066%20de%201947%20-%20Codigo%20Sanitario.pdf. Accessed 13 Aug 2013.

Asamblea Nacional de Panamá. 2010. *General de Transplantes de Componentes Anatómicos.* Ley 3 de 2 agosto 2010. Gaceta Oficial, 26468-B. http://www.gacetaoficial.gob.pa/pdfTemp/26468_B/25676.pdf. Accessed 13 Aug 2013.

Colegio Médico. 2012. *Código de Ética Panama 2003–2011.* http://www.hn.sld.pa/sites/default/files/upload/CÓDIGO%20DE%20ÉTICA%20COLEGIO%202011.pdf. Accessed 13 Aug 2013.

Contraloria de la Republica de Panamá. 2012. *Cuadro 421–02. Población Protegida por la Caja de Seguro Social Asegurados y Dependientes, Según Provincia y Comarca Indígena: Año 2011.* http://www.contraloria.gob.pa/inec/Publicaciones/Publicaciones.aspx?ID_SUBCATEGORIA=1&ID_PUBLICACION=503&ID_IDIOMA=1&ID_CATEGORIA=1. Accessed 13 Aug 2013.

Decreto de Gabinete. 1970. *Por el Cual se Establecen los Requisitos para Obtener la Idoneidad y el Libre Ejercicio de la Medicina y Otras Profesiones Afi nes.* 196 del 24-06-1970. Gaceta Oficial 16639. http://docs.panama.justia.com/federales/decretos-de-gabinete/decreto-degabinete-196-de-1970-jul-3-1970.pdf. Accessed 13 Aug 2013.

Martinez, J.C. 2011. *El Turismo Médico en Panama.* http://www.panamaqmagazine.com/2011_May/Medical_tourism_QT_2011_pg1_spanish.html. Accessed 13 Aug 2013.

Ministerio de Salud. 2000. *Programa de Salud Sexual y Reproductiva.* http://www.minsa.gob.pa/programa/programa-salud-sexual-y-reproductiva. Accessed 13 Aug 2013.

Sbwire. 2013. *PlanetHospital announced today that it has started offering surrogacy in Mexico forstraight and gay clients.* http://www.sbwire.com/press-releases/planethospital-announced-today-that-it-has-started-offering-surrogacy-in-mexico-for-straight-and-gay-clients-219420.htm. Accessed 13 Aug 2013.

Soto, G. 2012. *Instituto Gorgas aplaza proyecto de fertilidad. Panama America* http://www.panamaamerica.com.pa/content/instituto-gorgas-aplaza-proyecto-de-fertilidad. Accessed 4 June 2015.

World Health Organization (WHO). 2000. *Programa de Salud Sexual y Reproductiva.* http://www.who.int/reproductivehealth/es/. Accessed 13 Aug 2013.

7.9 Case 3: Compulsory Treatment for Injection Drug Use after Incarceration

Paul Christopher
Department of Psychiatry and Human Behavior, Warren Alpert Medical School
Brown University
Providence, RI, USA
e-mail: paul_christopher@brown.edu

Dora M. Dumont
Division of Community, Family Health and Equity
Rhode Island Department of Health
Providence, RI, USA

Josiah D. Rich
Department of Medicine, Warren Alpert Medical School
Brown University
Providence, RI, USA

This case is presented for instructional purposes only. The ideas and opinions expressed are the authors' own. The case is not meant to reflect the official position, views, or policies of the editors, the editors' host institutions, or the authors' host institutions.

7.9.1 Background

Injection drug use is a major public health problem, with an estimated 3.5 million users in the United States (Armstrong 2007) and 15.9 million users worldwide (Mathers et al. 2008). Between 24 and 36 % of U.S. adults addicted to heroin pass through the criminal justice system each year (Rich et al. 2005). Compared with the general population, injection drug users have higher rates of HIV, tuberculosis, hepatitis B and C, and sexually transmitted diseases (Baussano et al. 2010; Nelson et al. 2011; Weinbaum et al. 2005). Injection drug use contributes to correctional and community-level transmission of these conditions and threatens public safety because users frequently engage in criminal behaviors to support their drug use.

In the United States, more than two million people are incarcerated (Glaze and Parks 2012), and an estimated 70–80 % of U.S. inmates have at least one substance abuse problem (Karberg and James 2005; National Center on Addiction and Substance Abuse at Columbia University 1998). At least 40 % of state and federal inmates injected drugs in the month before their arrest (National Center on Addiction and Substance Abuse at Columbia University 1998). Moreover, 95 % of drug users return to drug use within 3 years of release from prison (Marlowe 2006). Compared with the general population, prisoners are nearly 13 times more likely to die of any cause in the 2 weeks after their release and 129 times more likely to die from an overdose (Binswanger et al. 2007).

Rates of incarceration are also substantially higher among minority groups, with African American males being more than 6 times as likely, and Hispanics males more than 2.5 times as likely, to be incarcerated than white males (Carson and Sabol 2012). African Americans and Hispanics also experience higher rates of conviction for drug-related offenses than whites (Carson and Sabol 2012) despite comparable rates of injection drug use between whites and Hispanics and lower rates among African Americans (Substance Abuse and Mental Health Services Administration 2007).

Although inmates make up only 0.8 % of the U.S. population, about 22–31 % of Americans with HIV, 40 % with tuberculosis, and 29–43 % with chronic hepatitis C pass through the correctional system each year (Hammett et al. 2002; Weinbaum et al. 2005). In the general community and prison population, minority groups bear a disproportionately high burden of new HIV infections and hepatitis, particularly among injection drug users (Blankenship et al. 2005; Centers for Disease Control and

Prevention 2013; Estrada 2002). Successful strategies to limit the spread of infectious disease, therefore, need to include interventions with effective substance abuse treatment that target minority groups, particularly anyone with a criminal background.

Correctional programs that link prisoners to treatment for substance abuse and related illnesses upon reentry to the community may reduce risky behaviors that contribute to high post-release mortality rates, bring much-needed care to a vulnerable and medically and socially disenfranchised population, and interrupt transmission of infectious diseases to the broader community. However, despite the lack of widespread access to such services during and after incarceration, perhaps the greatest obstacle to effectively treating drug users is poor motivation. In the United States, 95 % of people with untreated substance abuse fail to recognize the need for treatment (Substance Abuse and Mental Health Services Administration 2012). When people with substance abuse do present for care, it is often because of external, coercive pressure (Fagan 1999). Indeed, coercive strategies have long been used for treating individuals with substance abuse who do not otherwise seek help (Nace et al. 2007; Sullivan et al. 2008). One common argument in favor of coerced treatment is that it restores autonomy to people who have lost their ability to control their addiction (Caplan 2006). Another reason coercion may be necessary, in at least the initiation phase of treatment, is because permanent cognitive deficits can result from extended drug use (Sullivan et al. 2008).

The World Health Organization has concluded that legally coerced treatment is justified if due process and effective and humane treatment are assured (United Nations 2010). Still, although compulsory substance abuse treatment is frequently used for *pretrial* offenders, studies find little evidence that it reduces subsequent drug use (Perry et al. 2009). Indeed, findings are largely mixed about whether legally coerced substance abuse treatment—irrespective of a person's criminal justice involvement—works in different settings (Klag et al. 2005). Similarly, there are inconsistent findings on the effectiveness of coerced drug treatment in the U.S. criminal justice setting and concerns about a lack of experimental controls in those studies that suggest relative efficiency (Hough 2002; Marlowe 2006; Zhang et al. 2013).

Several reviews conclude that coerced treatment is certainly more effective than no treatment (Hough 2002; Kelly et al. 2005; Marlowe 2006). Emerging data suggest that coercive substance abuse treatment for *parolees* reduces rates of reincarceration; however, data are lacking on whether other clinical outcomes are improved (Zhang et al. 2013).

7.9.2 Case Description

You serve as the director of Substance Abuse Services (SAS) in a western state in the United States. Rates of substance abuse, particularly injection drug use, are higher than the national average. Several large cities in your state have among the highest rates in the country. SAS shares data and conducts collaborative research with the Department of Correction (DOC) and other state agencies within the Department of Health (DOH), of which SAS is a branch. Your research efforts have identified needle sharing among former prisoners, most of whom are members of minority groups, as the source of most new community cases of HIV and hepatitis B and C. You also found that more than half of these infected prisoners do not continue treatment when released and have high rates of reincarceration.

Following aggressive implementation of a statewide prison-based screening and treatment program for infectious diseases, your state has experienced a marked drop in prevalence of these diseases among prisoners. However, for three straight years rates have increased steadily and disproportionately among injection drug users, with rates rising faster among minorities.

To confront this problem, you have successfully worked with representatives from the DOC to offer methadone maintenance programs to opioid-dependent prisoners and have hired reentry specialists to help parolees get treatment for substance abuse and infectious diseases upon release. Unfortunately, to date, only 10–15 % of recently released prisoners who are eligible for these voluntary services have used them.

The governor has issued a directive to think creatively and foster better interagency collaboration so programs can be developed to reach the other 85–90 % of recently released prisoners who inject drugs or have infectious illnesses. You have been appointed to a task force along with other high-level representatives of state agencies, including the DOH, DOC, Department of Parole, and Department of Mental Health, to identify and implement other potential solutions. One suggested policy option is to establish compulsory post-release substance abuse treatment as a condition of parole that would be linked with voluntary infectious disease screening and treatment. Your own interagency research suggests a high rate of transmission of HIV and hepatitis B and C from needle sharing with former prisoners who have been incarcerated multiple times and have not been treated successfully. Accordingly, the target population would be recently released prisoners who have two or more incarcerations and at least one drug-related conviction, a history of injection drug use, and either HIV or hepatitis.

7.9.3 Discussion Questions

1. Given your research findings that most new community cases of HIV and hepatitis B and C result from needle sharing with former prisoners, most of whom are minorities, how would you defend or object to this policy proposal given it will disproportionately subject minority groups to compulsory treatment as a condition of their parole.
2. If such compulsory drug treatment for prison releases is shown to have little impact on community rates of infectious disease, what effect would the program need to have on recently released prisoners for you to support its use? Given a parolee's vulnerable status in society, would you support the program if it reduced criminal recidivism alone? If not, what other outcomes are important to you and why? Would outcomes have to be clinical, or could outcomes reflect a parolee's well-being or functioning in society?
3. What are the ethical implications of implementing (and funding) compulsory treatment for released prisoners in a community where availability of (or funding for)

voluntary treatment is currently inadequate? To what extent does lack of access to voluntary services (and other social determinants of health such as income and education) contribute to the need for compulsory treatment, particularly among people who are vulnerable to substance use, incarceration, and infectious disease?

4. Public resources and facilities are already in place to provide involuntary treatment for certain health conditions (e.g., tuberculosis and mental illness). Suppose that some mental health advocates object to the proposal to introduce compulsory drug treatment by arguing that it would divert funds from treating people with serious mental illness, including those with criminal histories. People with serious mental illness, they contend, constitute a far more vulnerable prison group, many of whom have co-occurring substance abuse problems. If true, how will your thinking about the case be influenced? Why?
5. Suppose someone argues that the compulsory treatment program under consideration is another example of society's punitive approach to managing substance abuse. To what extent do you agree or disagree with this argument? Why?

References

Armstrong, G.L. 2007. Injection drug users in the United States, 1979–2002: An aging population. *Archives of Internal Medicine* 167(2): 166–173.

Baussano, I., B.G. Williams, P. Nunn, M. Beggiato, U. Fedeli, and F. Scano. 2010. Tuberculosis incidence in prisons: A systematic review. *PLoS Medicine* 7(12): e1000381.

Binswanger, I.A., M.F. Stern, R.A. Deyo, et al. 2007. Release from prison—A high risk of death for former inmates. *New England Journal of Medicine* 356(2): 157–165.

Blankenship, K.M., A.B. Smoyer, S.J. Bray, and K. Mattocks. 2005. Black-white disparities in HIV/AIDS: The role of drug policy and the corrections system. *Journal of Health Care for the Poor and Underserved* 16(4 suppl B): 140–156.

Caplan, A.L. 2006. Ethical issues surrounding forced, mandated, or coerced treatment. *Journal of Substance Abuse Treatment* 31(2): 117–120.

Carson, E.A., and W.J. Sabol. 2012. Prisoners in 2011. *Bureau of Justice Statistics*. NCJ 239808. Washington, DC: U.S. Department of Justice, Office of Justice Programs. http://www.bjs.gov/content/pub/pdf/p11.pdf. Accessed 7 May 2013.

Centers for Disease Control and Prevention. 2013. *HIV surveillance report: Diagnoses of HIV infection in the United States and dependent areas, 2011*, vol. 23. http://www.cdc.gov/hiv/library/reports/surveillance/2011/surveillance_Report_vol_23.html. Accessed 21 May 2015.

Estrada, A.L. 2002. Epidemiology of HIV/AIDS, hepatitis B, hepatitis C, and tuberculosis among minority injection drug users. *Public Health Reports* 117(suppl 1): S126–S134.

Fagan, R. 1999. The use of required treatment for substance abusers. *Substance Abuse* 20(4): 249–261.

Glaze, L.E., and E. Parks. 2012. Correctional populations in the United States, 2011. *Bureau of Justice Statistics Bulletin* NCJ 239972. http://www.bjs.gov/content/pub/pdf/cpus11.pdf. Accessed 23 Jan 2014.

Hammett, T.M., M.P. Harmon, and W. Rhodes. 2002. The burden of infectious disease among inmates of and releases from US correctional facilities, 1997. *American Journal of Public Health* 92(11): 1789–1794.

Hough, M. 2002. Drug user treatment within a criminal justice context. *Substance Use & Misuse* 37(8–10): 985–996.

Karberg, J.C., and D.J. James. 2005. Substance dependence, abuse, and treatment of jail inmates, 2002. *Bureau of Justice Statistics: Special Report.* NCJ 209588. Washington, DC: U.S. Department of Justice, Office of Justice Programs. http://www.bjs.gov/content/pub/pdf/sdatji02.pdf. Accessed 7 May 2013.

Kelly, J.F., J.W. Finney, and R. Moos. 2005. Substance use disorder patients who are mandated to treatment: Characteristics, treatment process, and 1- and 5-year outcomes. *Journal of Substance Abuse Treatment* 28(3): 213–223.

Klag, S., F. O'Callaghan, and P. Creed. 2005. The use of legal coercion in the treatment of substance abusers: An overview and critical analysis of thirty years of research. *Substance Use & Misuse* 40(12): 1777–1795.

Marlowe, D.B. 2006. Depot naltrexone in lieu of incarceration: A behavioral analysis of coerced treatment for addicted offenders. *Journal of Substance Abuse Treatment* 31(2): 131–139.

Mathers, B.M., L. Degenhardt, B. Phillips, et al. 2008. The global epidemiology of injecting drug use and HIV among people who inject drugs: A systematic review. *Lancet* 372(9651): 1733–1745.

Nace, E.P., F. Birkmayer, M.A. Sullivan, et al. 2007. Socially sanctioned coercion mechanisms for addiction treatment. *The American Journal on Addictions* 16(1): 15–23.

National Center on Addiction and Substance Abuse at Columbia University. 1998. *Behind bars: Substance abuse and America's prison population.* http://www.casacolumbia.org/addictionresearch/reports/substance-abuse-prison-system-2008. Accessed 7 May 2013.

Nelson, P.K., B.M. Mathers, B. Cowie, et al. 2011. Global epidemiology of hepatitis B and hepatitis C in people who inject drugs: Results of systematic reviews. *Lancet* 378(9791): 571–583.

Perry, A.E., Z. Darwin, C. Godfrey, et al. 2009. The effectiveness of interventions for drug-using offenders in the courts, secure establishments and the community: A systematic review. *Substance Use & Misuse* 44(3): 374–400.

Rich, J.D., A.E. Boutwell, D.C. Shield, et al. 2005. Attitudes and practices regarding the use of methadone in US state and federal prisons. *Journal of Urban Health* 82(3): 411–419.

Substance Abuse and Mental Health Services Administration. 2007. *The NSDUH report: Demographic and geographic variations in injection drug use.* Rockville: Substance Abuse and Mental Health Services Administration. http://www.oas.samhsa.gov/2k7/idu/idu.pdf. Accessed 7 May 2013.

Substance Abuse and Mental Health Services Administration. 2012. *Results from the 2011 National Survey on Drug Use and Health: Summary of national findings*, NSDUH Series H-44, HHS Publication No. (SMA) 12–4713. Rockville: Substance Abuse and Mental Health Services Administration. http://www.samhsa.gov/data/nsduh/2k11results/nsduhresults2011.htm. Accessed 7 May 2013.

Sullivan, M.A., F. Birkmayer, B.K. Boyarsky, et al. 2008. Uses of coercion in addiction treatment: Clinical aspects. *American Journal on Addictions* 17(1): 36–47.

United Nations. 2010. *From coercion to cohesion: Treating drug dependence through health care, not punishment.* New York: United Nations Office on Drugs and Crime. http://www.unodc.org/docs/treatment/Coercion_Ebook.pdf. Accessed 7 May 2013.

Weinbaum, C.M., K.M. Sabin, and S.S. Santibanez. 2005. Hepatitis B, hepatitis C, and HIV in correctional populations: A review of epidemiology and prevention. *AIDS* 19(suppl 3): S41–S46.

Zhang, S.X., R.E. Roberts, and A.E. Lansing. 2013. Treatment or else: Coerced treatment for drug involved California parolees. *International Journal of Offender Therapy and Comparative Criminology* 57(7): 766–791.

7.10 Case 4: Unanticipated Vulnerability: Marginalizing the Least Visible in Pandemic Planning

Carrie Bernard
Department of Family and Community Medicine
University of Toronto
Toronto, ON, Canada

Department of Family Medicine McMaster University
Hamilton, ON, Canada
e-mail: carrie.bernard@utoronto.ca

Maxwell J. Smith
Dalla Lana School of Public Health and the Joint Centre for Bioethics
University of Toronto
Toronto, ON, Canada

Frank Wagner
Department of Family and Community Medicine, Faculty of Medicine
University of Toronto
Toronto, ON, Canada

Toronto Central Community Care Access Centre and
the University of Toronto Joint Centre for Bioethics
Toronto, ON, Canada

This case is presented for instructional purposes only. The ideas and opinions expressed are the authors' own. The case is not meant to reflect the official position, views, or policies of the editors, the editors' host institutions, or the authors' host institutions.

7.10.1 *Background*

Influenza is a common respiratory pathogen that affects the nose, throat, bronchi and lungs. The virus is spread through droplets and small particles when people cough or sneeze. Though influenza regularly affects people worldwide, the emergence of novel influenza virus subtypes has the potential to cause a pandemic (World Health Organization [WHO] 2008). In such a case, the population's low immunity can lead the virus to spread rapidly with high rates of sickness and death. Although no one can predict when a pandemic will strike, attack rates of 25–45 % have been suggested with mortality rates varying greatly depending on the virulence of the strain (WHO 2010).

With a virulent strain of pandemic influenza, many patients will become extremely ill, and their need for specialized treatment and intensive care may exceed resources. In addition, front-line health care workers will face great risk of becoming ill, dwindling human resources further and straining the health care system (WHO 2008; University of Toronto Joint Center for Bioethics 2005). In anticipation of these human and physical resource shortages, hospitals, public health agencies, and states have created plans to prepare for an influenza pandemic. Such plans typically include health services, public health measures, priority setting, and resource allocation and usually direct surveillance, preparedness, and response (WHO 2010).

Pandemic plans typically aim to minimize serious illness and overall deaths, but more comprehensive plans also refer to special needs of vulnerable groups. The term "vulnerable," however, often is left undefined, and, if specified (e.g., the elderly), it usually refers to increased biological or medical risk of succumbing to or transmitting pandemic influenza (Uscher-Pines et al. 2007). Few plans refer to vulnerability in social or economic terms (Uscher-Pines et al. 2007). This lack of specificity raises questions about whether (and how) special consideration ought to differ for vulnerable conditions, such as being homeless, being immunocompromised, or living in a remote community. Even when plans do mention such vulnerabilities, have decision makers or practitioners consulted the people in these categories about their needs in such situations? (Uscher-Pines et al. 2007) More importantly, has anyone reconciled the aim of minimizing sickness and death with the oft competing aim of meeting the needs of the vulnerable?

Meeting the needs of the most vulnerable while being mindful of health equity and social justice has been a long-standing tradition of public health (Beauchamp 1976; Krieger and Birn 1998). In particular, public health interventions targeting the social determinants of health have been heralded as an effective way to combat systemic inequities that lead to disparities in health outcomes (Wilson 2009). However, some challenge the notion of vulnerability as a static condition that can be predefined. Broadly defined categories of vulnerability can exclude people not traditionally seen as vulnerable (such as health care workers), while including people thought to be vulnerable who, with the right supports, can actually participate in the emergency response (e.g., retired older adults) (Mastroianni 2009). Considering and doing something about the context-specific needs of those who might be most vulnerable during a pandemic, can easily become a complex, ethically fraught task.

A further complication is that the interventions taken in response to a pandemic can unintentionally render some people more vulnerable (Mastroianni 2009). Most pandemic influenza plans, for example, seem to focus on hospitals, directing attention to managing intensive care unit (ICU) bed and equipment shortages and distributing resources in high-acuity settings. Such plans often call for redeploying workers from community settings to hospital settings. Because many of these workers already work part-time in the community and hospital sectors, this option is appealing. But if workers are shifted from community health care settings to hospitals, people in the community who depend on these workers may become vulnerable from the intervention.

7.10.2 Case Description

It has been 1 week since the World Health Organization officially declared the presence of an influenza pandemic. Person-to-person spread has been confirmed in several Canadian cities, and emergency rooms in your large metropolitan city overflow with influenza patients. Because routine cases usually fill the medical floors and intensive care units to capacity, there is concern that the surge of influenza admissions will overwhelm resources. To set priorities and possibly reallocate resources within the health care system, the regional health authority has called a meeting in anticipation of the surge in admissions. As the lead of the local health emergency management program, you are asked to attend.

A couple of hours before the meeting, you listen to a call on your answering machine from Julia, a friend and the director of the local community care access center (home care agency). This is the largest center in the region, employing 600 and subcontracting 20,000 health and community service workers through other agencies. Professional services that are subcontracted include in-home nursing, occupational therapy, physiotherapy, social work, speech and language therapy, and nutritionists; nonprofessional services include personal support workers and health care aids and attendants who assist with activities of daily living.

Having become aware of the upcoming meeting with the regional health authority, Julia wonders why no one from the community-based organizations that care for people in home settings has been asked to attend. She appreciates the media focus on the available ventilators and ICU beds in local hospitals, but she is concerned with the lack of attention on vulnerable populations in the community. She has heard rumors of plans to reallocate some nursing and personal support workers from community settings to acute care hospitals and asks if officials have considered that such a move may require some people, who normally manage their illness at home, to be hospitalized. Convinced that someone representing the community should attend priority-setting discussions, she urges you to advocate for such a presence.

Thinking on various levels about how you would respond to the message even as you plan for the meeting, you are particularly struck by how such decisions could adversely affect Julia herself. Her multiple sclerosis is serious enough to require the daily assistance of a personal support worker to help her get from home to her office.

7.10.3 Discussion Questions

1. In what ways does this case challenge conventional notions of who might be considered vulnerable during a pandemic?
2. What does Julia's exclusion from the meeting say about the attitude towards vulnerable populations at the administrative level?

3. How might a decision to shift financial and personnel resources from the community to the hospital setting deepen the health and social inequities that many vulnerable populations already face?
4. Would it be fair for Julia to ask her community workers to work more hours because the needs of the community have increased? What if the workers feel safer working away from the gravely ill at the hospital and prefer to increase community work at the expense of hospital work?
5. If the workers remain in their communities with their patients, it could mean they are able to help fewer members of the population than if they attended their shifts at the hospital. What is more important, treating more people or giving priority to the vulnerable or less privileged?
6. Do those who develop pandemic plans have a responsibility to identify people whose vulnerability might increase during a pandemic? If so, how should planners identify these people?
7. The document you received before the meeting indicated that one of the discussion topics will be priority setting, particularly the scarce resource of ventilators. The document proposes that a physical disability should disqualify a person from having access to a ventilator. How do you balance the need for rationing scarce acute care resources, like ventilators, with social justice values that advocate for the respect and consideration of those who are vulnerable due to systematic social disadvantage? How will you discuss this matter with Julia?
8. In light of Julia's message, how would you begin to identify systemic barriers that limit the inclusion of vulnerable populations in planning for a pandemic? How would you involve these populations in determining if barriers exist that may significantly limit their access to essential health services available to other populations during a pandemic?

References

Beauchamp, D.E. 1976. Public health as social justice. *Inquiry* 13(1): 3–14.

Krieger, N., and A.E. Birn. 1998. A vision of social justice as the foundation of public health: Commemorating 150 years of the spirit of 1848. *American Journal of Public Health* 88(11): 1603–1606.

Mastroianni, A.C. 2009. Slipping through the net: Social vulnerability in pandemic planning. *Hastings Center Report* 39(5): 11–12.

University of Toronto Joint Centre for Bioethics. 2005. *Stand on Guard for Thee: Ethical considerations in preparedness planning for pandemic influenza.* http://jcb.utoronto.ca/people/documents/upshur_stand_guard.pdf. Accessed 24 June 2015.

Uscher-Pines, L., P.S. Duggan, J.P. Garoon, R.A. Karron, and R.R. Faden. 2007. Planning for an influenza pandemic: Social justice and disadvantaged groups. *Hastings Center Report* 37(4): 32–39.

Wilson, J. 2009. Justice and the social determinants of health: An overview. *Public Health Ethics* 2(3): 210–213.

World Health Organization (WHO). 2008. *Addressing ethical issues in pandemic influenza planning: Discussion papers*. http://www.who.int/csr/resources/publications/cds_flu_ethics_5web.pdf. Accessed 8 May 2013.

World Health Organization (WHO). 2010. *Pandemic influenza preparedness and response: A WHO guidance document*. http://whqlibdoc.who.int/publications/2009/9789241547680_eng.pdf. Accessed 8 May 2013.

7.11 Case 5: Can Asylum Seeking Be Managed Ethically?

Karin Johansson Blight
The Policy Institute
Kings College London
London, UK
e-mail: karin.johansson_blight@kcl.ac.uk

This case is presented for instructional purposes only. The ideas and opinions expressed are the author's own. The case is not meant to reflect the official position, views, or policies of the editors, the editors' host institutions, or the author's host institution.

7.11.1 Background

Migration is a challenge managed against the backdrop of international accords and the social and historic circumstances peculiar to each country. The 1948 *Universal Declaration of Human Rights* (UDHR) states "everyone has the right to seek and to enjoy in other countries asylum from persecution" (United Nations 1948, Article 14). In 1951, the newly established International Organization for Migration (IOM) began promoting "humane and orderly migration for the benefit of all," affirming that all migration can be managed (IOM 2013). The United Nations (U.N.) estimated 221 million migrants worldwide in 2010 (U.N. 2013). EUROSTAT estimated 1.7 million immigrants, including forced migrants, in the European Union (EU) in 2011 (EUROSTAT 2014).

Sweden, a Nordic country that joined the EU in 1995, has a long tradition of monitoring the health of its residents. For example, its National Institute of Public Health, the National Board of Health and Welfare, and Statistics Sweden monitor public health trends, and a national center monitors suicide and mental illness (the National Centre for Suicide Research and Prevention of Mental Ill-Health). "Health on equal terms" is a political priority in Sweden that aligns with the country's strongly egalitarian and multicultural traditions dating back more than 300 years (Linell et al. 2013; Westin 2000, 2006). However, social contingencies throughout Sweden's history have put pressure on these values and traditions. For example, poor harvests and famine in the mid- to late-1800s triggered extensive emigration, virtually closing borders when emigration ended in the 1930s. In the 1940s, the borders reopened first for refugees from neighboring countries, then, in the 1950s–1960s, for labor immigrants from European countries. From the 1970s onward, the focus shifted to family reunification of migrants and refugees from outside the EU. According to Statistic Sweden's figures from 2012, of its 9.6 million population, about 15 % are foreign born (Statistics Sweden 2013). The Swedish Migration Board (SMB) suggests that 16 % of residencies granted in 2012 were on refugee, protection, humanitarian, or similar grounds (including temporary grounds) (SMB 2014).

The term migration management (MM) was coined in the 1990s, although the MM field originated in the 1950s (Widgren 1994). The rise of MM coincided with a time when several factors, including the mechanisms of colonialism and the Cold War, worked to control and minimize global migration. But other factors also influenced MM, such as resettlements after World War II; efforts to safeguard rights of refugees and migrant workers rights led by international organizations (e.g., the International Labour Organization, the United Nations High Commissioner for Refugees and the International Organization for Migration); and regional initiatives that removed immigration barriers to improve national economies (e.g., the Organisation for Economic Co-operation and Development and the Treaty of Rome). In the mid-1970s to mid-1980s, Western countries jointly attempted to harmonize entry controls, efforts that the third pillar of the EU's 1993 Maastricht Treaty later incorporated (Maastricht Treaty 1992).

Policies enacted since this treaty have focused on deterring unwanted migrants, arguably to the detriment of human rights and refugee protections (Fekete 2001). By 2002, experts suggested that reducing unwanted and unauthorized immigration could increase public support for integration assistance for foreign residents in Western countries (Martin and Widgren 2002). But this focus on reduction had the side effect of criminalizing "unwanted" migrants. By implying that unwanted migrants could pose a national security threat, policy instruments such as the 2006 Schengen Borders Code may have fed xenophobic tendencies (Schengen Borders Code 2010). Article 5 in the code includes, for example, a statement about entry conditions for short-stay, third-country nationals, that they are not "… considered to be a threat to public policy, internal security, public health, or the international relations of any of the Member States." At any rate, such increased deterrence and control measures do restrict access to work, housing, health care, and independent legal advice, and even separates families (Johansson Blight et al. 2009). Not surprisingly, detention policies harm health with disproportionately high rates of poor mental health, suicide, and self-harm amongst detainees (Silove et al. 2000; Cohen 2008). Moreover, evidence suggests that such controls have resulted in the rejection of asylum claims of torture survivors and people with severe health problems (Steel et al. 2006; Migration Court of Appeal 2007; Johansson Blight 2015). The evidence also suggests that controls led to children suffering due to exacerbated vulnerability in detention and to unaccounted deaths of forced migrants at Western country borders (Grewcock 2009; Steel et al. 2011). These injustices prompted repeated appeals to national law, the UDHR, and the Convention on the Rights of the Child and calls for change to relevant World Medical Association (WMA) documents such as the Geneva and Lisbon declarations (Hunt 2007; Bodegård 2014; Johansson Blight 2014; Johansson Blight et al. 2014).

An especially poignant example of the health challenges found among asylum seekers, especially children, is the condition known as pervasive arousal withdrawal syndrome (PAWS) (Bodegård 2014). This condition presents as pervasive loss of functioning and profound social withdrawal and apathy (Söndergaard et al. 2012; Envall 2013; Bodegård 2014; Johansson Blight 2014; Johansson Blight et al. 2014). Few children show signs of severe PAWS upon arrival in Sweden; however, routine data on incidence and prevalence are lacking (Envall 2013). Surveys conducted in the past 10 years have identified anywhere from 30 to 424 children with this condition (Envall 2013). Common predictors include exposure to severe persecution, human rights abuses or other traumatic experiences in the country of origin, and the prospect of deportation to countries with poor human rights records. Other signs of distress include suicide attempts (Johansson Blight 2014). PAWS commonly affects health and functioning gradually, over time rendering a child unresponsive and unable to eat or drink without support, which makes the condition life-threatening. Unfortunately, the required health assessment of asylum seekers is insufficient for detecting PAWS in its early stages (Johansson Blight 2014). Typically, static measures of health (such as the use of yes/no check boxes) are used, and life events such as discrimination, traumatizing episodes, or prolonged stress carry little weight in the health evaluation process requested by the migration authorities. From a health perspective, broader and more culturally appropriate assessments are recommended instead, such as illness narratives, family medical history taking, and recording of past and present social contexts (Bhugra et al. 2010). If adopted, more cases of PAWS could be identified, prevented, and treated. No cases of children dying with PAWS have been reported in Sweden, but there has been no systematic follow-up of children deported from Sweden (Envall 2013).

7.11.2 Case Description

The Swedish Migration Board (SMB), the ultimate authority on deportation of asylum seekers, announced it no longer deports children with PAWS. After this announcement, however, the media reported on a rejected asylum seeker, a 14-year-old Roma girl[1] with the condition, deported with her family to their country of origin (Edquist 2013; Myhrén 2013). During deportation, the girl who had lost all ability to function, was being fed through a feeding tube, and was unresponsive to pain. Upon arrival at their home country, the family was refused entry due to the girl's advanced illness and was eventually forced to return to Sweden.

A family friend in Sweden said that widespread persecution of Roma people in the family's home country had restricted the 14-year-old girl's life. For example, the girl had never attended school because her parents feared she would be ostracized, teased, ridiculed, or even physically hurt. The friend explained that the symptoms of

[1]The Roma people are an ethnic group who trace their origin to the Indian subcontinent, sometimes referred to as gypsies.

severe PAWS began the previous month after Swedish police visited the family's home in Sweden.

According to the SMB, the police who enforced the deportation reported that when they first visited the family, the girl was attending school, and although said to be somewhat shy and withdrawn, she appeared relatively healthy. A routine health assessment of asylum seekers to assess barriers to enforcing deportation found no medical or other reason to impede deportation. This claim conflicted with the statement of a therapist working for a human rights organization, who said he had informed the SMB about the girl's history of discrimination, trauma, and her state of complete function loss, which included her inability to communicate and engage in social interaction. In their defense, police say they followed standard procedures and stand by the initial assessment regarding deportation, which prompted no grounds for halting deportation.

Upon returning to Sweden, the family was detained in an immigration facility, where the father at first was separated from the family. At the time of the media reports, the family had been reunited and was awaiting a new SMB decision on whether they should again be deported.

You are a member of a commission established to decide the outcome of this case and come up with ways to improve the asylum and deportation system. Other members of the commission include medical officers, public health officials, lawyers, and former immigration officials.

7.11.3 Discussion Questions

1. Who are the main stakeholders and organizations in this case? What are their primary interests and obligations?
2. What bearing does vulnerability or increased risk of harm have on public health's obligation to prevent or mitigate harm to an individual? What impact should legal status have on that obligation?
3. What are the goals of the asylum and deportation process, and what are the values that drive these goals? How should these values be prioritized?
4. What decision would you make in this case?
5. Based on your prioritization of values, what recommendations would you make to improve the asylum and deportation system?

References

Bhugra, D., T. Craig, and K. Bhui (eds.). 2010. *Mental health of refugees and asylum seekers*. Oxford: Oxford University Press.

Bodegård, G. 2014. Comment on the paper 'Pervasive Refusal Syndrome (PRS) 21 years on – A reconceptualization and renaming' by Ken Nunn, Bryan Lask and Isabel Owen, invited commentary. *European Child & Adolescent Psychiatry* 23: 179–181.

Cohen, J. 2008. Safe in our hands? A study of suicide and self-harm in asylum seekers. *Journal of Forensic and Legal Medicine* 15(4): 235–244.

Edquist, K. 2013. *Utvisad Apatisk Flicka Tillbaka i Sverige, P4 Dalarna.* (*Deported Girl with Apathy Back in Sweden, P4 Dalarna.*) Sveriges Radio. http://sverigesradio.se/sida/artikel.aspx?programid=161&artikel=5500968. Accessed 2 June 2015.

Envall, E. 2013. *Barn med Uppgivenhetssyndrom, En Vägledning för Personal inom Socialtjänst och Hälso- och Sjukvård.* (*Children with Depressive Devitalisation, Guidance for Social and Health Care Personnel.*) Socialstyrelsen. (The National Board of Health and Welfare.) ISBN 978-91-7555-051-0. http://www.socialstyrelsen.se/publikationer2013/2013-4-5. Accessed 2 June 2015.

EUROSTAT. 2014. *Further Eurostat information, main tables, immigration (TPS00176).* http://epp.eurostat.ec.europa.eu/statistics_explained/index.php/Migration_and_migrant_population_statistics. Accessed 2 June 2015.

Fekete, L. 2001. The emergence of xeno-racism. *Race & Class* 43(2): 23–40.

Grewcock, M. 2009. *Border crimes. Australia's war on illicit migrants*, Sydney Institute of Criminology Series. The Institute of Criminology Series 29. Sydney: Institute of Criminology Press.

Hunt, P. 2007. *Implementation of General Assembly Resolution, 60/251 of 15 March 2006, entitled "Human Rights Council": Report of the Special Rapporteur on the Right of Everyone to the Enjoyment of the Highest Attainable Standard of Physical and Mental Health. Addendum: Mission to Sweden.* District General. Fourth Session, Item 2 of the provisional agenda, A/HRC/4/28/Add.2, 28 February, Human Rights Council, United Nations.

International Organization for Migration (IOM). 2013. *About IOM.* http://www.iom.int/about-iom. Accessed 29 May 2015.

Johansson Blight, K. 2014. Medical doctors commissioned by institutions that regulate and control migration in Sweden: Implications for public health ethics, policy and practice. *Public Health Ethics* 7(3): 239–252. (First published online August 8, 2014. doi:10.1093/phe/phu020).

Johansson Blight, K. 2015. Questioning fairness in Swedish asylum decisions. *State Crime* 4(1): 52–76.

Johansson Blight, K., S. Ekblad, F. Lindencrona, and S. Shahnavaz. 2009. Promoting mental health and preventing mental disorder among refugees in Western Countries. *International Journal of Mental Health Promotion* 11(1): 32–44.

Johansson Blight, K., E. Hultcrantz, A. D'Orazio, and H.P. Søndergaard. 2014. The role of the health care services in the asylum process. In *Nordic work with traumatised refugees: Do we really care*, ed. G. Overland, E. Guribye, and B. Lie, 300–315. Newcastle upon Tyne: Cambridge Scholars Publishing. ISBN (13): 978-1-4438-6136-6.

Linell, A., M.X. Richardson, and S. Wamala. 2013. The Swedish national public health policy report 2010. *Scandinavian Journal of Public Health* 41(suppl 10): 3–56.

Maastricht Treaty. 1992. *The Maastricht Treaty: Final Act and Declarations.* http://www.eurotreaties.com/maastrichtext.html. Accessed 2 June 2015.

Martin, P., and J. Widgren. 2002. International migration: Facing the challenge. *Population Bulletin* 57(1). Washington, DC: Population Reference Bureau.

Migration Court of Appeal. 2007. *Domstol: Migrationsöverdomstolen, Avgörandedatum 2007-06-25.* (Court: Migration Court of Appeal, Date of Deliberation: 2007-06-25.) Lagen.nu. https://lagen.nu/dom/mig/2007:35. Accessed 2 June 2015.

Myhrén, L. 2013. *Avvisad Flicka Skickades Tillbaka: "För Sjuk." Nyheter.* (*Deported Girl Was Sent Back: "Too ill."* News.), Ekot, Sveriges radio. http://sverigesradio.se/sida/artikel.aspx?programid=83&artikel=5502575. Accessed 2 June 2015.

Schengen Borders Code. 2010. *Schengen Borders Code*, ACT. Regulation (EC) No 562/2006 of the European Parliament. http://europa.eu/legislation_summaries/justice_freedom_security/free_movement_of_persons_asylum_immigration/l14514_en.htm. Accessed 2 June 2015.

Silove, D., Z. Steel, and C. Watters. 2000. Policies of deterrence and the mental health of asylum seekers. *Journal of the American Medical Association* 284(5): 604–611.

Söndergaard, H.P., M.M. Kushnir, B. Aronsson, P. Sandstedt, and J. Bergquist. 2012. Patterns of endogenous steroids in apathetic refugee children are compatible with long-term stress. *BMC Research Notes* 5: 186.

Statistics Sweden. 2013. *Summary of population statistics 1960–2012*. Statistics Sweden. http://www.scb.se/en/. Accessed 2 June 2015.

Steel, Z., D. Silove, R. Brooks, S. Momartin, B. Alzuhairi, and I. Susljik. 2006. Impact of immigration detention and temporary protection on the mental health of refugees. *The British Journal of Psychiatry* 188(1): 58–64.

Steel, Z., B.J. Liddell, C.R. Bateman-Steel, and A.B. Zwi. 2011. Global protection and the health impact of migration interception. *PLoS Medicine* 8(6): e1001038.

Swedish Migration Board (SMB). 2014. *Översikt av Beviljade Arbets—och Uppehållstillståndåren 2005–2014 (Förstagångstillstånd)*. (*Granted Work—and Resident Permits Year 2005–2014 [First Time Permissions]*.) http://www.migrationsverket.se/info/793.html. Accessed 2 June 2015.

United Nations (U.N.). 1948. *The universal declaration of human rights*. http://www.un.org/en/documents/udhr/index.shtml. Accessed 2 June 2015.

United Nations, Department of Economic and Social Affairs, Population Division. 2013. *Trends in international migrant stock: The 2013 revision – Migrants by destination and origin*. (United Nations database, POP/DB/MIG/Stock/Rev.2013/Origin).

Westin, C. 2000. *The effectiveness of settlement and integration policies towards immigrants and their descendants in Sweden*, International Migration Papers, 34. Geneva: Migration Branch, International Labour Office.

Westin, C. 2006. Sweden: Restrictive immigration policy and multiculturalism. *Migration Information Source: The Online Journal of the Migration Policy Institute*. http://www.migrationinformation.org/usfocus/display.cfm?ID=406. Accessed 2 June 2015.

Widgren, J. 1994. *Multilateral co-operation to combat trafficking in migrants and the role of international organizations*. Paper presented at the eleventh seminar of the IOM on International Response to Trafficking in Migrants and the Safeguarding of Migrant Rights, Geneva, 26–28 October.

7.12 Case 6: Tuberculosis Screening, Testing, and Treatment among Asylum Seekers

Christopher W. McDougall
Institute of Health Policy, Management and Evaluation,
and Joint Centre for Bioethics
University of Toronto
Toronto, ON, Canada
e-mail: christopher.mcdougall@utoronto.ca

This case is presented for instructional purposes only. The ideas and opinions expressed are the author's own. The case is not meant to reflect the official position, views, or policies of the editors, the editors' host institutions, or the author's host institution.

7.12.1 Background

Tuberculosis (TB), an airborne transmissible bacterial infection that most commonly affects the lungs, has been dubbed "the greatest killer in history" and one of "humankind's worst enemies" (Selgelid 2008). TB is typically contracted after prolonged close exposure to the coughing and sneezing of people with active infections.

Although only 5–10 % of people who are infected (but who are not HIV positive) become sick or infectious at some point during their lives, untreated TB kills about two-thirds of those it does infect, despite the availability of effective medicines since the 1950s (World Health Organization [WHO] 2012). Since 1995, the WHO standard for treatment has been directly observed therapy, short-course (DOTS), which involves people watching patients swallowing their pills. Treatments delivered through DOTS are inexpensive and 95 % effective, although 6–9 months may be required to cure ordinary active or latent strains of the infection (Minion et al. 2013).

Inconsistent or partial treatment—when patients do not take their medicines regularly for the required period because they start to feel better, because doctors and health workers prescribe the wrong treatment regimens, or because drug supply is unavailable due to cost or unreliable due to lack of regulation—has led to TB strains that resist one or more first-line drugs (i.e., those most effective and least likely to cause adverse side effects). Drug-resistant TB has been documented in every country surveyed (WHO 2012). A particularly dangerous form of drug-resistant TB is multidrug-resistant TB (MDR-TB), defined as the disease caused by TB bacilli resistant to at least isoniazid and rifampicin, the two standard anti-TB drugs. Curing MDR strains of the bacteria is much less effective (with a 30–40 % failure rate in Canada, slightly better than the global average of 52 %, according to Minion et al. 2013), costs much more, produces reactions that diminish compliance, and may take as long as 20–24 months (Public Health Agency of Canada. 2014). MDR-TB accounts for 1.2 % of all TB cases in Canada, for example, and typically costs five times as much ($250,000 vs $47,290 per patient) (Public Health Agency of Canada 2014; Menzies et al. 2008).

TB has retained dramatically high levels of incidence, prevalence, and morbidity and mortality worldwide, especially in developing countries, because social, political, and economic factors (rather than simply biological ones) play key roles in infectious disease patterns. Recent global estimates put the numbers at 15 million active, and perhaps 2 billion latent (asymptomatic) infections, with 9 million new infections yearly, and 1.5 to 2 million deaths per year (95 % of which occur in sub-Saharan Africa and Asia) (WHO 2012). TB is the world's leading cause of preventable death among young adults, and the leading cause of death among those who are HIV positive, since the infection tends to affect and progress quickly in those whose immune systems are compromised by other conditions, particularly HIV but also measles, malaria, or alcoholism. TB is thus often referred to as a "classic social disease" and a "disease of poverty" because of its association with overcrowding, malnutrition, stress, destitution, and rapid social change. TB has also been dubbed the forgotten plague because it rarely affects the wealthy, who are largely insulated from exposure (Kim et al. 2005; Ryan 1993). Thus, although TB was extremely common in eighteenth- and nineteenth-century England throughout the industrial revolution, infection rates declined substantially when housing, sanitation, nutrition, and labor conditions improved and endemic infections all but disappeared in developed countries well before effective drugs were widely available (Selgelid 2008).

TB, though relatively uncommon in Canada today with around 1,600 cases reported annually, is costly ($58 million in direct costs, and $74 million total related expenditure, in Canada in 2004) (Menzies et al. 2008), frequently results in hospital admission, and retains an 11 % mortality rate (Greenaway et al. 2011). Foreign-born persons account for 65 % of active TB, although they make up only 20 % of the population. Up to half of recent immigrants and refugees to Canada are estimated to harbor latent TB and are thus at risk of progressing to active infection, and TB in refugee populations is about double that in other classes of immigrant populations (Greenaway et al. 2011). Those most at risk domestically are the urban homeless and aboriginal communities, followed by residents of long-term care and correctional facilities, and then the staff who work in such institutions (Public Health Agency of Canada 2014).

The cornerstone of TB ethics, according to the WHO, is the protection of individuals and communities through the proper treatment of infected individuals (active and latent) and the prevention of new infections. These goals are said to rely on the promotion of key values including social justice and equity, solidarity, the common good, autonomy, reciprocity, effectiveness, subsidiarity, participation, and transparency and accountability (WHO 2010). The WHO also stresses, in cases where involuntary isolation or detention measures are implemented, the importance of using the least restrictive means necessary to achieve public health goals, as set forth in the Siracusa Principles. These principles require states to ensure that such interventions are proportional to the risk of public harm, necessary and relevant to protecting the public good, and applied without discrimination (WHO 2010).

7.12.2 Case Description

On a chilly gray autumn morning, Canadian Coast Guard officials take into custody 77 people (66 men, and 11 boys between 8 and 16 years of age) after their vessel, suspected to have been abandoned by human smugglers, is found adrift off the northwest Pacific coast. All immediately claim refugee status and are transferred to a provincial prison, the nearest facility judged sufficiently secure to detain them, review their claims, and physically examine them per immigration procedures. Overcrowding at the criminal correction center, already an issue, becomes severe with the addition of these individuals, many of whom are housed four or five to cells designed for only two people, and often in portable trailers parked in the prison yard. The asylum seekers are subject to the same institutional rules as criminal detainees: they must wear prison uniforms and are significantly restricted in making or receiving telephone calls (Nakache 2011). The federal Refugee Protection Division and provincial health authorities jointly appoint you as a member of an ad hoc local public health unit task force responding to the situation.

Canadian immigration law requires asylum seekers in the country to undergo a medical examination, including screening to assess potential burden of illness, linked to ongoing surveillance or clinical actions only for TB, syphilis, and HIV (Gushulak et al. 2011; Gardam et al. 2014). Within 48 h, medical examinations and chest X-ray results suggest active TB in four of the new detainees: two adults and two brothers ages 6 and 11. Based on their overall health conditions and patient histories (to the extent that these can be verifiably ascertained under the circumstances) and TB epidemiology in the region of origin, the medical team strongly suspects all four to be infected with MDR-TB, and cultures are thus ordered. The tests will take 2 weeks before results can confirm the presence of drug-resistant strains (6 weeks are needed to confirm negative cultures).

The Canadian Immigration and Refugee Protection Act (IRPA) (Government of Canada 2001) and accompanying regulations (Government of Canada 2013) stipulate that people likely to be a danger to public health or a "public charge" (defined as likely to make excessive demands on health or social services but likely unable or unwilling to support themselves) may be deemed inadmissible for refugee status. However, considerable discretionary power, particularly for children and others in need of protection, is built into the law and related regulations, and initial decisions by immigration officers are generally subject to appeal (Bailey et al. 2005; Greenaway et al. 2011). Section 249 of the IRPA regulations, moreover, sets out special requirements for minor refugee claimants, including the duty to consider the availability of local childcare arrangements, of segregated spaces in detention centers, and of education, counseling, and recreational services (Government of Canada 2013).

7.12.3 Discussion Questions

1. Although all 77 refugee claimants have been screened for TB, they have not been tested for TB. Given the journey and conditions just endured by this group on board the cramped vessel, should the task force advise local public health authorities to test all claimants for active or latent TB? Why or why not?
2. What recommendations should the task force make concerning ongoing detainment conditions? What information should be provided to the current residents and staff of the regional corrections center?
3. Given the clinicians' conclusions, should second-line TB treatment be immediately offered to the four affected refugees? If they refuse treatment, should treatment be compelled? How and why?
4. When news breaks locally of the TB status of the two young brothers, community leaders of the same ethnic background offer to shelter the boys and oversee their treatment. Discuss the relevance of the principle of "least restrictive means" to such a scenario, and indicate when or whether local public health authorities should consider community care and support approaches to MDR-TB treatment.
5. Three months into their detainment, the claims of several refugees are rejected. Hunger strikes and violence among the detainees ensue. How should the task force respond?
6. Consider a scenario in which the status of one of the two adults suspected of being infected by MDR-TB is subsequently confirmed and the patient is denied refugee status as well. What are the costs and risks of the repatriation of MDR-TB cases

compared with standard TB cases? Do the task force, public health authorities, and provincial or federal authorities have any obligations under such a scenario?
7. How should the goals of public health and those of immigration policy be balanced?

References

Bailey, T., T. Caulfield, and N. Ries (eds.). 2005. *Public health law and policy in Canada.* Markham: LexisNexis Canada.

Gardam, M., M. Creatore, and R. Deber. 2014. Danger at the gates? Screening for tuberculosis in immigrants and refugees. In *Case studies in Canadian health policy and management*, 2nd ed, ed. R.B. Deber and C.L. Mah. Toronto: University of Toronto Press.

Government of Canada. 2001. *Immigration and Refugee Protection Act.* (S.C. 2001, c. 27). http://laws.justice.gc.ca/eng/acts/i-2.5/. Accessed 22 Jan 2014.

Government of Canada. 2013. *Immigration and Refugee Protection Regulations.* (SOR/2002-227). http://laws-lois.justice.gc.ca/eng/regulations/SOR-2002-227/. Accessed 22 Jan 2014.

Greenaway, C., A. Sandoe, B. Vissandjee, et al. 2011. Tuberculosis: Evidence review for newly arriving immigrants and refugees. *Canadian Medical Association Journal* 183(12): E939–E951. doi:10.1503/cmaj.090302.

Gushulak, B.D., K. Pottie, J. Hatcher Roberts, et al. 2011. Migration and health in Canada: Health in the global village. *Canadian Medical Association Journal* 183(12): E952–E958. doi:10.1503/cmaj.090287.

Kim, J.Y., A. Shakow, K. Mate, et al. 2005. Limited good and limited vision: Multidrug-resistant tuberculosis and global health policy. *Social Science & Medicine* 61: 847–859.

Menzies, D., M. Lewis, and O. Oxlade. 2008. Costs for tuberculosis care in Canada. *Canadian Journal of Public Health* 99(5): 391–396.

Minion, J., V. Gallant, J. Wolfe, F. Jamieson, and R. Long. 2013. Multidrug and extensively drugresistant tuberculosis in Canada 1997–2008: Demographic and disease characteristics. *PLoS ONE* 8(1): e53466. doi:10.1371/journal.pone.0053466.

Nakache, D. 2011. *The human and financial cost of detention of asylum-seekers in Canada.* UN High Commissioner for Refugees commissioned report. http://www.socialsciences.uottawa.ca/sites/default/files/public/dvm/eng/documents/dnakache-finalreport-december2011.pdf. Accessed 3 June 2013.

Public Health Agency of Canada. 2014. *Canadian tuberculosis standards*, 7th ed. Ottawa: Minister of Public Works and Government Services Canada. http://strauss.ca/OEMAC/wpcontent/uploads/2013/11/Canadian_TB_Standards_7th-edition_English.pdf. Accessed 9 June 2015.

Ryan, F. 1993. *The forgotten plague: How the battle against tuberculosis was won—And lost.* Boston: Little, Brown.

Selgelid, M. 2008. Ethics, tuberculosis and globalization. *Public Health Ethics* 1(1): 10–20.

World Health Organization (WHO). 2010. *Guidance on ethics of TB prevention, care and control.* Geneva: World Health Organization. http://whqlibdoc.who.int/publications/2010/9789241500531_eng.pdf. Accessed 3 June 2013.

World Health Organization (WHO). 2012. *Tuberculosis, Fact Sheet No. 104.* Geneva: World Health Organization. http://www.who.int/mediacentre/factsheets/fs104/en/index.html. Accessed 3 June 2013.

Chapter 8
International Collaboration for Global Public Health

Eric M. Meslin and Ibrahim Garba

8.1 Introduction

There is a long tradition of global collaboration in biomedicine and public health. Examples range from medical outposts in rural communities run by foreign missionaries (Good 1991) to the early infectious disease programs of the Rockefeller Foundation (Fosdick 1989) and from medical services and training programs for indigenous populations set up by colonial authorities (Marks 1997) to the Pan American Health Organization (PAHO) established by a collective of sovereign governments (Cueto 2007).

Two complementary sets of factors provide context for understanding collaboration in global public health: first, the factors that inform globalization generally and global *health* specifically; second, the factors that shape ethical standards for global health programs generally and global health *research* specifically. Good examples of both factors are reflected in this chapter's case studies.

The opinions, findings, and conclusions of the authors do not necessarily reflect the official position, views, or policies of the editors, the editors' host institutions, or the authors' host institutions.

E.M. Meslin, PhD (✉)
Indiana University Center for Bioethics, Indianapolis, IN, USA
e-mail: emeslin@iu.edu

I. Garba, MA, JD, LLM
Indiana University Center for Bioethics, Indianapolis, IN, USA

Public Health Law Program, Office of State, Tribal, Local, and Territorial Support,
Centers for Disease Control and Prevention, Atlanta, GA, USA

D.H. Barrett et al. (eds.), *Public Health Ethics: Cases Spanning the Globe*,
Public Health Ethics Analysis 3, DOI 10.1007/978-3-319-23847-0_8

8.2 The Rise of Globalization and Global Health

Collaboration in global health, as we know it today, began taking shape after World War II when new laws and institutions were established to govern relations among countries. The war's end was marked by efforts to establish a body that would facilitate peaceful relations among member countries. In 1945, the United Nations (U.N.) was established "to save succeeding generations from the scourge of war" and to "promote social progress and better standards of life" (U.N. 1945). Various U.N. agencies were set up to realize these goals—most prominently the World Health Organization (WHO), founded in 1948 "to act as the directing and coordinating authority on international health work" (WHO 1948).[1] Yet even as these institutions were being established, their ability to encourage international collaboration was hampered in two ways.

First, most low- and middle-income countries (LMICs), which bear the bulk of today's global disease burden, were under colonial rule for the first decade of the U.N.'s existence. Hence, these countries were unrepresented in the new organization. In later years, the principle of self-determination (i.e., the right of "peoples" to govern themselves and choose their developmental priorities) and the efforts of nationalist movements secured political independence and membership in the international community. In effect, the governments of these countries were authorized under international law to represent their populations in relations with other governments, thereby enabling equitable partnerships, even in matters of health.

Second, the escalation of the Cold War in the founding years of the U.N. introduced ideological rivalries into its workings. These rivalries often impeded coordinated actions involving health. For example, the 1950s and 1960s were marked by the superpowers' competitive attempts to eradicate specific (often communicable) diseases (e.g., the United States targeted malaria while the Soviet Union focused on smallpox) (WHO 2008b). This selective, disease-specific vertical approach conflicted with the realization in the 1970s that primary health care was a vital component of a national health system. The latter approach defined "health" broadly, recognizing it as a right and acknowledging the impact of socioeconomic factors on wellness (WHO 1978). The emphasis on primary health care became critical for governments of newly independent countries faced with the task of expanding health systems that under colonial rule had catered to a narrow, privileged segment of the population (WHO 2008a). However, ideological disputes over government's role in society and the policies of the International Monetary Fund (IMF), which favored privatization of certain public services (Stuckler and Basu 2009), neglected the primary health care approach (WHO 2008b). The Cold War also influenced patterns of global health collaboration, particularly among members of feuding coalitions that continued to support ideologic allies (Feldbaum et al. 2010).

[1] Other U.N.-affiliated agencies not directly related to health but influencing collaboration in public health include the International Monetary Fund, World Bank, and World Trade Organization.

The fall of the Berlin Wall in 1989 and the collapse of the Soviet Union shortly thereafter marked the end of the Cold War. These events led more countries to adopt liberal and capitalist principles. Other developments—advances in communications (most notably, the Internet) and greater trade and travel across borders—intensified exchanges among national communities. Collectively referred to as *the process of globalization*,[2] these changes altered the global context for public health collaboration.

On the one hand, the absence of a drawn-out ideological battle led to constructive deliberation and global action in public health. For example, in 2000, all members of the U.N. General Assembly declared their commitment to achieving eight objectives (the Millennium Development Goals) by 2015—half of which pertained to health. Also significant were widespread efforts to address the HIV/AIDS epidemic through such mechanisms as the Joint United Nations Programme on HIV/AIDS (UNAIDS)[3] and the more recently established Global Fund to Fight AIDS, Tuberculosis and Malaria.[4]

On the other hand, the growing influence of liberal and capitalist principles in the global environment of the 1990s affected the extent to which governments (especially those of LMICs) were involved and able to collaborate in public health. These changes included

> … an increasing reliance upon the free market; a significant growth in the influence of international financial markets and institutions in determining national policies; cutbacks in public sector spending; the privatization of functions previously considered to be the exclusive domain of the state; and the deregulation of a range of activities with a view to facilitating investment and rewarding entrepreneurial initiative. These trends serve to reduce the role of the state in economic affairs, and at the same time increase the role and responsibilities of private (non-state) actors, especially those in corporate business, but also those in civil society…. (WHO 2002)

Generally associated with neoliberal principles, the changes discussed above have reduced governments' public policy role. These developments notwithstanding, there remain compelling arguments for deliberate and sustained engagement by governments in the interest of global public health. Three are discussed below.

8.2.1 Collective Health

The first argument is that even with their reduced profile in national health systems, governments continue to bear primary responsibility for population health. Individual citizens can take responsibility for personal health, but certain health

---

[2] Definitions of globalization vary by disciplinary focus. Richard Labonté (2004) describes globalization as "a process by which nations, businesses, and people are becoming more connected and interdependent across the globe through increased economic integration and communication exchange, cultural diffusion (especially of Western culture), and travel."

[3] See http://www.unaids.org/en/

[4] See http://www.theglobalfund.org/en/

benefits (e.g., clean air, safe roads, potable water) can be secured only through organized, collective efforts generally involving the exercise of public authority. As such, in the interest of global health, a country's public health institutions should be robust—equipped to protect population health, reduce disease, and administer programs that save money and lives (Frieden and Koplan 2010). This case needs to be made for LMICs especially; otherwise, neoliberal principles guiding globalization may further weaken emergent, poorly governed, or underfunded health systems.

Indeed, the exercise (or failure) of public authority influence all ethical issues presented by the cases in this chapter. In Jensen and Gaie's case, an LMIC government has neither passed legislation nor provided support that would effectively prevent discrimination against citizens seeking HIV services. In Zinner's case, an international aid worker must make difficult decisions about who gets preventive HIV/AIDS treatment in an African community characterized by a neglected, poorly funded health system. In Timms' case, a physician encounters an ethical challenge brought about by the underdeveloped health infrastructure in India, the government's lax enforcement of research regulations, and the substantial influence of large foreign pharmaceutical companies on national policy. In List and Boyd's case, a foreign researcher must decide whether there is an ethical obligation to expose an African government's avoidable failure to prevent a TB medication stock-out. Under question in Millum's case is the degree to which both the U.N. (as a collective body of governments carrying out a humanitarian intervention) and the Haitian government (as the provider of health infrastructure for its citizens) can be held morally or legally liable for a cholera outbreak. In Al-Faisal, Hussain, and Sen's case, a public health expert testifying before a U.N. Commission must weigh in on the extent to which (1) foreign governments are obliged to minimize harm to the health of Syrians and Iraqis when applying sanctions and (2) Syrian and Iraqi governments are obliged to conduct a foreign policy that does not jeopardize the health of their citizens. A U.S.-based researcher grapples in Lee, Kleinfeld, and Glassford's case with the question of whether she can ethically justify publishing a paper based on data obtained from two African countries whose governments have neither institutional review boards nor national research guidelines.

8.2.2 Coordination

The second argument favoring active engagement of governments in national health systems is their longstanding ability to enter binding legal agreements with each other and other stakeholders. A government's continued involvement is indispensable to shaping broad-based and sustainable solutions to the challenges of global public health. The broad scope of a government's responsibilities (and authority associated with performing these responsibilities) enables it to coordinate public health efforts involving public, private, and civic institutions. The importance of governmental involvement was crystallized in the words of former WHO Director General, Gro Harlem Brundtland, as the 2003 WHO Framework Convention on

Tobacco Control was being drafted: "Tobacco control cannot succeed solely through the efforts of individual governments, national NGOs (nongovernmental organizations), and media advocates. We need an international response to an international problem" (Bodansky 1999). Tackling one of the world's leading causes of preventable death (i.e., smoking), the Framework Convention adopts a comprehensive strategy that has been signed by the governments of 168 countries.[5]

With completion of the human genome and development of various technologies to use it, interest in DNA repositories has surged (Kaye et al. 2009). The development and increasing use of biorepositories of DNA, tissues, and other biological materials in institutions worldwide present far-reaching ethical challenges. Some challenges, such as those resulting from the collection and use of dried blood spots (Hendrix et al. 2013) or from regular surveillance like the U.S. Centers for Disease Control and Prevention (CDC) HIV surveillance projects, are recurrent and familiar.[6] When specimens must be shared in the context of collaborative public health emergency response and planning, the challenges can take on greater urgency. Such emergency collaborative sharing has occurred with virus strains for pandemic influenza planning[7] and with the sequencing of the SARS coronavirus jointly undertaken by researchers from Canada, Hong Kong, Taipei, the United States, and Vietnam during the global outbreak (Tong et al. 2004). Similarly, the sharing of data and health information has long been a source of ethical and legal commentary and is widely viewed as desirable ethical behavior with demonstrable scientific benefit (Committee on National Statistics 1985; Benkler and Nissenbaum 2006).

8.2.3 *Accountability*

The third argument supporting government engagement in global public health is based on democratic theory. Put simply, a country's citizens can hold their governments accountable for failure to meet health commitments. In contrast to governments that are accountable to their entire populations, NGO stakeholders in global health answer to narrower constituencies (i.e., corporations to their stockholders, NGOs to their funders, and foreign health organizations to their home governments). Because public health is of general concern, a level of accountability is essential for the entire health system to function properly. The involvement of governments is, therefore, critical both to ensure the widest participation possible in formulating health policies and to sustain such policies despite shifting interests or diminishing profits of partners.

Setting aside the issue of relative advantages or demerits, the diminished role of governments in global public health—especially governments of LMICs—creates

[5] See http://www.who.int/fctc/signatories_parties/en/index.html

[6] See http://www.cdph.ca.gov/programs/aids/Pages/TOASurv.aspx

[7] See http://www.ip-watch.org/2013/05/27/world-health-assembly-pandemic-flu-framework-clears-committee/

room for others to enter the field. Entrants include public institutions (e.g., international intergovernmental bodies, governments of emerging economies); NGOs (e.g., development and relief agencies, academic health partnerships, faith-based initiatives); private entities (e.g., corporations, philanthropies, individuals); and hybrid entities that pool resources and expertise from public, nongovernmental, and private stakeholders (e.g., The Global Fund to Fight AIDS, Tuberculosis and Malaria). Each entrant to the global health environment plays a unique role. Some take direct action by providing care, some facilitate and leverage the work of others, and some effect change in policies to cultivate better and closer collaboration. All undertake some form of partnership activity.

Essentially, rather than being merely an instrument of foreign policy and diplomacy or a means to technical aid between governments, collaboration in health has grown into a global endeavor involving many actors and stakeholders (Elmendorf 2010). The declining role of governments in public policy presents special challenges for global public health, and the proliferation of stakeholders makes the formation of partnerships more demanding and critical. As such, effective ethical frameworks that can serve as guides for planning and also as arbiters between competing values are indispensable.

8.3 Ethics Frameworks for Global Health

Complementing this political history has been an equally comprehensive set of approaches, each of which provides a moral foundation for defending actions, policies, and decisions in global health. Foremost among these are principle-based approaches, human-rights frameworks, and social determinants of health (SDH), although other approaches have been suggested (Ruger 2009).

8.3.1 Principles and Benchmarks

The debate arising from the 1997 AIDS Clinical Trial Group Study 076 (ACTG-076) to reduce maternal–fetal transmission of HIV served many purposes. Among the most useful was the attention focused on how ethical arguments are applied to substantive problems in global health (Lurie and Wolfe 1997; Varmus and Satcher 1997). Until then, most bioethical reflection had concentrated on domestic topics, aside from revisions to the *Declaration of Helsinki* and other documents. ACTG-076, however, energized discussion about, among other things, the nature of ethical obligations and commitments to groups, countries, and regions—whether of researchers to research participants, of science to society, or sponsors to host countries (Shapiro and Meslin 2001). Accusations of parachute research and double standards abounded, leading many to rethink the applicability of accepted ethical principles and practices and to consider new contexts. They also questioned whether researchers, sponsors, or governments owed any continuing obligation of care to research participants at the end of a study. The bioethics principles developed over three decades by Beauchamp and Childress (2009) provided a formidable foundation upon which debates about research and health care could be played out—even in the face of critiques about their adequacy and sufficiency as moral theory (Clauser and Gert 1990). Other principles have been recommended by scholars (Lavery et al. 2007) and organizations (United Nations Educational, Scientific and Cultural Organization [UNESCO] 2005), but even proponents of principle-based approaches recognized that more was needed to meet challenges in emerging areas of science (e.g., public health genomics and transborder studies) (Lavery et al. 2007; Emanuel et al. 2008; Macklin 2008).

Indeed, early in the tenure of the National Bioethics Advisory Commission (NBAC) that later reported on the ethics of clinical trials (NBAC 2001), Ezekiel Emanuel proposed that the Commission review the *Belmont Report* principles. He urged the Commission to adopt a new principle to its canon of bioethics, namely a principle of *community* to accommodate ethical issues arising from the recruitment of groups. Although the Commission did not adopt this principle, Emanuel's proposal has since emerged as one of several benchmarks for assessing ethical acceptability of clinical research in developing countries (Emanuel et al. 2004). More relevantly, the concept of community engagement and participation has taken on a greater role in discussions about the importance of partnerships.

The cases by Timms and by Lee, Kleinfeld, and Glassford illustrate the utility of using ethical principles to frame the unique challenges of global collaboration in biomedical research. Timms raises a critical issue about whether a multinational pharmaceutical company conducting clinical trials in an LMIC is responsible for harms sustained by research participants during its investigations. The ACTG-076 debate has broadened the question of accountability, recognizing that impoverished and poorly educated populations living with underdeveloped regulatory, health, and social service infrastructures must prompt reassessment of a multinational trial sponsor's ethical obligations. Such reassessment has focused, naturally, on measures that prevent exploitation of vulnerable and desperate individuals in LMICs (e.g., appropriate informed consent, vigilant recruitment practices). But it has also raised the question of whether foreign sponsors and researchers have an ethical obligation to the host community or country supplying the large and diverse recruitment pool at comparatively lower cost.

In the case described by Lee, Kleinfeld, and Glassford, a researcher must determine, apart from questions of scientific validity and potential health utility, whether proper informed consent was obtained in the acquisition of data and tissue samples being used for research on which she has been invited to collaborate. These data and specimens were gathered using various consent methods from six African countries, none of which had ethics review boards or national research guidelines. Her collaborator assures her that the consent modalities applied, though varying widely, were appropriate to the settings in which they were used. In deciding whether to coauthor an article based on acquired data, the researcher must consider how (or whether) the requirements of informed consent, a foundational principle of ethical research, can be met in different global settings, particularly those characterized by cultural or linguistic differences, low health literacy, and absence of regulatory infrastructure.

8.3.2 Human Rights

Human rights constitute a compelling ethical framework for global collaboration. Based on an ethical vision discernable in early Greco-Roman writings, these principles matured in the work of such social contract theorists as Thomas Hobbes, Jean-Jacques Rousseau, and John Locke. The modern view of human rights presupposes that all persons, simply for being human, have inherent dignity. This dignity constitutes the normative foundation for people having certain inalienable rights. The terms *inherent* and *inalienable* mean such dignity and rights belong to people naturally and are, certainly, *not bestowed* by a political authority. According to human rights theory, a political authority has no ethical basis for arbitrarily depriving individuals of these rights (not having granted such rights in the first place). But because some needs are common and not all goals can be met individually, people choose to surrender certain rights to a public authority established to ensure these ends are realized. Hence, a government

> … exists to ensure the well-being of the individuals who give up certain rights in exchange for certain protections and benefits […]. The same applies to the community they jointly establish. From this analysis, the traditional roles of government include such things as collective security, the administration of justice, the protection of property and […] the promotion of the public's health…. (Meslin and Garba 2011)

This theoretical sketch provides a backdrop to the 1948 U.N. *Universal Declaration of Human Rights* (UDHR), the ethical cornerstone of the human rights system since the end of World War II. Using human dignity as its starting point, the UDHR codifies a unified ethical vision for preserving a peaceful and just international order while also emphasizing "social progress and better standards of life" (U.N. 1948). Correspondingly, the UDHR contains rights that are broadly political (e.g., fair trial, free speech, freedom of religion) and others that focus on economic and social conditions (e.g., housing, education, health).

As discussed previously, however, the Cold War introduced ideological rivalries into the U.N., rifts that split the unified ethical vision of the UDHR into two treaties: the International Covenant on Civil and Political Rights (ICCPR) (U.N. 1966a) and the International Covenant on Economic, Social and Cultural Rights (ICESCR) (U.N. 1966b).[8] The two treaties reflected the priorities of the opposing sides—the ICCPR advocated by the U.S.-led capitalist alliance and the ICESCR championed by the U.S.S.R.-led communist bloc. Having two treaties hindered the deployment of human rights as an effective ethical framework for health collaboration during the latter half of the twentieth century.

---

[8] Article 12 of the ICESCR codifies the right to health.

As the Cold War abated, the global community adopted a more holistic approach to human rights, including the right to health. This was captured in the 1993 U.N. Vienna Declaration and Programme of Action, a document that reaffirmed human rights as "universal, indivisible, and interdependent and interrelated" (U.N. 1993). The Vienna Declaration laid the foundation for the creation of the Office the United Nations High Commissioner for Human Rights (OHCHR), an agency that oversees the promotion and protection of human rights throughout the U.N. system. Moreover, the U.N. Human Rights Council (HRC),[9] through its special procedures, appoints independent experts (or "special rapporteurs")[10] to report on areas of concern, including such health-related themes as food, physical and mental health, adequate housing and extreme poverty, and healthy and sustainable environments.[11] As noted previously, this holistic approach was also reflected in the adoption of the Millennium Development Goals (most of which are related to health) and exemplified in the coordinated approach to tackling HIV/AIDS. The health and human rights movement, which gained traction during the global discussion on sexual and reproductive health, firmly took root once health professionals responded to the peculiar challenges of treating HIV-positive people facing discrimination (Gruskin et al. 2007; Mann 1997).

Quite apart from the scarcity of fiscal resources that often plague LMIC governments, other challenges preclude adopting an integrated approach to the right to health. For example, a long-standing argument is that the right to health as codified in the International Covenant on Economic, Social and Cultural Rights attaches to individuals and is, hence, unsuited for effectively achieving public health objectives, goals that by definition focus on population health (Meier 2006). In addition, the proliferation of non-state actors in global health mentioned earlier (e.g., relief agencies, academic health partnerships, corporations, philanthropies) make coordination and accountability about the right to health more demanding. By and large, governments are the sole entities authorized to sign health-related human rights treaties such as the ICESCR. International treaties typically have mechanisms for ensuring that signatories fulfill legal commitments. But as discussed earlier, the diminishing role of governments in national policy and the increasing privatization of public services under globalization (WHO 2002) mean that treaty law will likely play a correspondingly smaller role in global health collaboration. Although the influx of new non-state actors allows stakeholders to partner in innovative ways to address challenges in global health, the stability and accountability of international human rights law remains a valuable asset in a constantly evolving field.

Most cases in this chapter feature ethical issues that are illuminated but sometimes complicated by the human rights framework. In Jensen and Gaie's case, human rights potentially impede a public health strategy for controlling the spread of HIV/AIDS. The case calls for a public health official to balance the human rights

[9] Until 2006, the U.N. Commission on Human Rights

[10] The Human Rights Council also uses working groups.

[11] For special procedures of the Human Rights Council, see http://www.ohchr.org/EN/HRBodies/SP/Pages/Welcomepage.aspx

of individuals (possibly suffering discrimination and stigma-related violence under routine or mandatory testing policies) against the health of the community, which, arguably, is better served by precisely such testing regimes.

A distinguishing mark of globalization is the increased influence of transnational businesses on the policies of LMIC governments. Timms' case illustrates the impact of this development. Given the economic and political clout of transnational businesses, there are continuing discussions on the extent of their human rights obligations (Weissbrodt and Kruger 2003; Ratner 2001). In this case, even if the pharmaceutical company conducting research in India is not directly bound by a human rights treaty, is it obliged to comply with human rights norms on some other basis (e.g., national laws, industry standards, corporate codes of conduct)?

In 2011, the U.N. Human Rights Council endorsed the *Guiding Principles on Business and Human Rights*, a document outlining what has come to be known as the U.N. "Protect, Respect and Remedy" framework. *Guiding Principles* recognizes governments' duty to *protect* human rights, acknowledges corporate responsibility to *respect* human rights, and requires governments to ensure that people harmed within their jurisdiction have access to effective judicial and nonjudicial *remedies*.

List and Boyd's case questions how one's freedom of expression (Article 19, ICCPR) affects public health. Should one be allowed to use the free press to advocate on behalf of fellow citizens? Does the free press furnish a forum for an informed and representative discussion on public health policy? Are expatriate workers less likely than nationals to face official retaliation when they use media outlets to criticize government?

Conflict in the Balkans and killings in Rwanda in the early 1990s revived lively debate on the international community's obligation to intervene in internal affairs of member countries to defend human rights (Kardaş 2010; Chopra and Weiss 1992). Organizing international action to address human rights violations remains a perennial challenge—exemplified by the intractable situation in Syria following major pro-democracy protests in 2011. But ideological alliances and rivalries during the Cold War made consensus building around such interventions arduous (Eisner 1993). The Balkan and Rwandan conflicts and a growing atmosphere of cooperation in the face of global challenges (e.g., environmental degradation, climate change) contributed to an increase in peacekeeping and humanitarian operations organized by the international community. These operations, though designed to further human rights, sometimes undermined the target population's right to health.

Millum's case and that of Al-Faisal, Hussain, and Sen raise issues that result, paradoxically, from increasing adoption of the human rights framework as an international norm. Millum's case questions responsibility during a major cholera outbreak originating in a camp occupied by Nepali soldiers on a U.N. peacekeeping mission in the Caribbean. The Al-Faisal, Hussain, and Sen case considers how the health of vulnerable groups in Iraq and Syria is affected by economic sanctions imposed on the two countries' governments and shows how interventions intended to protect human rights can still have adverse health consequences.

Increasingly, human rights are being used to frame responses to global public health challenges (Adorno 2009; Mann 1997). Human rights are a pervasive transcultural and normative discourse. Issues once relegated to bioethics are now cast as human rights concerns (Adorno 2009; Faunce 2005). For example, UNESCO adopted three declarations that use human rights to frame health challenges: the Universal Declaration on the Human Genome and Human Rights (1997), the International Declaration on Human Genetic Data (2003), and the Universal Declaration on Bioethics and Human Rights (2005). Each declaration codifies the principle of informed consent—a principle at stake in the case cited by Lee, Kleinfeld, and Glassford and, to a lesser degree, the case by Timms. The cross-fertilization of concepts and concerns between bioethics and human rights is a salutary consequence of public health partnerships forged in an increasingly interconnected and complex world.

8.3.3 Social Determinants of Health

The social determinants of health (SDH) framework is based on social justice (Lee 2004). The guiding principle of SDH is *equity.* As with public health, SDH emphasizes population health and prevention. However, SDH goes beyond traditional public health approaches because, in addition to deploying interventions aimed at reducing population mortality and morbidity, SDH targets "the social context and conditions in which people live" (Blas et al. 2011). These contextual factors and conditions that affect health outcomes in a given population are called *social determinants of health.*[12] These include such factors as housing, education, transportation, employment, insurance coverage, and access to health care (Brennan Ramirez et al. 2008).

The SDH framework stands on 40 years of research demonstrating that clinical care alone cannot improve health outcomes unless social factors are addressed (WHO 2007). Statistical associations between social disadvantage and poor health became increasingly clear, impelling the inference that closing the gap in health status between populations required corresponding improvements in the social contexts of disadvantaged populations.

The ethical norm underlying efforts to eliminate these preventable health differences is the principle of equity. Health *in*equities are differences "socially produced; systematic in their distribution across the population; and unfair" (WHO 2007). On the other hand, health *equity* is "the absence of unfair and avoidable or remediable differences in health among population groups defined socially, economically, demographically, or geographically" (WHO 2007). These definitions highlight two aspects of SDH. First, the differences in health are not merely descriptive but prescriptive as well, implying an ethical obligation in favor of their elimination. Second, the focus on social context and conditions means that policy and action must be intersectoral, involving actors and spheres outside the health field (WHO 2007).

[12]The social determinants of health have also been characterized as "the conditions in which people live and work that affect their opportunities to lead healthy lives" (Labonté and Schrecker 2007).

Health disparities among populations in different parts of the world motivate public health interventions and assist the development of useful analytical tools for global health. A case in point would be the gaps in infant mortality rates and life expectancy between countries with strong economies and LMICs. These gaps provide moral stimulus for elimination and benchmarks for setting goals and assessing progress (e.g., the health-related Millennium Development Goals).

The SDH framework faces several challenges and limitations. Most people do not realize the impact of social and contextual factors on health outcomes. Political orientations and worldviews further impede the acceptance of SDH as a viable policy alternative (Gollust et al. 2009). Some argue that variations of SDH oversimplify the link between wealth and health, thereby failing to consider other causes of health disparities (Poland et al. 1998). Even though statistical links have been made between social context and ill health, scientific questions remain on the mechanisms that account for these associations. This is especially critical in the field of mental health, where attempts have been made to clarify associations between SDH and psychological well-being (Marmot et al. 1997; Bovier et al. 2004; Fisher and Baum 2010; Paananen et al. 2013).

Aside from the availability of HIV/AIDS health services and medication, the Jensen and Gaie case and Zinner case demonstrate how social factors affect health. In Jensen and Gaie, advocates of client-initiated voluntary testing (vigilant, rights-based) offer compelling reasons to minimize the potential for discrimination and stigma-related violence against people living with HIV. As the case points out, the risk of violence or discrimination is particularly high in LMIC societies where social, cultural, and legal protections are nonexistent or being developed.

Although HIV-positive status can have adverse social consequences, Zinner illustrates how social factors increase the risk of infection in the first place. In this case, an international anti-AIDS program administering pre-exposure prophylactic medication is deciding whether to budget small sums of money to educate young girls in the community. Investing in education should reduce their likelihood of getting infected in unequal liaisons with older men (sugar-daddy relationships) while creating openings in the program for other at-risk groups to participate. In effect, the program is considering medical intervention (i.e., a pre-exposure prophylactic drug) and social determinants of health (i.e., girl–child education) in making its allocation decisions.

Both Timms' and Lee, Kleinfeld, and Glassford's cases show how social determinants (e.g., gender, caste, economic status, literacy) influence the effectiveness of informed consent for vulnerable LMIC populations participating in drug research. Less direct but equally critical, these cases also show how geographic disparities in social conditions establish context for global health research. The challenge of ensuring that drug research is conducted ethically in LMICs derives from such contextual factors as greater disease burdens in these regions due to underdeveloped health systems, lax regulation of biomedical research due to ineffective governance structures, and economic and social vulnerability of most potential research participants (Barlett and Steele 2011).

In the context of SDH, empowerment "is inseparably linked to marginalized and dominated communities gaining effective control over the political and economic processes that affect their well-being" (WHO 2007). List and Boyd's case demonstrates how citizens of LMICs can use mass media to influence their governments on public health topics. A physician-national in an East African country fears retaliation if she talks to the media about a TB medication stock-out potentially due to government corruption and misuse of public funds. Her fears underscore the risks and responsibilities associated with the role of health workers as advocates for the socially and politically marginalized in their communities (Pérez and Martinez 2008; Farmer 2004; Geiger and Cook-Deegan 1993). Also pertinent from a global SDH perspective is the likelihood that an expatriate whistleblower, especially a citizen from a higher-income country, would not face as serious a risk.

8.4 Summary

The approaches and methods for collaborating in global public health are diverse—just like the cases in this chapter. These cases reflect the rich and multifaceted context for global public health while also emphasizing the role that different ethical standards (and the foundations for those standards) play. In so doing, the cases offer a fresh and innovative perspective on the ethics of public health.

References

Adorno, R. 2009. Human dignity and human rights as a common ground for a global bioethics. *Journal of Medicine and Philosophy* 34(3): 223–240.

Barlett, D.L., and J.B. Steele. 2011. Deadly medicine. *Vanity Fair*. 122. http://www.vanityfair.com/politics/features/2011/01/deadly-medicine-201101. Accessed 17 June 2015.

Beauchamp, T.L., and J.F. Childress. 2009. *Principles of biomedical ethics*, 6th ed. New York: Oxford University Press.

Benkler, Y., and H. Nissenbaum. 2006. Commons-based peer production and virtue. *Journal of Political Philosophy* 14(4): 394–419.

Blas, E., J. Sommerfeld, and A.S. Kurup (eds.). 2011. *Social determinants approaches to public health: From concept to practice*. Geneva: World Health Organization. http://whqlibdoc.who.int/publications/2011/9789241564137_eng.pdf. Accessed 17 June 2015.

Bodansky, D. 1999. *The framework convention/protocol approach*, Technical Briefing Series (Framework Convention on Tobacco Control, Paper 1, No. WHO/NCD/TFI/99). Geneva: World Health Organization. http://whqlibdoc.who.int/hq/1999/WHO_NCD_TFI_99.1.pdf. Accessed 17 June 2015.

Bovier, P.A., E. Chamot, and T.V. Perneger. 2004. Perceived stress, internal resources, and social support as determinants of mental health among young adults. *Quality of Life Research* 13(1): 161–170.

Brennan Ramirez, L.K., E.A. Baker, and M. Metzler. 2008. *Promoting health equity: A resource to help communities address social determinants of health*. Atlanta: U.S. Department of Health and Human Services, Centers for Disease Control and Prevention. http://www.cdc.gov/healthycommunitiesprogram/tools/pdf/SDOH-workbook.pdf. Accessed 17 June 2015.

Chopra, J., and T.G. Weiss. 1992. Sovereignty is no longer sacrosanct: Codifying humanitarian intervention. *Ethics & International Affairs* 6(1): 95–117.

Clauser, K.D., and B. Gert. 1990. A critique of principlism. *Journal of Medicine and Philosophy* 15(2): 219–236. doi:10.1093/jmp/15.2.219.

Committee on National Statistics, and National Research Council. 1985. In *Sharing research data*, ed. S.E. Fienberg, M.E. Martin, and M.L. Straf. Washington, DC: National Academy Press.

Cueto, M. 2007. *The value of health: A history of the Pan American Health Organization*. Washington, DC: Pan American Health Organization.

Eisner, D. 1993. Humanitarian intervention in the post-Cold War era. *Boston University International Law Journal* 11: 195–225.

Elmendorf, A.E. 2010. Global health: Then and now. *UN Chronicle* XLVII(2). http://unchronicle.un.org/article/global-health-then-and-now/. Accessed 17 June 2015.

Emanuel, E.J., D. Wendler, J. Killen, and C. Grady. 2004. What makes clinical research in developing countries ethical? The benchmarks of ethical research. *Journal of Infectious Diseases* 189(5): 930–937.

Emanuel, E., R. Grady, R. Crouch, C. Lie, F. Miller, and D. Wendler (eds.). 2008. *The Oxford textbook of clinical research ethics*. New York: Oxford University Press.

Farmer, P. 2004. *Pathologies of power: Health, human rights, and the new war on the poor*. Berkeley: University of California Press.

Faunce, T.A. 2005. Will international human rights subsume medical ethics? Intersections in the UNESCO Universal Bioethics Declaration. *Journal of Medical Ethics* 31(3): 173–178.

Feldbaum, H., K. Lee, and J. Michaud. 2010. Global health and foreign policy. *Epidemiologic Reviews* 32(1): 82–92.

Fisher, M., and F. Baum. 2010. The social determinants of mental health: Implications for research and health promotion. *Australian and New Zealand Journal of Psychiatry* 44(12): 1057–1063.

Fosdick, R.B. 1989. *The story of the Rockefeller Foundation*. New Brunswick: Transaction Books.

Frieden, T.R., and J.P. Koplan. 2010. Stronger national public health institutes for global health. *Lancet* 376(9754): 1721–1722.

Geiger, H.J., and R.M. Cook-Deegan. 1993. The role of physicians in conflicts and humanitarian crises. Case studies from the field missions of physicians for human rights, 1988 to 1993. *Journal of the American Medical Association* 270(5): 616–620.

Gollust, S.E., P.M. Lantz, and P.A. Ubel. 2009. The polarizing effect of news media messages about the social determinants of health. *American Journal of Public Health* 99(12): 2160–2167.

Good, C.M. 1991. Pioneer medical missions in colonial Africa. *Social Science & Medicine* 32(1): 1–10.

Gruskin, S., E.J. Mills, and D. Tarantola. 2007. History, principles, and practice of health and human rights. *Lancet* 370(9585): 449–455.

Hendrix, K.S., E.M. Meslin, A.E. Carroll, and S.M. Downs. 2013. Attitudes about the use of newborn dried blood spots for research: A survey of underrepresented parents. *Academic Pediatrics* 13(5): 451–457. doi:10.1016/j.acap.2013.04.010.

Kardaş, Ş. 2010. Examining the role of the UN Security Council in post-Cold War interventions. *USAK Yearbook of International Politics and Law* 3: 55–75.

Kaye, J., P. Boddington, and J. de Vries, et al. 2009. *Ethical, legal and social issues arising from the use of GWAS in medical research*. Report for the Wellcome Trust. http://www.wellcome.ac.uk/stellent/groups/corporatesite/@msh_peda/documents/web_document/wtx058032.pdf. Accessed 17 June 2015.

Labonté, R. 2004. Globalization, health, and the free trade regime: Assessing the links. *Perspectives on Global Development and Technology* 3(1): 47–72.

Labonté, R., and T. Schrecker. 2007. Globalization and social determinants of health: Introduction and methodological background (part 1 of 3). *Globalization and Health* 3(5): 1–10.

Lavery, J.V., C. Grady, E. Wahl, and E.J. Emanuel (eds.). 2007. *Ethical issues in international biomedical research: A casebook*. New York: Oxford University Press.

Lee, J. 2004. *Address by the Director-General at the Fifty-seventh World Health Assembly*. http://www.who.int/dg/lee/speeches/2004/wha57/en/index.html. Accessed 17 June 2015.

Luric, P., and S.M. Wolfe. 1997. Unethical trials of intervention to reduce perinatal transmission of the human immunodeficiency virus in developing countries. *New England Journal of Medicine* 337(12): 853–856.

Macklin, R. 2008. Global justice, human rights, and health. In *Global bioethics: Issues of conscience for the twenty-first century*, ed. R.M. Green, A. Donovan, and S.A. Jauss, 142–160. New York: Oxford University Press.

Mann, J.M. 1997. Medicine and public health, ethics and human rights. *Hastings Center Report* 27(3): 6–13.

Marks, S. 1997. What is colonial about colonial medicine? And what has happened to imperialism and health? *Social History of Medicine* 10(2): 205–219.

Marmot, M., C.D. Ryff, L.L. Bumpass, M. Shipley, and N.F. Marks. 1997. Social inequalities in health: Next questions and converging evidence. *Social Science & Medicine* 44(6): 901–910.

Meier, B.M. 2006. Employing health rights for global justice: The promise of public health in response to the insalubrious ramifications of globalization. *Cornell International Law Journal* 39: 711–777.

Meslin, E.M., and I. Garba. 2011. Biobanking and public health: Is a human rights approach the tie that binds? *Human Genetics* 130(3): 451–463.

National Bioethics Advisory Commission (NBAC). 2001. *Ethical and policy issues in international research: Clinical trials in developing countries*. https://bioethicsarchive.georgetown.edu/nbac/clinical/Vol1.pdf. Accessed 17 June 2015.

Paananen, R., T. Ristikari, M. Merikukka, and M. Gissler. 2013. Social determinants of mental health: A Finnish nationwide follow-up study on mental disorders. *Journal of Epidemiology and Community Health* 67(12): 1025–1031.

Pérez, L.M., and J. Martinez. 2008. Community health workers: Social justice and policy advocates for community health and well-being. *American Journal of Public Health* 98(1): 11–14.

Poland, B., D. Coburn, A. Robertson, and J. Eakin. 1998. Wealth, equity and health care: A critique of a "population health" perspective on the determinants of health. *Social Science & Medicine* 46(7): 785–798.

Ratner, S.R. 2001. Corporations and human rights: A theory of legal responsibility. *The Yale Law Journal* 111(3): 443–545.

Ruger, J.P. 2009. Global health justice. *Public Health Ethics* 2(3): 261–275.

Shapiro, H.T., and E.M. Meslin. 2001. Ethical issues in the design and conduct of clinical trials in developing countries. *New England Journal of Medicine* 345: 139–141.

Stuckler, D., and S. Basu. 2009. The International Monetary Fund's effects on global health: Before and after the 2008 financial crisis. *International Journal of Health Services* 39(4): 771–781.

Tong, S., J.R. Lingappa, Q. Chen, et al. 2004. Direct sequencing of SARS-coronavirus S and N genes from clinical specimens shows limited variation. *Journal of Infectious Diseases* 190(6): 1127–1131. doi:10.1086/422849.

United Nations (U.N.). 1945. *Charter of the United Nations*. http://www.un.org/en/documents/charter/. Accessed 17 June 2015.

United Nations. 1948. *The Universal Declaration of Human Rights*. http://www.un.org/en/documents/udhr/. Accessed 17 June 2015.

United Nations. 1966a. *International Covenant on Civil and Political Rights*. http://www.ohchr.org/EN/ProfessionalInterest/Pages/CCPR.aspx. Accessed 17 June 2015.

United Nations. 1966b. *International Covenant on Economic, Social and Cultural Rights*. http://www.ohchr.org/EN/ProfessionalInterest/Pages/CESCR.aspx. Accessed 17 June 2015.

United Nations. 1993. *Vienna Declaration and Programme of Action*. http://www.ohchr.org/en/professionalinterest/pages/vienna.aspx. Accessed 17 June 2015.

United Nations Educational, Scientific and Cultural Organization (UNESCO). 1997. *Universal Declaration on the Human Genome and Human Rights*. http://www.unesco.org/new/en/social-and-human-sciences/themes/bioethics/human-genome-and-human-rights/. Accessed 17 June 2015.

United Nations Educational, Scientific and Cultural Organization. 2003. *International Declaration on Human Genetic Data*. http://www.unesco.org/new/en/social-and-human-sciences/themes/bioethics/human-genetic-data/. Accessed 17 June 2015.

United Nations Educational, Scientific and Cultural Organization. 2005. *Universal Declaration on Bioethics and Human Rights*. http://portal.unesco.org/en/ev.php-URL_ID=31058&URL_DO=DO_TOPIC&URL_SECTION=201.html. Accessed 17 June 2015.

Varmus, H., and D. Satcher. 1997. Ethical complexities of conducting research in developing countries. *New England Journal of Medicine* 337: 1003–1005.
Weissbrodt, D., and M. Kruger. 2003. Norms on the responsibilities of transnational corporations and other business enterprises with regard to human rights. *American Journal of International Law* 97(4): 901–922.
World Health Organization (WHO). 1948. *Constitution of the World Health Organization*. http://www.who.int/governance/eb/who_constitution_en.pdf. Accessed 17 June 2015.
World Health Organization (WHO). 1978. *Declaration of Alma-Ata*. http://www.who.int/publications/almaata_declaration_en.pdf. Accessed 17 June 2015.
World Health Organization (WHO). 2002. *25 questions and answers on health and human rights*, Health and Human Rights Publication Series (No. 1). Geneva: World Health Organization. http://www.who.int/hhr/information/25%20Questions%20and%20Answers%20on%20Health%20and%20Human%20Rights.pdf. Accessed 17 June 2015.
World Health Organization (WHO). 2008a. Consensus during the Cold War: Back to Alma-Ata. *Bulletin of the World Health Organization* 86(10): 745–746.
World Health Organization (WHO). 2008b. Primary health care comes full circle: An interview with Dr. Halfdan Mahler. *Bulletin of the World Health Organization* 86(10): 747–748.
World Health Organization Commission on Social Determinants of Health. 2007. *A conceptual framework for action on the social determinants of health (Discussion paper draft)*. Geneva: World Health Organization. http://www.who.int/social_determinants/resources/csdh_framework_action_05_07.pdf. Accessed 17 June 2015.

8.5 Case 1: The Ethics of HIV Testing Policies

Kipton E. Jensen
Department of Philosophy and Religion
Morehouse College
Atlanta, GA, USA
e-mail: kipton.jensen@morehouse.edu

Joseph B.R. Gaie
Department of Theology and Religious Studies
University of Botswana
Gaborone, Botswana

This case is presented for instructional purposes only. The ideas and opinions expressed are the authors' own. The case is not meant to reflect the official position, views, or policies of the editors, the editors' host institutions, or the authors' host institutions.

8.5.1 Background

The global public health community has significantly advanced our understanding of the biology of the human immunodeficiency virus (HIV) and developed reliable diagnostic tests and effective antiretroviral treatments. Despite these advancements, the rate of prevalence and transmission, especially in low- and middle-income countries, remains alarmingly high. HIV prevention, often considered better than a cure, remains the mainstay of our collective response to the epidemic. By all accounts, HIV testing plays a pivotal role in treatment and prevention, yet in low- or middle-income countries, only 10 % of those who have been exposed to HIV infection may have access to counseling and testing (UNAIDS/WHO 2004; Centers for Disease Control and Prevention 2012). In general, HIV testing policies range from voluntary or client-initiated counseling and testing to provider-initiated approaches (e.g., routine testing, mandatory HIV screening). Most policy makers and health workers have promoted voluntary HIV testing, although routine HIV counseling and testing increasingly is being adopted. Notably, however, the global health community has adamantly discouraged mandatory HIV testing (UNAIDS/WHO 2004).

Resource-poor countries may be unable or unwilling to ensure social and medical infrastructures adequate for safeguarding the human rights of people seeking services. As a result, global health officials have encouraged countries to adopt voluntary or client-initiated counseling and testing policies opposed to routine or provider-initiated policies. Even in settings in which voluntary counseling and testing is readily available, few people take advantage of these services. Stigmatization persists as an obstacle to HIV counseling and testing, which, by all accounts, is vital to effectively treat people living with HIV and AIDS and to reduce further infection.

Many public health ethicists recommend that policy makers and health workers carefully consider the ethical consequences of routine testing policies, especially for people in locales that lack protections against discrimination and stigma-related violence (Rennie and Behets 2006). To protect individuals against HIV-related discrimination and threat of violence, advocates of the human-rights approach vigilantly oppose the application of standard methods of disease control, which include mandatory testing and partner notification. But this vigilant rights-based approach to HIV prevention, an approach that Bayer (1991) labelled AIDS exceptionalism, can undermine society's ability and indeed responsibility to control the epidemic. And although public health officials are a minority, some argue for mandatory HIV testing (Schuklenk and Kleinsmidt 2007), seeing it as the only way to control the HIV epidemic. Failure to apply standard methods of disease control, some argue, devalues public health and social justice (Frieden et al. 2005; De Cock et al. 2002). By treating HIV/AIDS differently than other infectious diseases, AIDS exceptionalism may inadvertently increase stigmatization rather than reduce it (De Cock et al. 2002). Proponents of testing point to its potential to reduce stigma by raising awareness, preventing transmission, expanding treatment, and empowering individuals (Crepaz et al. 2004).

HIV testing policy recommendations from the global international public health community can also challenge if not undermine the authority of the indigenous knowledge system or indigenous ethical codes (Chilisa 2005; Dube 2006; Jensen and Gaie 2010). These recommendations typically stipulate ethical preconditions within voluntary HIV testing policies, such as strict confidentiality, informed consent, and competent pre- and post-test counseling. Some argue that preconditions constitute a Western approach that blocks local efforts to control the epidemic. Although many believe that the context of provider-initiated HIV testing preserves "sufficient voluntariness," others have criticized this approach. Critics maintain that opting-out from provider-initiated HIV testing differs significantly from client-initiated or voluntary HIV counseling and testing (Kenyon 2005). In either case, all agree, medical practitioners and policy makers cannot guarantee ideal or even adequate social and institutional support services (Weiser et al. 2006).

These disputes are by no means merely theoretical. In Botswana, for example, policy has shifted within the past 5 years from a client-initiated to a provider-initiated or routine HIV diagnostic counseling and testing strategy (Botswana Ministry of Health 2012). More recently, in response to a parliamentary-approved public health bill presently being contested as unconstitutional (Botswana Network on Ethics, Law and HIV/AIDS 2012), the debate has shifted to whether certain conditions render mandatory testing ethically permissible.

8.5.2 Case Description

The Minister of Health of a sub-Saharan nation has asked you, a public health official and physician from a Western country, to recommend an effective HIV testing policy. The sub-Saharan nation is among the hardest hit by the HIV epidemic (e.g., the HIV prevalence rate among pregnant women aged 15–49 is >25 %). In this resource-poor nation, people with HIV and AIDS are commonly stigmatized despite national campaigns to reduce stigma. Even if the nation were to adopt a policy of voluntary HIV counseling and testing, more than 50 % of people living with HIV and AIDS are unaware of their serostatus. Although HIV treatment is currently unavailable, international donors have promised to provide free or inexpensive antiretroviral therapies (ART).

You have sought the input of your colleagues in global public health only to discover they are contentiously divided. Some vigorously oppose enhanced HIV testing policies that would move from voluntary to routine HIV testing to protect the community against discrimination or stigma-related violence. They also oppose in principle Western-based interventions, which, they say, undermine traditional loci of authority and indigenous systems of medical knowledge. Other colleagues insist that human rights-based approaches undermine public health's ability, as well as responsibility, to control the HIV epidemic. They are for moving beyond client-initiated approaches and vigorously support mandatory HIV testing. These colleagues feel that the only way to control the HIV epidemic is to apply the standard methods of disease control.

Given these divergent views, you hope to be able to recommend a HIV policy that strikes a balance between the Hippocratic ideal of doing no harm and the equally compelling mandate to protect if not improve public health.

8.5.3 Discussion Questions

1. How might an emphasis on protecting human rights in HIV prevention reduce the importance of public health and social justice?
2. Is opting in, or not opting out, as part of the routine testing strategy, ethically equivalent to acquiring consent within a voluntary testing site? What are the

necessary and sufficient conditions, ethical or otherwise, for "adequate information" or "sufficient voluntariness" in cases of HIV testing?
3. Is there an ethical conflict between one's duty, whether as a physician or a public health official, whether as the minister of health or simply as a person, to adopt what are considered to be effective methods of controlling disease, e.g., HIV, and the obligation to respect indigenous knowledge systems and approaches to public health? If there is a conflict, which duty should take precedent?
4. What policy would you recommend under these circumstances? And what ethical principles guided your recommendation?
5. How would your recommendation provide, if at all, protections against discrimination and stigma-related violence?

References

Bayer, R. 1991. Public health policy and the AIDS epidemic: An end to HIV exceptionalism? *New England Journal of Medicine* 324(21): 1500–1504.

Botswana Ministry of Health. 2012. *Routine HIV Testing (RHT)*. Gaborone, Botswana: Department of HIV and AIDS Prevention & Care.

Botswana Network on Ethics, Law and HIV/AIDS. 2012. *Public health bill shocking and regressive*. Press Release, December 6. http://www.bonela.org/index.php?option=com_k2&view=item&Itemid=223&id=104:06-december-2012. Accessed 17 July 2013.

Centers for Disease Control and Prevention. 2012. *Strategic plan, division of HIV/AIDS prevention (2011–2015)*. http://www.cdc.gov/hiv/pdf/policies_DHAP-strategic-plan.pdf. Accessed 23 Jan 2014.

Chilisa, B.C. 2005. Educational research within postcolonial Africa: A critique of HIV/AIDS research in Botswana. *International Journal of Qualitative Studies in Education* 18(6): 659–684.

Crepaz, N., T.A. Hart, and G. Marks. 2004. Highly active antiretroviral therapy and sexual risk behavior: A meta-analytic review. *Journal of the American Medical Association* 292(2): 224–236.

De Cock, K.M., D. Mbori-Ngacha, and E. Marum. 2002. Shadow on the continent: Public health and HIV/AIDS in Africa in the 21st century. *Lancet* 360(9326): 67–72.

Dube, M.W. 2006. Adinkra! Four hearts joined together: On becoming healing-teachers of African indigenous religion/s in HIV & AIDS prevention. In *African women, religion, and health: Essays in honor of Mercy Amba Ewudziwa Oduyoye*, ed. I.A. Phiri and S. Nadar, 131–156. Maryknoll: Orbis Books.

Frieden, T.R., M. Das-Douglas, S.E. Kellerman, and Henning K. J. 2005. Applying public health principles to the HIV epidemic. *New England Journal of Medicine* 353(22): 2397–2402.

Jensen, K., and J.B. Gaie. 2010. African communalism and public health policies: The relevance of indigenous concepts of personal identity to HIV/AIDS policies in Botswana. *African Journal of AIDS Research* 9(3): 297–305. doi:10.2989/16085906.2010.530187.

Kenyon, K. 2005. Routine HIV testing: A view from Botswana. *Health and Human Rights* 8(2): 21–23.

Rennie, S., and F. Behets. 2006. Desperately seeking targets: The ethics of routine HIV testing in low income countries. *Bulletin of the World Health Organization* 84(1): 52–57.

Schuklenk, U., and A. Kleinsmidt. 2007. Rethinking mandatory HIV testing during pregnancy in areas with high HIV prevalence rates: Ethical and policy issues. *American Journal of Public Health* 97(7): 1179–1183.

UNAIDS/WHO. 2004. *UNAIDS/WHO policy statement on HIV testing*. Geneva: World Health Organization. http://www.who.int/ethics/topics/en/hivtestingpolicy_who_unaids_en_2004.pdf. Accessed 17 July 2013.

Weiser, S.D., M. Heisler, K. Leiter, et al. 2006. Correction: Routine HIV testing in Botswana: A population-based study on attitudes, practices, and human rights concerns. *PLoS Medicine* 3(10), e395. doi:10.1371/journal.pmed.0030395.

8.6 Case 2: Just Allocation of Pre-exposure Prophylaxis Drugs in Sub-Saharan Africa

Susan Zinner
School of Public and Environmental Affairs
Indiana University Northwest
Gary, IN, USA
e-mail: szinner@iun.edu

This case is presented for instructional purposes only. The ideas and opinions expressed are the author's own. The case is not meant to reflect the official position, views, or policies of the editors, the editors' host institutions, or the author's host institutions.

8.6.1 Background

During the summer of 2012, the U.S. Food and Drug Administration (FDA) announced the approval of Truvada (emtricitabine/tenofovir disoproxil fumerate) for use in pre-exposure prophylaxis programs (PrEP) for people at high risk of HIV infection (FDA 2012). After successful use of antiretroviral therapy (ART) drugs to treat HIV/AIDS-infected populations, researchers found that daily prophylactic use of these drugs in uninfected individuals who engaged in high-risk activities was also effective in reducing their risk of HIV/AIDS. The U.S. Centers for Disease Control and Prevention (CDC) noted that PrEP could reduce HIV rates for men having sex with men if those at high risk of HIV infection were targeted and if PrEP was used as part of a comprehensive set of preventive services, including regular monitoring of HIV status, adherence, and risk behaviors (CDC 2011). Candidates for Truvada should first be tested for HIV to ensure that they are in fact HIV negative before beginning the PrEP program.

This innovative prophylactic approach to reducing the likelihood of contracting HIV holds great promise. One study found that Truvada reduced the risk of HIV infection 42 % compared with men taking placebos and having sex with other men (Grant et al. 2010), whereas a second study found that risk fell by up to 75 % compared with serodiscordant couples taking placebos (Baeten et al. 2012). However, Truvada is associated with some side effects, including nausea and vomiting (CDC 2011) and possible decreases in bone mineral density (Grigsby et al. 2010).

Furthermore, Truvada is contraindicated for anyone with decreased kidney function. Regular testing of kidney function is recommended for those people taking this medication (CDC 2011).

Truvada has been tested only in serodiscordant couples—not in women. Its efficacy in the general population of women, in sex workers, and in young girls in sugar-daddy relationships (i.e., young girls in unequal relationships with older males) is unknown.

Sub-Saharan Africa has been hit especially hard by HIV/AIDS. An estimated two-thirds of people affected by HIV worldwide are concentrated in this area, although significant variations exist in different parts of the continent (Kalipeni et al. 2004). Unfortunately, the distribution and availability of ART drugs have exposed the inadequacies of some African national health systems, such as the negative effects of a long-neglected health sector, economic challenges, declining public expenditures, and decentralized funding (Schneider et al. 2006).

Many international aid groups help fund public health programs, including programs to reduce the spread of HIV/AIDS. Programs such as PEPFAR (The United States President's Emergency Plan for AIDS Relief), the Global Fund, the World Bank, the United Nations, and the Gates Foundation have all contributed large sums of money for this purpose.

African groups at high risk of contracting new infections (and thus good potential candidates for PrEP) include sex workers, men having sex with men, serodiscordant couples, and girls in sexual sugar-daddy relationships. The latter group poses specific ethical issues. These girls, typically teenagers, may be coerced into sexual relationships with men old enough to be their fathers or even grandfathers through the offering of gifts or money. These sugar daddies generally engage in multiple sexual relationships, possibly with a spouse and several young women, while putting the girls at risk of HIV. Every averted case of HIV increases economic productivity, lowers the risk of social unrest, strengthens the labor force, and improves the investment climate (Over 2011).

8.6.2 Case Description

You are the head of an international anti-AIDS effort currently stationed in a community of 40,000 in sub-Saharan Africa, where the HIV prevalence rate is 21 %. You have received funding from different world organizations, including some based in the United States. Your organization is piloting the use of Truvada in populations that are at high risk of HIV. The organizations funding this project will allow you and the two health workers assigned to assist you to make all allocation decisions.

The cost of Truvada for one patient is about $500 per year. Those living in this community are poor, and none could afford this drug without the existence of your program. Many populations in the community are at high risk of HIV infection, including homosexual and bisexual men who routinely engage in sex with other men, girls in sugar-daddy relationships, sex workers, and serodiscordant couples. You have been given enough Truvada to treat and monitor 100 patients for a year.

The funding organizations have indicated that they are likely to provide more Truvada if you find its use results in no or few new infections during the year among the 100 selected patients. The community of 40,000 people include the following:

- 80 men who have sex with other men;
- 80 girls in sugar-daddy relationships;
- 40 sex workers; and
- 30 serodiscordant couples (60 people; noninfected partner receives Truvada while the infected partner is not medically eligible for ART).

One challenge you face is that many feminist organizations and child health advocates are pressuring you to include all girls in the group because ample research shows that girls in sugar-daddy relationships are relatively powerless and cannot ask their partners to wear a condom, virtually ensuring that these girls will become infected. There is some evidence, however, that simply paying girls a small amount of money to attend school (and thus dramatically reducing the possibility of these relationships) is cost effective. If you adopt this approach, you could use the Truvada for the other groups. You may need to consider whether to request more money from the funding organizations if you adopt this approach. One of your organization's goals is to respect cultural norms and beliefs if the health of those at risk of HIV/AIDS is not jeopardized. You have been asked to allocate the PrEP drugs in your community.

8.6.3 Discussion Questions

1. What role should the community play as you make your allocation decisions? How do you remain culturally sensitive when implementing this program?
2. Create a rubric to help you consider each group for inclusion in the PrEP program. What factors will you weigh in making allocation decisions? If you do not pick an entire group, what criteria do you use to select individuals in that group? How would your criteria differ if you were distributing ART drugs to infected individuals (and not to those who are at risk but not infected)?
3. What role should the likelihood of patient adherence play in your allocation decision? Keep in mind that patients are expected to take their medication daily on a strict time schedule.
4. How will you determine if your program is successful? How will you determine whether your allocation decisions are just and fair?

References

Baeten, J.M., D. Donnell, P. Ndase, et al. 2012. Antiretroviral prophylaxis for HIV prevention in heterosexual men and women. *The New England Journal of Medicine* 367(5): 399–410. doi:10.1056/NEJMoa1108524.

Centers for Disease Control and Prevention (CDC). 2011. Interim guidance: Preexposure prophylaxis for the prevention of HIV infection in men who have sex with men. *Morbidity and*

Mortality Weekly Report 60(3): 65–68. http://www.cdc.gov/mmwr/preview/mmwrhtml/mm6003a1.htm. Accessed 5 May 2013.

Food and Drug Administration (FDA). 2012. *FDA approves first drug for reducing the risk of sexually acquired HIV infection.* FDA News Release July 16. http://www.fda.gov/NewsEvents/Newsroom/PressAnnouncements/ucm312210.htm. Accessed 15 May 2013.

Grant, R.M., J.R. Lama, P.L. Anderson, et al. 2010. Preexposure chemoprophylaxis for HIV prevention in men who have sex with men. *The New England Journal of Medicine* 363(27): 2587–2599. doi:10.1056/NEJMoa1011205.

Grigsby, I.F., L. Pham, L.M. Mansky, R. Gopalakrishnan, and K.C. Mansky. 2010. Tenofovir-associated bone density loss. *Therapeutics and Clinical Risk Management* 6: 41–47.

Kalipeni, E., S. Craddock, and J. Ghosh. 2004. Mapping the AIDS pandemic in Eastern and Southern Africa: A critical overview. In *HIV & AIDS in Africa: Beyond epidemiology*, ed. E. Kalipeni, S. Craddock, J.R. Oppong, and J. Ghosh, 58–69. Malden: Blackwell Publishing.

Over, M. 2011. *Achieving an AIDS transition: Preventing infections to sustain treatment.* Washington, DC: Center for Global Development.

Schneider, H., D. Blaauw, L. Gilson, N. Chabikuli, and J. Goudge. 2006. Health systems and access to antiretroviral drugs for HIV in Southern Africa: Service delivery and human resources challenges. *Reproductive Health Matters* 14(27): 12–23.

8.7 Case 3: Drug Trials in Developing Countries

Olinda Timms
Department of Health and Humanities
St. Johns Research Institute
Bangalore, Karnataka, India
e-mail: olindatimms@gmail.com

This case is presented for instructional purposes only. The ideas and opinions expressed are the author's own. The case is not meant to reflect the official position, views, or policies of the editors, the editors' host institutions, or the author's host institutions.

8.7.1 Background

Clinical trials outsourced to India offer, in addition to business opportunities for clinical research management, the prospect of health infrastructure development and collaborative research. Since 2005, drug trials in India have increased as foreign drug companies eagerly take advantage of the favorable research environment (British Broadcasting Corporation [BBC] News 2006; Russia Today 2010; Overdorf 2011; John 2012). These advantages include highly qualified English-speaking doctors, a large and diverse population, and lower costs and relative freedom from burdensome regulations for privately funded research trials (World Health Organization 2008). As a result, clinical research organizations working on behalf of pharmaceutical companies frequently approach doctors in private or government practice to recruit patients for drug trials, often offering attractive payouts per recruit and promising coauthorship and publication credits as incentives.

For vast sections of its demographic, India grapples with inadequate access to health services and high rates of infant mortality and communicable diseases (Government of India Planning Commission 2011). Only a small slice of the population can afford the high-end private and corporate hospital care in urban pockets of the nation. Though extremely deferent to physicians, the Indian population is insufficiently informed about the risks and benefits of clinical trials. Illiterate, impoverished, and unaware of the implications of participation, many drug trial recruits are vulnerable to exploitation (Srinivasan and Nikarge 2009). With limited health care options, some gladly enroll in a drug trial, considering themselves fortunate to receive medical attention, food, and compensation for local travel. Such circumstances compromise the intent behind freely giving informed consent.

The media has drawn attention to several high-profile cases. These involved poor people from lower castes who enrolled in drug trials without adequate consent, resulting in severe adverse effects, including death (Lloyd-Roberts 2012). Citing data for 2005–2012, the BBC reported that 2,000 clinical trials took place in India. The death count among people enrolled in these clinical trials was 288 in 2008, 637 in 2009, 668 in 2010, and 438 in 2011 (Lloyd-Roberts 2012). The media also raised concerns about inadequate regulation of private trials, inconsistent application of informed consent requirements, and irregularities in ethics reviews (The Hindu 2011; The Indian Express 2012).

Although officials have been responsive to these concerns, their efforts still leave the vulnerable unprotected. In 2000, the Ministry of Health and Family Welfare established legal guidelines regulating the conduct of research in India that align with international guidelines on research ethics including the International Conference on Harmonisation of Good Clinical Practice (ICH-GCP) (1996), the Declaration of Helsinki (World Medical Association 2008) and Council for International Organizations of Medical Sciences (CIOMS) guidelines (2002). The Indian Council of Medical Research also developed guidelines specifically for clinical trials (2006). Further, the Drugs and Cosmetics Rules were amended to require review and registration of trials and to compensate trial participants or their families in the event of an adverse event (Government of India 2005). Unfortunately, adverse events go grossly underreported. Few recruits receive compensation, and hardly any investigations result in convictions for unethical research practices.

8.7.2 Case Description

Sharada, a 45-year-old woman of a low social caste in an impoverished town in India, lives on less than 2 U.S. dollars a day. She has access only to the government hospital system that provides free health care to underserved citizens. Complaining of chest pains, she is taken to the nearest government hospital and diagnosed with heart and renal failure. Pharmakon, a multinational pharmaceutical company, happens to be conducting a trial for a drug that has renal-protective effects in cardiac failure. From a colleague serving as a site investigator for this trial, Sharada's cardiologist hears that pilot testing of the drug has shown promising results. But he also learns that his colleague's compensation is tied to the number of subjects he enrolls in the study. Worse, Pharmakon has a history of enrolling patients without ensuring they fully understand they will be participating in a research project. Despite misgivings about this history and his colleague's financial incentive to enroll patients, Sharada's cardiologist recommends that she enroll in the drug trial. He emphasizes that enrollment offers the only way to obtain an expensive drug necessary to save her life that would otherwise be unaffordable. Given the family's lack of education, he is uncertain how much they understood, yet they seem grateful for the prospect of immediate care and treatment. While on this medication, Sharada develops cardiac arrhythmias, is taken off the drug, and is discharged from the hospital in a few days. Almost a month later, she succumbs to cardiac arrest at home. Soon thereafter, the high number of serious drug-related complications forces discontinuation of the drug trial.

8.7.3 Discussion Questions

1. Who are the stakeholders in this case, what is at stake for each of them, and what values does each bring to the situation?
2. What are the risks and benefits of enrolling impoverished, uneducated patients living in developing countries in clinical drug trials? What are the barriers to obtaining true informed consent from these patients, and what can be done to overcome these barriers?
3. What are the ethical implications of tying a researcher's compensation to the number of subjects enrolled? Should this practice be permitted?
4. Are multinational pharmaceutical companies that benefit from cost-effective drug trials in developing countries obligated to improve the lives of people living in those countries?
5. Who should be held responsible for adverse events due to a drug trial conducted by a multinational company in a country where there is limited health insurance, no social security, and poor enforcement of regulations? What international or grassroots efforts might help ensure accountability for adverse events?

References

British Broadcasting Corporation News. 2006. *Drug trials outsourced to Asia.* April 22. http://news.bbc.co.uk/2/hi/south_asia/4932188.stm. Accessed 27 June 2013.

Council for International Organizations of Medical Sciences (CIOMS). 2002. *For biomedical research involving human subjects.* http://www.cioms.ch/publications/layout_guide2002.pdf. Accessed 27 June 2013.

Government of India. 2005. *Drugs and cosmetics rules: Schedule Y.* http://dbtbiosafety.nic.in/act/Schedule_Y.pdf. Accessed 23 Jan 2014.

Government of India Planning Commission. 2011. *Report of the working group on National Rural Health Mission (NRHM) for the Twelfth Five Year Plan (2012–2017).* New Delhi: Government of

India. http://planningcommission.nic.in/aboutus/committee/wrkgrp12/health/WG_1NRHM.pdf. Accessed 27 June 2013.

Indian Council of Medical Research. 2006. *Ethical guidelines for biomedical research on human participants.* New Delhi: Indian Council for Medical Research. http://icmr.nic.in/ethical_guidelines.pdf. Accessed 27 June 2013.

International Conference on Harmonisation of Good Clinical Practice (ICH-GCP). 1996. *International Conference on Harmonisation of Technical Requirements for Registration of Pharmaceuticals for Human Use. Good clinical practice.* http://ichgcp.net/. Accessed 27 June 2013.

John, S. 2012. Trial and error: India can attract 5–10% of the global market for drug trials. *Times of India*, October 22. http://timesofindia.indiatimes.com/business/india-business/Trial-and-Error-India-can-attract-5-10-of-the-global-market-for-drug-trials/articleshow/16910327.cms. Accessed 27 June 2013.

Lloyd-Roberts, S. 2012. Have India's poor become human guinea pigs? *BBC News Magazine*, November 1. http://www.bbc.co.uk/news/magazine-20136654. Accessed 27 June 2013.

Overdorf, J. 2011. India: Deadly drug trials. *GlobalPost*, June 19. http://www.globalpost.com/dispatch/news/regions/asia-pacific/india/110618/india-health-drug-trials. Accessed 27 June 2013.

Russia Today. 2010. India becomes global drug trial ground for pharmaceuticals. October 23. http://rt.com/news/india-drug-trial-pharma/. Accessed 27 June 2013.

Srinivasan, S., and S. Nikarge. 2009. *Ethical concerns in clinical trials in India: An investigation.* Mumbai: Centre for Studies in Ethics and Rights. http://www.fairdrugs.org/uploads/files/Ethical_concerns_in_clinical_trials_in_India_An_investigation.pdf. Accessed 27 June 2013.

The Hindu. 2011. Opinion/editorial: A shockingly unethical trial. May 15. http://www.thehindu.com/opinion/editorial/a-shockingly-unethical-trial/article2021657.ece. Accessed 27 June 2013.

The Indian Express. 2012. 10 die per week in drug trials in India. July 8. http://indianexpress.com/article/india/regional/10-die-per-week-in-drug-trials-in-india/. Accessed 27 June 2013.

World Health Organization (WHO). 2008. Clinical trials in India: Ethical concerns. *Bulletin of the World Health Organization* 86(8): 581–582. doi:10.2471/BLT.08.010808.

World Medical Association. 2008. *Declaration of Helsinki—Ethical principles for medical research involving human subjects.* http://www.wma.net/en/30publications/10policies/b3/index.html. Accessed 27 June 2013.

8.8 Case 4: Ethical Issues in Responding to International Medication Stock-Outs

Justin List
Robert Wood Johnson/VA Clinical Scholars Program
University of Michigan
Ann Arbor, MI, USA
e-mail: justin.list@gmail.com

Andrew Boyd
Department of Medicine, Section of Hospital Medicine
Columbia University
New York, NY, USA

This case is presented for instructional purposes only. The ideas and opinions expressed are the authors' own. The case is not meant to reflect the official position, views, or policies of the editors, the editors' host institutions, or the authors' host institutions.

8.8.1 Background

The World Health Organization (WHO) maintains a list, updated every 2 years, of medications it considers essential—medications that a given country should have on hand to distribute to its citizens (WHO 2015). In functioning health systems, the intent is to have essential medicines of assured quality available at all times in adequate amounts, in appropriate dosage forms, and at an affordable price (WHO 2015). Among those medications are treatments for tuberculosis (TB), a ubiquitous, slow-growing bacteria that kills 1.4 million people annually (WHO 2012).

Control of TB requires the availability of medication for months of treatment. Procurement of TB medication requires an intact and predictable supply chain. Ideally, ministries of health in low-income countries forecast accurately the number and types of medications needed to treat the local burdens of disease. Then governments typically purchase medications to store in a central facility for regional distribution. Inefficiencies in drug supply forecasting; stocking practices; storage capabilities; transportation capacity; and timely funding, procurement, and delivery can lead to a breakdown in a supply chain.

One barrier to TB control in low-resource countries, as well as in the United States, is intermittent unavailability of TB medication, an occurrence known as a stock-out (Centers for Disease Control and Prevention 2013). Medication stock-outs often result in delayed treatment, an increased risk of drug resistance in incompletely treated people, and the potential for untreated or incompletely treated people to infect others. Stock-outs occur for different reasons, including budget constraints, poor drug procurement policies and distribution networks, and political corruption slowing drug availability (Stop Stock-outs Campaign 2010).

Although 80 % of national ministries of health reporting to WHO have an uninterrupted supply of first-line TB medications, 45 % of the 20 highest-burden countries report stock-outs (WHO 2009). More recently, 14 countries experienced anti-TB drug stock-outs in 2011 (Stop TB Partnership 2011). To contend with recurrent stock-outs, the Stop TB Partnership provides technical support and drug procurement avenues to resource-poor nations through its Global Drug Facility (GDF) and Green Light Committee (GLC) (Stop TB Partnership 2011). Although GDF and GLC are essential players in ensuring at-risk nations have adequate drug supplies, both are limited in how quickly they can respond to stock-outs.

Advocacy groups and nongovernmental organizations can generate widespread public attention in hope of quicker resolution of stock-outs. A paucity of literature covers the ethical roles of expatriate health workers in stock-outs. The model of "ethics of engaged presence" in health practice for expatriate health workers in low-income countries may offer a framework of solidarity with local people (Hunt et al.

2012). This nondirective framework broadly centers on the moral dimensions of expatriate involvement in humanitarian health work undertaken with local individuals. Still, limited ethical guidelines exist for expatriates who seek to enter foreign political and social forays to affect change—leaving the problem of essential TB medication stocks-outs unresolved.

8.8.2 *Case Description*

You are a visiting researcher in an East African country investigating TB case-finding detection strategies in an urban area. This country has one of the highest TB burdens in the world. Its government funds the national medical stores to stock anti-TB drugs per WHO's essential medication list. On occasion, you work in the TB clinic at the local hospital treating TB patients, some of whom have multidrug-resistant TB. You know that your research participants are guaranteed TB drugs through your study's funding. Potential participants who do not qualify for the study but have active TB infection are referred to a local clinic.

After months living and working in this country, you learn that many of the urban and rural clinics carry an inadequate supply of anti-TB medications. You speak with local doctors about the anti-TB drug shortage. They are frustrated and speculate as to why there have been stock-outs. Some suspect corruption and misuse of funds by the ministries of finance and health are to blame. Others blame drug manufacturers for unreliable supplies.

You search for drug stock-outs in this country using Internet search engines and come across stock-outs for other drugs but find no mention of anti-TB drug stock-outs. You return to a weekly clinic meeting and note that the news has not covered the stock-outs your colleagues are experiencing at their clinics. You ask if any of them will push the ministry of health to fix the shortage. One physician says he heard that the ministry will "provide the TB drugs again shortly." You suggest that one of the physicians contact someone from a media outlet to raise attention. After a period of silence, a physician says she fears that the government will somehow retaliate if this issue is raised.

After further conversations with colleagues, you decide to attract media attention to this issue. Your local colleagues support you, even saying they will provide you with data about the stock-out. Contacts in your U.S.-based sponsoring organization feel ambivalent about your working with the media to raise attention but will not prohibit it so long as you do not mention your affiliation.

You decide to contact an international health and human rights organization about the stock-out, and its staff puts you in touch with a local partner organization. The local partner wants you to speak, along with local human rights advocates, at a stock-out conference and interview with newspaper reporters. Despite your wanting to help those dependent on the national drug supply for their TB treatment, you are conflicted about your participation and its possible repercussions. Before committing, you tell the local partner that you need to think the matter through thoroughly.

8.8.3 Discussion Questions

1. What are some risks and benefits of your involvement with the stock-out conference and contact with the media? What ethical concepts should inform your decision? Would your decision change if your colleagues or sponsoring organization urged you to say nothing?
2. How does your limited understanding of local institutional hierarchy and governance inform your ethical analysis of whether or not to engage in advocacy around stock-outs? If you conclude you should engage, are there ways to do so besides public testimony?
3. Does it matter ethically if the stock-out pertained to antimalarial medications; that is, a medication outside your research area (TB medication)? Why or why not?
4. In terms of perceptions and consequences from the media and government ministries, how might your public reporting of the stock-out differ from a local official reporting it? What different types of impact might result from each? How might your ability to work with local health professionals in the future be affected if you report the alleged stock-out?
5. Knowing that you have ready access to anti-TB medication for research participants, should you broaden the inclusion criteria to allow more patients to receive guaranteed treatment? Why or why not?
6. Should you attempt to bring the stock-out to the attention of the global health international community by inviting members of the international media to the stock-out conference? If not, why not? If so, what approaches might international and local nongovernmental organizations, World Health Organization departments, and patient advocacy groups employ to effectively publicize and resolve stock-outs? If not, why not?
7. Do you have an ethical duty to report the stock-out if local health officers will not do so?

Acknowledgements Dr. List thanks staff members of the National Institutes of Health/Fogarty International Clinical Research Scholars program, Physicians for Human Rights, and Action Group for Health, Human Rights and HIV/AIDS (AGHA-Uganda) for advice on this case study's content. Both authors thank the leadership of the Yale/Stanford Johnson & Johnson Global Health Scholars Program for training medical residents in ethics before their clinical work assignments in Rwanda.

References

Centers for Disease Control and Prevention. 2013. Interruptions in supplies of second-line antituberculosis drugs—United States, 2005–2012. *Morbidity and Mortality Weekly Report.* http://www.cdc.gov/mmwr/preview/mmwrhtml/mm6202a2.htm. Accessed 24 Mar 2013.

Hunt, M.R., L. Schwartz, C. Sinding, and L. Elit. 2012. The ethics of engaged presence: A framework for health professionals in humanitarian assistance and development work. *Developing World Bioethics.* doi:10.1111/dewb.12013.

Stop Stock-outs Campaign. 2010. *What are stock-outs?* http://stopstockouts.org/stop-stock-outscampaign/what-are-stock-outs/. Accessed 28 Dec 2012.
Stop TB Partnership. 2011. *Global drug facility annual report 2011.* http://www.stoptb.org/assets/documents/gdf/whatis/GDF_Annual_Report_2011_web_lowres.pdf. Accessed 28 Dec 2012.
World Health Organization (WHO). 2009. *Global tuberculosis control 2009: Epidemiology, strategy, financing*, 37. Geneva: World Health Organization.
World Health Organization (WHO). 2012. *Global tuberculosis report 2012: Executive summary.* http://apps.who.int/iris/bitstream/10665/75938/1/9789241564502_eng.pdf. Accessed 3 June 2015.
World Health Organization (WHO). 2015. *Essential medicines.* http://www.who.int/topics/essential_medicines/en/. Accessed 24 June 2015.

8.9 Case 5: Transmitting Cholera to Haiti

Joseph Millum
Clinical Center Department of Bioethics and Fogarty International Center
National Institutes of Health
Bethesda, MD, USA
e-mail: joseph.millum@nih.gov

This case is presented for instructional purposes only. The ideas and opinions expressed are the author's own. The case is not meant to reflect the official position, views, or policies of the editors, the editors' host institutions, or the author's host institutions.

8.9.1 Background

Cholera is caused by infection with *Vibrio cholerae* bacteria, which colonize the small intestine and produce cholera toxin. The disease is characterized by sudden onset of severe, watery diarrhea and vomiting. Left untreated, cholera rapidly leads to dehydration and shock. Severe cholera can be fatal in more than 50 % of cases. Prompt treatment reduces the case fatality rate to less than 1 % (Boore et al. 2008). Treatment primarily addresses the loss of fluids: patients should be aggressively treated with oral rehydration solution or, if severely dehydrated, through intravenous fluids. Treatment with antibiotics shortens the course of the disease.

Cholera is transmitted through contaminated food or water. In developing countries, where most infections and deaths occur, inadequate sanitation is frequently the cause of the spread of *V. cholerae*, as untreated fecal matter from cholera sufferers leaks into the water supply. Each year, 3–5 million cases of cholera occur, leading to about 120,000 deaths (Harris et al. 2012).

Cholera is endemic in more than 50 countries. In many places, cholera outbreaks are seasonal—flaring up during the rainy season and dying down again during dry periods. Outbreaks can be prevented or contained by properly treating sewage, promoting rigorous hygiene practices, and sterilizing drinking water. Two oral cholera vaccines are commercially available but not included in most cholera control programs, although the World Health Organization (WHO) recommends them for use in outbreaks and for high-risk populations (WHO 2010). Before 2010, Haiti had not experienced cholera for at least a century.

Haiti, a country of ten million people, occupies the western portion of the island of Hispaniola in the Caribbean. Although its per capita gross domestic product (GDP) is about $1,200 (Central Intelligence Agency 2012),[13] a tiny elite controls most of the country's wealth. With 80 % of the population living below the poverty line, Haiti is the lowest-ranked country in the Americas on the United Nations (U.N.) Human Development Index (UNDP 2011). The economy depends heavily on remittances from Haitians working abroad and on foreign aid.

Life expectancy in Haiti is 62 years, while infant mortality is 52 per 1,000 live births (UNDP 2011). Sixty-four percent of Haitians have access to an improved water source (i.e., one that is protected from outside contamination), but just 26 % have access to improved sanitation (i.e., a facility that separates human excreta from human contact) (WHO/UNICEF 2013). Communicable diseases, including HIV/AIDS, tuberculosis, diarrheal diseases, and malaria remain substantial causes of disability and death. There are severe shortages of physicians, nurses, hospital beds, and essential medicines. About 6 % of GDP is spent on health, of which three-quarters is private expenditure. Out-of-pocket spending on health care is extremely high (UNDP 2011).

Haiti has a long history of political instability, characterized by multiple coups, foreign interference and occupation, and extended periods of dictatorship, notably under François Duvalier (Papa Doc) and his son Jean-Claude Duvalier (Baby Doc) between 1957 and 1986. Following a coup in 2004, the U.N. stationed peacekeepers in Haiti. The U.N. Stabilization Mission in Haiti (MINUSTAH) has been in Haiti ever since.

In January 2010, a magnitude 7.0 earthquake struck Haiti. Hundreds of thousands of people died and up to a million were left homeless. International aid agencies, donor governments, and nongovernmental organizations (NGOs) mobilized rapidly in response, and substantial amounts of money and aid were promised to assist in rebuilding.

8.9.2 Case Description

In mid-October 2010, upstream of the Artibonite River, a sudden rush of people began presenting at the local hospital with acute diarrhea, signaling the first cholera cases. People living nearby use the river extensively for washing, bathing, and drinking water; farmers downstream use it for irrigation. Within days, the spread of cholera to the Artibonite River Delta and settlements on the coast had overwhelmed local clinics and hospitals. The facilities lacked cholera cots that allow patients to defecate hygienically from their beds, while insufficient space for all patients prevented isolation of cholera victims. For the thousands of sufferers, the supply of

[13] Purchasing power parity in 2011 U.S. dollars.

doctors, nurses, and rehydration packs proved inadequate. The epidemic exploded across Haiti. Since cholera was not endemic, the population lacked immunity. Within months, thousands of people had died and hundreds of thousands had been sickened.

NGOs and some international donor agencies, including from the U.N., who were already in Haiti dealing with the aftermath of the earthquake, diverted resources to combat cholera. They distributed medical supplies, organized educational campaigns on cholera prevention, trucked clean drinking water and water purification tablets across the country, and worked with local hospitals to institute rigorous infection control measures.

The Haitian and international response to the cholera outbreak rapidly brought the case fatality rate from around 9 % to less than 1 %. Although the outbreak died down, the aid efforts failed to rectify the dire state of Haiti's water and sanitation infrastructure. During the rainy season, cases would spike again, exposing the difficulty of improving the Haitian health care system so that it could respond to new outbreaks without external assistance.

Haiti had been cholera-free for more than a century—so how had cholera got there? Almost as soon as the outbreak started, rumors circulated blaming U.N. peacekeepers. A contingent of soldiers from Nepal, where cholera is endemic, had arrived in October 2010. They were stationed at a camp on a tributary of the Artibonite River near where the outbreak began. Waste management at the base was rumored to be inadequate and had allowed sewage to flow into the river.

Initially, U.N. officials denied responsibility for bringing cholera to Haiti. But rumors and public protest persisted, fueled by independent investigations suggesting the camp as the source (Piarroux et al. 2011). Finally, the U.N. Secretary General convened an independent panel of experts charged with determining the source of the cholera outbreak. The panel completed its report in May 2011. It argued that the evidence from the Artibonite River's tributary system, the epidemiological timeline, and genetic analyses of Haitian *V. cholerae* bacteria indicated that the outbreak resulted from contamination of the river with feces carrying a strain of the current South Asian bacterium. Moreover, the report noted that the "haphazard" plumbing construction in the main toilet and showering area offered significant potential for cross-contamination, and that heavy rains could cause the open septic pit into which black water was deposited to overflow into the tributary (Cravioto et al. 2011).

The report offered a series of recommendations to prevent similar occurrences and concluded

> The introduction of this cholera strain as a result of environmental contamination with feces could not have been the source of such an outbreak without simultaneous water and sanitation and health care system deficiencies. These deficiencies, coupled with conducive environmental and epidemiological conditions, allowed the spread of the *Vibrio cholerae* organism in the environment, from which a large number of people became infected.
>
> The independent panel concludes that the Haiti cholera outbreak was caused by the confluence of circumstances as described above and was not the fault of, or deliberate action of, a group or individual (Cravioto et al. 2011).

Since the initial outbreak, more than 7,500 Haitians have died from cholera and more than 600,000 have been sickened. Subsequent independent genetic analysis confirmed that the Haitian strain was almost identical with the strain currently circulating in South Asia (Hendriksen et al. 2011).

Many commentators believe that the systemic deficiencies that enabled the outbreak are partly the fault of the Haitian government. It failed to take appropriate measures to protect its population from disease, such as improving drinking water and sanitation, investing in health care infrastructure, and so forth. The Independent Panel concluded that the introduction of cholera by the U.N. mission was therefore not the fault of the U.N. An alternative view is that multiple actors were at fault for this tragedy, including the Haitian government, the U.N., and foreign governments whose policies affect Haiti.

A distinct issue is whether and how the victims of the outbreak should be compensated. One option is to make compensation the responsibility of those at fault, although the difficulties in assigning fault may make this option challenging. An alternative is to establish a no-fault scheme that would compensate anyone affected, but determining who must pay is also problematic. Donors working on earthquake relief in Haiti, for example, arguably should not have to divert funds to remedy a problem they did not create. In November 2011, a legal suit was brought against the U.N. seeking compensation for the victims of the cholera outbreak (Sontag 2012). In February 2013, the U.N. invoked legal immunity against such suits and refused to provide compensation.

8.9.3 Discussion Questions

1. Which parties' interests are affected by the cholera outbreak? Which parties might have some responsibility to respond to the outbreak?
2. The U.N.'s Independent Panel of Experts concluded that "the Haiti cholera outbreak was caused by the confluence of circumstances … and was not the fault of, or deliberate action of, a group or individual." Assume that they are correct about the facts. Does it follow that no one is morally at fault? Explain why or why not.
3. Imagine that you are providing recommendations for compensating the victims of infectious disease outbreaks, like Haiti's. Should individual actors be held accountable, or should a no-fault compensation scheme be put in place? If the latter, who should provide compensation? Explain the reasons for your responses. (Douglas 2009 discusses "no-fault" compensation in another context.)
4. If the Haitian government has neglected its responsibilities to its citizens, does this make any difference to the help that international aid agencies should provide to Haiti? Explain why or why not.
5. One possible concern with seeking compensation for the people who contracted cholera is that it may have a "chilling effect" on international assistance. For example, if aid agencies believe they are at risk of being sued for unintentionally transmitting disease, they may be deterred from working in a country in the first place. Should the Haitian government or the lawyers representing the victims take this concern into account? Why or why not?

References

Boore, A., M. Iwamoto, E. Mintz, and P. Yu. 2008. Cholera and other vibrioses. In *Control of communicable diseases manual*, 19th ed, ed. D.L. Heymann, 113–127. Washington, DC: American Public Health Association.

Central Intelligence Agency. 2012. *The world factbook.* https://www.cia.gov/library/publications/the-world-factbook/. Accessed 29 May 2013.

Cravioto, A., C.F. Lanata, D.S. Lantagne, and G.B. Nair. 2011. *Final report of the independent panel of experts on the cholera outbreak in Haiti.* http://www.un.org/News/dh/infocus/haiti/UN-cholera-report-final.pdf. Accessed 29 May 2013.

Douglas, T. 2009. Medical injury compensation: Beyond 'no fault'. *Medical Law Review* 17(1): 30–51. doi:10.1093/medlaw/fwn022.

Harris, J.B., R.C. LaRocque, F. Qadri, E.T. Ryan, and S.B. Calderwood. 2012. Cholera. *Lancet* 379(9835): 2466–2476. doi:10.1016/S0140-6736(12)60436-X.

Hendriksen, R.S., L.B. Price, J.M. Schupp, et al. 2011. Population genetics of *Vibrio cholerae* from Nepal in 2010: Evidence on the origin of the Haitian outbreak. *mBio* 2(4): e00157–e001511. doi:10.1128/mBio.00157-11. http://mbio.asm.org/content/2/4/e00157-11.full.pdf+html. Accessed 29 May 2013.

Piarroux, R., R. Barrais, B. Faucher, et al. 2011. Understanding the cholera epidemic, Haiti. *Emerging Infectious Diseases* 17(7): 1161–1168.

Sontag, D. 2012. *In Haiti, global failures on a cholera epidemic. New York Times*, March 31.

United Nations Development Programme (UNDP). 2011. *Human development report 2011: Sustainability and equity: A better future for all.* http://hdr.undp.org/en/content/humandevelopment-report-2011. Accessed 29 May 2013.

WHO/UNICEF Joint Monitoring Programme (JMP) for Water Supply and Sanitation. 2013. *Data and estimates.* http://www.wssinfo.org/data-estimates/table/. Accessed 29 May 2013.

World Health Organization (WHO). 2010. Cholera vaccines: WHO position paper. *Weekly Epidemiological Record* 85(13): 117–128. http://www.who.int/wer/2010/wer8513.pdf?ua=1. Accessed 11 June 2015.

8.10 Case 6: Perilous Path to Middle East Peace: The Sanctions Dilemma

Waleed Al-Faisal
Department of Family and Community Medicine, Faculty of Medicine
Damascus University
Damascus, Syrian Arab Republic

Primary Health Care
Dubai Health Authority
Dubai, United Arab Emirates

Hamid Hussain
Faculty of Medicine
University of Baghdad
Baghdad, Iraq

Dubai Residency Training Program and Public Health Consultant
Dubai Health Authority
Dubai, United Arab Emirates
e-mail: hussainh569@gmail.com

Kasturi Sen
Global Public Health, Wolfson College (Common Room)
University of Oxford
Oxford, UK

This case is presented for instructional purposes only. The ideas and opinions expressed are the authors' own. The case is not meant to reflect the official position, views, or policies of the editors, the editors' host institutions, or the authors' host institutions.

8.10.1 Background

During the last century, public health practices have greatly improved the health of individuals and societies in the Middle East and North Africa (MENA) region through successful interventional programs like expanded immunization for children and universal salt iodization programs. The major challenge for public health in the twenty-first century is to simultaneously maintain and upgrade the infrastructure created to improve peoples' lives.

Currently, the MENA region faces multiple challenges to its public health achievements, one of which is the impact of sanctions being used against MENA countries to influence political behavior. Sanctions—defined as mostly economic but also political and military penalties introduced to alter political/military threats and behavior—are employed by the United States and other countries to discourage the proliferation of weapons of mass destruction and ballistic missiles, bolster human rights, end terrorism, thwart drug trafficking, discourage armed aggression, promote market access, protect the environment, and replace governments (Haass 1998). Sanctions often involve economic measures, such as restricting or eliminating foreign assistance, freezing countries' assets, imposing export and import limitations, and revoking most-favored-nation trade status (World Health Organization 2003).

Empirical evidence indicates that sanctions have profound long- and short-term public health impact on the health of citizens in the affected countries, with the greatest harm affecting the elderly, women, and children (Garfield 1999; Ali and Shah 2000). This impact goes far beyond problems with medical supplies or other health-specific resources. Public health services depend on a safe water supply, a functioning sanitation system, and a reliable power infrastructure; on availability of equipment such as ambulances, X-ray machines, and refrigerators for storing vaccines; on the public having resources to access health care (e.g., transportation, financial resources); and on human resources, the trained staff who use the equipment.

Two examples of the use of sanctions were those imposed by the United Nations (U.N.) against Iraq in the 1990s and against Syria beginning in 2011.

8.10.2 The Case of Iraq

To assess the health impact of the Iraq sanctions, the U.N. Children's Fund (UNICEF), in collaboration with the World Health Organization and local health authorities surveyed child health in Iraq during February through May 1999 (UNICEF 1999a, b). Between 1984 and 1989, infant mortality in Iraq was 47 per 1,000 live births (Ali and Shah 2000). In southern and central Iraq, the infant mortality rate almost tripled, rising to 108 per 1,000 live births during 1994 through 1999. The under-5 child mortality rate also drastically increased (more than doubled) from 56 to 131 per 1,000 live births for the same period (Ali and Shah 2000). Yet in the autonomous northern region of Iraq, infant mortality declined from 64 to 59 per 1,000 live births and under-5 mortality fell from 80 to 72 per 1,000 live births for the same period. These differences were attributed to better food and resource allocation due to Western support for an autonomous region and the nonapplication of universal sanctions (UNICEF 2002).

Other studies of the health impact of sanctions on Iraq have similar negative findings (Armijo-Hussein et al. 1991; Hurwitz and David 1992; Central Statistical Organization, Iraq 1996, 1997). Table 8.1 summarizes data from these studies and shows the change in health indicators once sanctions were imposed in 1990.

8.10.3 The Case of Syria

Since May 2011, economic sanctions against Syria significantly affected the exchange rate, devaluing its Syrian Lira (SL). The exchange rate of 45 SL for every U.S. dollar increased to more than 200 SL and had serious economic ramifications. The cost of living essentials such as gas, eggs, milk, bread, and cooking oil more than tripled over the past 2 years. At the same time, the purchasing power of

Table 8.1 Health status indicators before and after the 1990 sanctions against Iraq

Indicator	1985	1991	1996
Infant mortality rate	52	42	97
Under-5 mortality rate	64	42	126
Chronic malnutrition (%)	18	18	32
Stunting (%)	12	29	26
Maternal mortality per 100,000 births	–	121	294
Diarrhea episodes per child per year	–	3.8	14.4
Births below 2.5 Kg (%)	5–9	4.5	12

Note. A dash indicates that reliable data are not available

salaries was halved. Families, nearing starvation, were forced out of work, and more than 20 % of the working population was unable to purchase living essentials (Zarzar 2013; Food and Agriculture Organization of the United Nations 2013). The collapse of the exchange rate increased the cost of health services and of medicines. Despite the emphasis of sanctions on economic measures, they prevented entry of essential medical supplies into the country, including those for chronic diseases such as cancer, diabetes, and heart disease, which are not produced locally. Local drug production, an area in which Syria had been 90 % self-sufficient before the sanctions and conflict, largely collapsed. This opened channels for counterfeit drugs and corruption among those who smuggled supplies through the country's porous borders. The high cost of heating and electricity during 2 years of conflict compounded the adverse effects of Syria's extreme winter and summer temperatures. Most notably, the cold chain of vaccines were destroyed, contributing to the virtual collapse of the once successful vaccination programme (Al Faisal et al. 2012a, b). The combination of price increases, job losses, and lower salaries devastated families, especially those with children or members who were pregnant or elderly (United Nations Office for the Coordination of Humanitarian Affairs 2013). Millions of small businesses collapsed in Syria. Many were small-scale and home-based, run by women providing invaluable income to cope with price inflation and to purchase food, school books and uniforms for children, and essential medicines and emergency medical care.

8.10.4 *Ethical Considerations*

Before World War I, economic sanctions were considered acts of warfare that, like military sieges, inflicted suffering on entire populations. Viewed this way, economic sanctions appear ethically suspect from a number of perspectives. Sanctions violate the just war ban on targeting noncombatants, the Kant's philosophy not to use people as means to an end, and the negative right of populations not to be deprived of their means of subsistence (Gordon 1999; United Nations 2005). However, after World War I when the League of Nations was created, economic sanctions came to be viewed as a peaceful, diplomatic alternative to war that could prevent military intervention (Gordon 1999). This viewpoint holds that to justify sanctions, the benefits of avoiding the presumably far greater harms caused by war, civil war, or long-term political oppression must outweigh the harms sanctions impose on a populace. But this grim utilitarian calculus must also consider the probability of the success of sanctions, which generally is low. Pape (1997), for example, estimates that sanctions lead to political compliance less than 5 % of the time. More optimistically, Hufbauer et al. (2009) judge sanctions effective in 34 % of situations used. However, they stress that the success of sanctions depends on many factors including the purpose; the relative economic instability of the country receiving sanctions; whether the country receiving sanctions is part of a broad array of diplomatic, economic, military, and covert measures; and whether the sanctions are being imposed in the context of a broader international coalition (Hufbauer et al. 2009).

8.10.5 Case Description

You are a public health official from a country in the Middle East researching the impact of economic sanctions on the health of populations. You have seen first-hand the impact sanctions have had on vulnerable populations. You also have expertise in public health ethics and have written extensively about ethics in the use of economic sanctions. You have been invited by a United Nations commission to testify on the health impact of sanctions. The commission values your opinion on whether sanctions are ever ethical and justified.

8.10.6 Discussion Questions

1. What are the range of ethical considerations for and against the use of economic sanctions? Are there ways of imposing economic sanctions that can avoid forms of collective punishment and minimize subsequent adverse health impact on individuals and populations?
2. In extreme situations where many human lives are at stake, such as emergency disaster relief, doctors and public health officials often revert to simple utilitarian calculations of lives lost or saved (e.g., triage decisions). To what extent is the ethical logic surrounding economic sanctions similar or dissimilar to the ethical logic of emergency disaster relief?
3. Can economic sanctions be ethically justified
   (a) as an alternative to long-standing political oppression and human rights violations?
   (b) to prevent civil war?
   (c) to avert war?
   (d) to effect regime change?

References

Al Faisal, W., Y. Al Saleh, and K. Sen. 2012a. Syria: Public health achievements and sanctions. *The Lancet* 379(9833): 2241. doi:10.1016/S0140-6736(12)60871-X. http://www.thelancet.com/journals/lancet/article/PIIS0140-6736(12)60871-X/fulltext. Accessed 5 July 2013.

Al Faisal, W., K. Sen, and Y. Al Saleh. 2012b. Syria: Public health achievements and the effect of sanctions. *Indian Journal of Medical Ethics* 9(3): 151–153.

Ali, M.M., and I.H. Shah. 2000. Sanctions and childhood mortality in Iraq. *Lancet* 355(9218): 1851–1858. http://www.thelancet.com/journals/lancet/article/PIIS0140673600022893/. Accessed 4 July 2013.

Armijo-Hussein, N.A., E. Benjamin, R. Moodie, et al. 1991. The effect of the Gulf Crisis on the children of Iraq. *New England Journal of Medicine* 325(13): 977–980. doi:10.1056/NEJM199109263251330.

Central Statistical Organization, Iraq. 1996. *The 1996 Multiple Indicator Cluster Survey: A survey to assess the situation of children and women in Iraq. Final Report with Results from South/ Centre Governorates*. Iraq, UNICEF Ref IRQ/97/288, August.

Central Statistical Organization, Iraq. 1997. *The 1996 Multiple Indicator Cluster Survey: A survey to assess the situation of families in Iraq. Final Report with Results from Northern Governorates.* Iraq, UNICEF, Rep/97/166, May.

Food and Agriculture Organization of the United Nations. 2013. *Four million Syrians are unable to produce or buy enough food.* http://www.fao.org/news/story/en/item/179446/icode/. Accessed 6 July 2013.

Garfield, R. 1999. *The impact of economic sanctions on health and well being*, Relief and Rehabilitation Network, Paper 31, 1–4. London: Overseas Development Institute.

Gordon, J.A. 1999. A peaceful, silent, deadly remedy: The ethics of economic sanctions. *Ethics & International Affairs* 13(1): 123–142. doi:10.1111/j.1747-7093.1999.tb00330.x.

Haass, R.N. 1998. *Economic sanctions: Too much of a bad thing.* Brookings Policy Brief Series. http://www.brookings.edu/research/papers/1998/06/sanctions-haass. Accessed 21 Apr 2013.

Hufbauer, G.C., J.J. Schott, K.A. Elliott, and B. Oegg. 2009. *Economic sanctions reconsidered*, 3rd ed. Washington, DC: Peterson Institute for International Economics.

Hurwitz, M., and P. David. 1992. *The state of children's health in pre-war Iraq.* London: Centre for Population Studies, London School of Hygiene and Tropical Medicine.

Pape, R.A. 1997. Why economic sanctions do not work. *International Security* 22(2): 90–136.

United Nations. 2005. *Economic, social and cultural rights: Handbook for national human rights institutions*, Professional Training Series No. 12. New York: United Nations. http://www.ohchr.org/Documents/Publications/training12en.pdf. Accessed 8 July 2013.

United Nations Office for the Coordination of Humanitarian Affairs. 2013. *Syria Humanitarian Assistance Response Plan* (SHARP, 1 January–30 June 2013). http://www.unocha.org/cap/appeals/humanitarian-assistance-response-plan-syria-1-january-30-june-2013. Accessed 21 Apr 2013.

UNICEF. 1999a. Iraq surveys show 'humanitarian emergency.' *UNICEF Newsline.* August 12.

UNICEF. 1999b. *Questions and answers for the Iraq child mortality surveys.* August 16. http://www.casi.org.uk/info/unicef/990816qa.html. Accessed 9 Feb 2014.

UNICEF. 2002. *Nutritional Survey 2002: Overview of nutritional status of under-fives in South/Central Iraq.* http://www.casi.org.uk/info/unicef/0211nutrition.pdf. Accessed 9 Feb 2014.

World Health Organization (WHO). 2003. *Health situation in Iraq prior to March 2003.* WHO/EMRO: 5/2003: 47. Diaz, J., and R. Garfield. 2003. Iraq Watching Briefs: Health and Nutrition. http://www.google.ae/url?sa=t&rct=j&q=&esrc=s&frm=1&source=web&cd=1&ved=0CCcQFjAA&url=http%3A%2F%2Fwww.corpwatch.org%2Fdownloads%2FIraqiHealthWatching_Brief.doc&ei=Sxj3Ut7mCqip0AXUyoDwCg&usg=AFQjCNGKtg9iCFecdctGW6U-7Gt94E8Hnw&sig2=EB5Zjewajg3mr6F0pse29g. Accessed 9 Feb 2014.

Zarzar, A. 2013. The ballooning cost of living in Damascus. *Al-Akhbar.* http://english.al-akhbar.com/node/14624. Accessed 9 Feb 2014.

8.11 Case 7: Advancing Informed Consent and Ethical Standards in Multinational Health Research

Drew E. Lee
Department of Family Medicine
Advocate Lutheran General Hospital
Park Ridge, IL, USA
e-mail: drewleemd@gmail.com

Sarah A. Kleinfeld
Department of Psychiatry
Medstar Georgetown University Hospital
Washington, DC, USA

Rachel M. Glassford
School of Public Health and Health Services
George Washington University
Falls Church, VA, USA

This case is presented for instructional purposes only. The ideas and opinions expressed are the authors' own. The case is not meant to reflect the official position, views, or policies of the editors, the editors' host institutions, or the authors' host institutions.

8.11.1 Background

In the United States, regulations for informed consent largely came about during the 1950s through 1970s not only in response to unethical human experiments carried out in Nazi Germany, but also to those within U.S. borders (Beecher 1966). Experiments like the U.S. Public Health Service Tuskegee Syphilis Study (Jones 1981) prompted Congress to enact human research regulations, initially through the 1974 National Research Act. Subsequently, other research guidelines have been developed and revised (World Health Organization 2000; Council for International Organizations of Medical Sciences 2002; The International Conference on Harmonisation of Technical Requirements for Registration of Pharmaceuticals for Human Use 1996; World Medical Association 2008), fostering expansion of ethics commissions and review boards and making informed consent an integral component of health research (Meslin and Johnson 2008). Yet, half a century later, many countries still lack adequate human research regulations or regulatory authorities. These regulatory gaps leave research participants, their families, and communities at risk for great harm through sociocultural discrimination, research-related illness, disability, and death and post-experimental medical abandonment. In Nigeria, Pfizer tested an unapproved drug on infants and children (Abdullahi v. Pfizer Inc. 2002); in India, Johns Hopkins tested cancer drugs on patients without proper consent (Sharma 2001); and other such incidents have been reported (LaFraniere et al. 2000). Even the U.S. National Institutes of Health failed to produce consent forms for experiments on HIV-positive women in developing countries (Public Citizen 1998).

On a practical and ethical level, debate continues over human research and informed consent (Tri-Council 2010; Marshall 2008; Nuffield Council on Bioethics 2002). While some argue for a single ethical standard for human research (Lurie and Wolfe 1997; Angell 1997), others believe that imposing a global ethical standard irrespective of cultural differences would amount to ethical imperialism (Resnik 1998). *The New England Journal of Medicine* "has taken the position that it will not publish reports of unethical research regardless of their scientific merit" (Angell 1997). But like other scientific journals, it has found difficulty in determining what is unethical versus what is culturally appropriate research in different settings.

There are many challenges to obtaining informed consent. Some involve illiteracy; noncomprehension of information; language and communication barriers; or unfamiliarity with certain scientific, medical, or ethical concepts. Other challenges are attributable to complex sociocultural, psychological, or structural elements, such as shared decision making by community members, rather than by an individual (Marshall 2000, 2008). Some studies, however, take the stance that such challenges do not preclude an individual's ability to understand or voluntarily participate in research studies (Pace et al. 2003). Consequently, in order to ensure that research participation is voluntary, it is important to safeguard a participant's right to refuse or withdraw from a study at any time.

One practical solution to obtaining appropriate consent is by implementing culturally acceptable methods such as oral consent, video documentation, or community meetings (Tri-Council 2010; Nuffield Council on Bioethics 2002; Dawson and Kass 2005). Another is to require foreign researchers to receive dual approval through a local review board and their own institutional review board (IRB) (World Health Organization 2000; Council for International Organizations of Medical Sciences 2002; Tri-Council 2010). Nevertheless, multinational collaborations in research, especially those originating in regions that lack adequate research regulations, can be problematic because research "approval" may not provide adequate protections.

De-identified data and information[14] pose an additional complication for obtaining proper informed consent. These can include "x-rays, endoscopic images, images of organs or tissues taken during an autopsy, still or video recordings of surgical procedures, and microscopic images" (Tranberg et al. 2003). As long as these remain de-identified, researchers need not obtain informed consent (European Union 1995; U.S. Department of Health and Human Services 2009; National Institutes of Health 2007). However, in countries lacking adequate research ethics infrastructures, waiving informed consent is problematic at several levels. First, verifying if appropriate consent was obtained becomes virtually impossible. Second, the lack of consent can be medically dangerous for research participants and have legal repercussions for researchers (Flory et al. 2008). Finally, it can complicate the research process by compromising the utility of research samples and data (Wendler 2008).

Continued globalization, international development and increased accessibility to data through electronic medical records and online databases will increase multinational human research. As multinational research becomes more common, the need to find appropriate ethical standards and informed consent policies will become more urgent. Ultimately, the goal of such standards and policies should be to ensure that research participants and their information are safeguarded at the origin and throughout every step of the research process.

[14] De-identification involves stripping data and information of personal identifiers (e.g. names, addresses, birth dates, photos, or any unique identifiers), such that an individual's identity remains anonymous and cannot be retraced.

8.11.2 Case Description

You are an infectious disease specialist working at a university in a high-income country and are interested in researching cervical cancer in immunocompromised patients. Because you collaborate regularly with colleagues worldwide, other researchers commonly seek your input. An African colleague e-mails you for advice on a multinational cervical cancer study she is conducting with several other researchers in seven different African countries. This study began 3 years ago to address the local population's health needs and has been funded by local hospitals and organizations. This colleague, a public health professional, has compiled the research data in an online database. The information she sends you includes an electronic copy of the preliminary report, de-identified data set, and pathology slides of cervical specimens. After reviewing her preliminary findings, you agree that her research could positively impact the health outcomes of individuals in her community.

Excited by this initial review, your colleague invites you to coauthor an upcoming manuscript on the study. You carefully review the methods section of the preliminary report, focusing on how consent was obtained. In one research country, consent was provided via video documentation; in two others, it was obtained through a standardized consent form; and in a fourth, through verbal consent of male community leaders *before* seeking consent from individual participants, a practice in line with local cultural norms. For the remaining three countries, no consent documentation exists.

You follow-up with your colleague about the various consent methods. She indicates that none of the countries involved in the project have IRBs or national research guidelines, but that consent methods were typical for research projects in these countries. Regarding the three countries lacking consent documentation, she believes that some form of consent was obtained from the research participants, although she lacks supporting evidence.

Although the information you received was de-identified, you wonder about the lack of uniformity in the consent process but attribute it to respect for differing cultural norms. Based on all information provided, you believe the research has scientific merit and the data collected is scientifically valid. You also believe the study should be published, as it could significantly improve the health of the region and advance future research.

8.11.3 Discussion Questions

1. Who would you turn to in your institution for guidance regarding your involvement in the research, coauthorship of the manuscript, and other contributions to this research study?
2. What are some appropriate ways to obtain informed consent when conducting research in areas with culture or language different from yours? Name some pros and cons to each approach.

3. Does the use of multiple methods to obtain consent raise questions about the reliability of the data or validity of the research project? Without confirmation of informed consent, would you consider the publication of this research study to be scientific misconduct?
4. What are some appropriate ways to obtain informed consent for research conducted in countries with different consent standards and requirements? Are there instances when one set of requirements should take priority over another?
5. Given the multiple methods used to obtain consent, are you willing to coauthor your colleague's paper? Why or why not?

References

Abdullahi v. Pfizer, Inc., ("Abdullahi I"). 2002. U.S. Dist. LEXIS 17436 (S.D.N.Y., 17 Sep).

Angell, M. 1997. The ethics of clinical research in the Third World. *New England Journal of Medicine* 337(12): 847–849.

Beecher, H.K. 1966. Ethics and clinical research. *New England Journal of Medicine* 274(24): 1354–1360.

Council for International Organizations of Medical Sciences. 2002. *International ethical guide lines for biomedical research involving human subjects*. Geneva: Collaboration with the World Health Organization. http://www.cioms.ch/publications/layout_guide2002.pdf. Accessed 3 Jan 2013.

Dawson, L., and N.E. Kass. 2005. Views of US researchers about informed consent in international collaborative research. *Social Science & Medicine* 61(6): 1211–1222.

European Union. 1995. *Directive 95/46/EC of the European Parliament and of the Council on the protection of individuals with regard to the processing of personal data and on the free movement of such data*. http://ec.europa.eu/justice/policies/privacy/docs/95-46-ce/dir1995-46_part1_en.pdf. Accessed 3 Jan 2013.

Flory, J.H., D. Wendler, and E.J. Emanuel. 2008. Empirical issues in informed consent for research. In *The Oxford textbook of clinical research ethics*, ed. E.J. Emanuel, C. Grady, R.A. Crouch, K. Lie, F.G. Miller, and D. Wendler, 645–660. Oxford: Oxford University Press.

International Conference on Harmonisation of Technical Requirements for Registration of Pharmaceuticals for Human Use. 1996. *The ICH Harmonised tripartite guideline: Guideline for good clinical practice*. http://www.ich.org/fileadmin/Public_Web_Site/ICH_Products/Guidelines/Efficacy/E6/E6_R1_Guideline.pdf. Accessed 3 Jan 2013.

Jones, J.H. 1981. *Bad blood: The Tuskegee syphilis experiment*. New York: Free Press.

LaFraniere, S., M.P. Flaherty, and J. Stephens. 2000. The dilemma: Submit or suffer 'Uninformed Consent' is rising ethic of the drug test boom. *The Washington Post*. http://www.washingtonpost.com/wp-dyn/content/article/2008/10/01/AR2008100101150.html. Accessed 27 Mar 2013.

Lurie, P., and S.M. Wolfe. 1997. Unethical trials of intervention to reduce perinatal transmission of the human immunodeficiency virus in developing countries. *New England Journal of Medicine* 337(12): 853–856.
Marshall, P.A. 2000. Informed consent in international health research: (1) Cultural influences on communication, (2) The protection of confidentiality. In *Biomedical research ethics: Updating international guidelines*, ed. A. Consultation, R.J. Levine, S. Gorovitz, and J. Gallagher, 100–134. Geneva: World Health Organization.
Marshall, P.A. 2008. "Cultural competence" and informed consent in international health research. *Cambridge Quarterly of Healthcare Ethics* 17(2): 206–215.
Meslin, E.M., and S. Johnson. 2008. National bioethics commissions and research ethics. In *The Oxford textbook of clinical research ethics*, ed. E.J. Emanuel, C. Grady, R.A. Crouch, R.K. Lie, F.G. Miller, and D. Wendler, 187–197. Oxford: Oxford University Press.
National Institutes of Health. 2007. *How can covered entities use and disclose protected health information for research and comply with the Privacy Rule?* http://privacyruleandresearch.nih.gov/pr_08.asp. Accessed 3 Jan 2013.
Nuffield Council on Bioethics. 2002. *The ethics of research related to healthcare in developing countries*. London: Nuffield Council on Bioethics. http://www.nuffieldbioethics.org/wp-content/uploads/2014/07/Ethics-of-research-related-to-healthcare-in-developing-countries-I.pdf. Accessed 3 Jan 2013.
Pace, C., C. Grady, and E.J. Emanuel. 2003. *What we don't know about informed consent*. http://www.scidev.net/en/opinions/what-we-dont-know-about-informed-consent.html. Accessed 14 Apr 2013.
Public Citizen. 1998. *Health group fi les suit over NIH experiments on HIV-positive women in developing countries*. http://www.citizen.org/pressroom/pressroomredirect.cfm?ID=241. Accessed 27 Mar 2013.
Resnik, D.B. 1998. The ethics of HIV research in developing nations. *Bioethics* 12(4): 286–306.
Sharma, D.C. 2001. Johns Hopkins and RCC face drug trial allegations. *Lancet Oncology* 2(9): 530.
Tranberg, H.A., B.A. Rous, and J. Rashbass. 2003. Legal and ethical issues in the use of anonymous images in pathology teaching and research. *Histopathology* 42(2): 104–109.
Tri-Council. 2010. *Tri-Council policy statement: Ethical conduct for research involving humans*. Canadian Institutes of Health Research, National Sciences and Engineering Research Council of Canada, and Social Sciences and Humanities Research Council of Canada. http://www.ethics.gc.ca/pdf/eng/tcps2/TCPS_2_FINAL_Web.pdf. Accessed 3 Jan 2013.
U.S. Department of Health and Human Services. 2009. *Title 45 (Public Welfare), Code of Federal Regulation, Part 46 (Protection of Human Subjects)*. http://www.hhs.gov/ohrp/policy/ohrpregulations.pdf. Accessed 3 Jan 2013.
Wendler, D. 2008. Research with biological samples. In *The Oxford textbook of clinical research ethics*, ed. E.J. Emanuel, C. Grady, R.A. Crouch, R.K. Lie, F.G. Miller, and D. Wendler, 290–297. Oxford: Oxford University Press.
World Health Organization (WHO). 2000. *Operational guidelines for ethics committees that review biomedical research*. http://www.who.int/tdr/publications/documents/ethics.pdf. Accessed 3 Jan 2013.
World Medical Association. 2008. *Declaration of Helsinki*. http://www.wma.net/en/30publications/10policies/b3/. Accessed 3 Jan 2013.

Chapter 9
Public Health Research

Drue H. Barrett, Leonard W. Ortmann, Natalie Brown, Barbara R. DeCausey, Carla Saenz, and Angus Dawson

9.1 Introduction

Having a scientific basis for the practice of public health is critical. Research leads to insight and innovations that solve health problems and is therefore central to public health worldwide. For example, in the United States research is one of the ten essential public health services (Public Health Functions Steering Committee 1994). The *Principles of the Ethical Practice of Public Health*, developed by the Public Health Leadership Society (2002), emphasizes the value of having a scientific basis

---

The opinions, findings, and conclusions of the authors do not necessarily reflect the official position, views, or policies of the editors, the editors' host institutions, or the authors' host institutions.

D.H. Barrett, PhD (✉) • L.W. Ortmann, PhD
Office of Scientific Integrity, Office of the Associate Director for Science,
Office of the Director, Centers for Disease Control and Prevention, Atlanta, GA, USA
e-mail: dbarrett@cdc.gov

N. Brown, MPH
Human Research Protections Office, Office of Scientific Integrity, Office of the Associate Director for Science, Office of the Director, Centers for Disease Control and Prevention, Atlanta, GA, USA

B.R. DeCausey, MPH, MBA
Clinical Research Branch, Division of Tuberculosis Elimination, National Center for HIV/AIDS, Viral Hepatitis, STD, and TB Prevention, Centers for Disease Control and Prevention, Atlanta, GA, USA

C. Saenz, PhD
Regional Program on Bioethics, Office of Knowledge Management, Bioethics, and Research, Pan American Health Organization, Washington, DC, USA

A. Dawson, PhD
Center for Values, Ethics and the Law in Medicine, Sydney School of Public Health, The University of Sydney, Sydney, Australia

D.H. Barrett et al. (eds.), *Public Health Ethics: Cases Spanning the Globe*, Public Health Ethics Analysis 3, DOI 10.1007/978-3-319-23847-0_9

for action. Principle five specifically calls on public health to seek the information needed to carry out effective policies and programs that protect and promote health.

This chapter presents ethical issues that can arise when conducting public health research. Although the literature about research ethics is complex and rich, it has at least two important limitations when applied to public health research. The first is that much of research ethics has focused on clinical or biomedical research in which the primary interaction is between individuals (i.e., patient-physician or research participant-researcher). Since bioethics tends to focus on the individual, the field of research ethics often neglects broader issues pertaining to communities and populations, including ethical issues raised by some public health research methods (e.g., the use of cluster randomized trials to measure population, not just individual, effects). However, if our discussion of public health research ethics begins by examining public health activities, it becomes apparent that the process of gaining consent involves more than individuals. We must consider that communities bear risks and reap benefits; that not only individuals but also populations may be vulnerable; and that the social, political, and economic context in which research takes place poses ethical challenges. Public health research, with its focus on intervention at community and population levels, has brought these broader ethical considerations to researchers' attention, demonstrating how ethics guidance based on biomedical research may limit, if not distort, the ethical perspective required to protect human subjects.

The second limitation has to do with how guidelines and regulations are conceived and used. As described in Chaps. 1 and 2 of this casebook, research ethics has mostly evolved out of concern for research abuses. Consequently, the intent of many guidelines and regulations is to strengthen the ethical practice of research with human subjects. These ethical guidance documents include the *Nuremberg Code* (1947); the *Universal Declaration of Human Rights* (United Nations 1948); the *Declaration of Helsinki* (World Medical Association 1964, last revised in 2013); and two documents developed by the Council for International Organizations of Medical Sciences (CIOMS) in collaboration with the World Health Organization (WHO): *International Ethical Guidelines for Biomedical Research Involving Human Subjects* (CIOMS 2002) and the *International Ethical Guidelines for Epidemiological Studies* (CIOMS 2009). In the United States, the primary ethical guidance for protecting human subjects is Title 45, Part 46, of the Code of Federal Regulations (U.S. Department of Health and Human Services 2009). The ethical principles of respect for persons, beneficence, and justice have often framed the discussion on ethical conduct of research with human subjects. These principles were first articulated by the U.S. National Commission for the Protection of Human Subjects of Biomedical and Behavioral Research (1979) in the *Belmont Report* and expanded upon by Beauchamp and Childress (1979) in *Principles of Biomedical Ethics*.

Such guidelines and regulations often represent a consensus on landmark issues and show ways to consider ethical issues. However, consensus documents can pose obstacles if used uncritically with overgeneralized rules applied blindly. For example, such documents seem to assume that the randomized controlled trial is the gold standard of research methodology, obscuring the fact that all research methods may raise ethical issues. In addition, it is debatable whether these guidelines adequately capture community- and population-oriented values and issues central to public health (Verweij and Dawson 2009). A general concern is that overreliance on guidance documents encourages a legalistic or compliance approach to ethics, rather than encouraging reflection and analysis (Coughlin et al. 2012). Coughlin and colleagues argue that to be successful, research oversight needs to focus on moral judgment and reflection, not on strict rule-like adherence to regulations documented on a checklist. Though formal training in ethics is desirable, moral judgment and discernment are developed by making ethical judgments. This highlights a problem inherent in research oversight. Review of research protocols requires scientific and ethical expertise. However, members of ethics review committees are often unpaid and uncompensated for service time and are frequently asked to perform review duties in addition to their normal work. This lack of regard for their service often results in considerable turnover among committee members and does not allow sufficient time for new members to develop moral discernment. Review of research protocols for human subjects should include consideration of the wider ethical implications of the research and not just focus on compliance with ethics regulations. When inappropriate, guidance should be adapted or even set aside.

Chapter 1 of this casebook provides an account of public health ethics that builds upon the disciplines of both ethics and public health. Following a similar approach, this chapter advances a view of public health research ethics that builds upon concepts of research ethics and public health research. As a result, many ethical issues discussed apply to all health research, including public health research. However, once we examine public health examples, we see that something beyond the traditional resources of current research regulations is needed. We will discuss these ethical issues by reflecting upon traditional research tenets and studying their limitations in a public health context. We will conclude by illustrating via the case studies included in this chapter how ethical challenges arise in public health research. It is impossible to closely analyze all possible ethical issues that may arise either in health research or public health research; thus our intent is to highlight some of the major ethical challenges and considerations.

9.2 What Is Different About Public Health Research?

The community and population perspective of public health, especially when addressing health issues in resource-poor contexts or in marginalized populations, frequently brings ethical challenges into focus. In public health, research typically occurs outside of the controlled environment that is characteristic of biomedical research. Instead, in public health, research often occurs in real world settings in a particular social, political, and economic context. It may involve interventions with whole communities or populations impacted by catastrophic public health emergencies.

9.2.1 Can Public Health Research Be Clearly Distinguished from Public Health Practice?

Distinguishing between public health *practice* and public health *research* is challenging. Many of the tools and methods are similar. Both involve systematic collection and analysis of data that may lead to generalizable knowledge. Public health research can take forms ranging from descriptive approaches (e.g., correlational studies and cross-sectional surveys) to analytic epidemiologic approaches (e.g., case control studies and cohort studies, including clinical trials). These same approaches can characterize methods for collecting information as part of public health practice.

A common way to define research is on the basis of its goal to develop generalizable knowledge. For example, the *International Ethical Guidelines for Biomedical Research Involving Human Subjects* (CIOMS 2002) defines research as "… a class of activity designed to develop or contribute to generalizable knowledge. Generalizable knowledge consists of theories, principles or relationships, or the accumulation of information on which they are based, that can be corroborated by accepted scientific methods of observation and inference." Similarly, in the United States, research is defined as "…a systematic investigation, including research development, testing and evaluation, designed to develop or contribute to generalizable knowledge" (U.S. Department of Health and Human Services 2009).

In jurisdictions with legal requirements governing research activities, such as the United States, determining what is and is not research becomes critical. Sometimes, however, the line between research and practice-related activities is blurry. One way to identify if an activity is research is to look at intent. The primary intent of public health research is to yield generalizable knowledge. Key characteristics of public health research include (1) benefits beyond the needs of the study participants, (2) collection of data exceeding what is needed to care for study participants, and (3) generation of knowledge with relevance outside the population from which data were collected. In contrast, the primary intent of activities that constitute public health practice are to "… prevent or control disease or injury and improve health, or to improve a public health program or service …" (Centers for Disease Control and Prevention [CDC] 1999, 2010). Key characteristics of public health practice include (1) benefits that focus on activity participants, (2) collection of data needed to improve the activity or the health of the participants, and (3) generation of knowledge that does not go beyond the scope of the activity (CDC 1999, 2010).

Some researchers suggest that the difficulty in distinguishing public health research from public health practice emerges from a deeper conceptual issue relating to the impossibility of satisfactorily defining "research" and related categories (Fairchild and Bayer 2004). For example, public health surveillance might involve identical interventions and risks for public health research as for practice. This has led many public health professionals to call for reorienting ethical review around an activity's level of risk, which applies to activities in both public health research and practice (Willison et al. 2014). Jurisdictions that do not yet have legal structures or have more flexibility to govern research activities than the United States might have an advantage. Whereas other jurisdictions might need to modify their approach to correlate ethical review with risk instead of on whether something falls under a slippery concept such as research.

9.3 Ethical Considerations for Protecting the Public during Health Research

This section outlines core aspects of research ethics and not only explains their relevance to public health, but also delves into why research ethics principles might need to be applied differently to public health research than to biomedical research.

9.3.1 Informed Consent

Informed consent is often treated as the primary means of protecting research participants. Although informed consent can be defined in different ways, it is foremost an active agreement made by someone with the capacity to understand, on the basis of relevant information, and in the absence of pressure or coercion. The common ethical justification for seeking informed consent is an appeal to the notion of autonomy, which holds that individuals have values and preferences and thus should voluntarily decide whether to participate in research. However, gaining consent can result from a more direct appeal to beneficence or to general welfare. Many research ethics guidelines and regulations require an interactive process between the investigator and research participant to best provide information and ensure comprehension.

Some potential research participants will always lack capacity to look after their own interests (e.g., children, people with dementia, the unconscious) and thus cannot provide consent. To protect people with diminished autonomy, informed consent is usually obtained from a parent, guardian, or legal representative. While it is clear that research participants with diminished capacity need extra protection, empirical evidence shows that even research participants with full cognitive capacity may not understand information presented as part of the consent process (Dawson 2009). For this reason, informed consent cannot be the only mechanism for protecting research participants. For instance, a research ethics committee can protect participants by assessing risks and benefits. Requiring approval by a research ethics committee might be considered a paternalistic judgment, but not an obviously wrong one (Garrard and Dawson 2005; Miller and Wertheimer 2007). Research ethics committees routinely consider waiving informed consent. This is true in public health research where the risk can be less than in biomedical research. Reliance on the judgments of research ethics committees presupposes that members have a high level of professional trustworthiness and have the skills for ethical deliberation and analysis.

Cultural or social influences can challenge the ideal model of informed consent when conducting public health research. Marshall (2007) provides an excellent overview of challenges with obtaining informed consent, especially in resource-poor settings. These challenges include cultural and social factors that affect comprehension, communication of risks, and decisional authority for consent to do research. Language barriers and low literacy, mistaken beliefs about the benefits of participation, especially when access to health care is limited, and the need to communicate complex scientific information may reduce comprehension of study procedures, benefits, and risks. Marshall (2007) emphasizes the importance of engaging community leaders and soliciting and considering the opinions of community residents when identifying project goals and procedures and establishing consent processes. She notes that in many communities, relying solely on individual consent may not be culturally appropriate. In these situations, adding family or community consent is fitting.

Some research cannot be conducted if the standards of autonomous informed consent are always applied. A good example is emergency research when unconscious victims of head trauma may be randomized to different promising treatments, but the relative effectiveness of each treatment option is unknown. Some countries allow such research via waivers of informed consent if relevant conditions are met (e.g., minimal risk, and the research could not otherwise be carried out) (U.S. Department of Health and Human Services 2009). A public health research method for which it sometimes may be appropriate not to seek informed consent is the cluster randomized trial. By design, a cluster randomized trial compares interventions that target a group (i.e., social entity such as village or town, or a population). Various characteristics of these clusters are matched to ensure a robust comparison of interventions (including no intervention). In some cluster trials, obtaining individual informed consent can seem prohibitively expensive, damaging to achieving study goals, or even impossible to attain (Sim and Dawson 2012; McRae et al. 2011b). Where consent is impossible to attain, is it right to require it at the expense of not doing the research? Attempts have been made to justify research without first attaining individual consent by appealing to an ethics committee for review, soliciting viewpoints from the community about whether the research is acceptable, or even seeking some form of community consent.

Dickert and Sugarman (2005) make a distinction between community consent and community consultation. Consent means seeking *approval*, whereas consultation means seeking *ideas and opinions*. They note, however, that this distinction gets blurred in practice, and that community consultation should not be approached as a box to check off without scrutinizing the input. They identify four ethical goals for any community consultation: enhanced protection, enhanced benefits, legitimacy, and shared responsibility. Adherence to these goals may ensure that risks are identified and protections put into place; that the research benefits not only the researchers, but also the participants and communities being studied; and that the legitimacy of the findings is increased. However, this does not constitute a direct parallel to the individual model of informed consent described previously. Community consent involves meeting with legitimate community representatives empowered to permit researchers to conduct studies involving community members (Weijer and Emanuel 2000; Dickert and Sugarman 2005). The involvement of community representatives in public health research is most clearly seen in community-based participatory research (CBPR). In CBPR, authorities are involved at all levels of research—from initiation of ideas and projects through data collection, analysis and interpretation, and use of research findings to prompt community change (Flicker et al. 2007).

9.3.2 *Risk/Benefit Analysis*

A central concern for research ethics is the weighing of expected benefits against possible harms. The commonly employed criteria for assessing risk to human subjects who participate in health research are that risks are minimized and reasonable in relation to the anticipated benefits. For example, one can argue that procedures used in research are justifiable when already being used for diagnosis or treatment and the risks are proportional to the importance of the knowledge reasonably expected to result from the research. However, one problem in such a determination is the uncertainty of all judgments about risks and benefits. Such determinations have to be made carefully and fairly and on the basis of the best possible evidence.

Research participants may encounter several types of risks. One obvious risk is physical harm, which may include discomfort, pain, or injury from interventions such as drug regimens or medical procedures. Another risk is psychological harm. Research participants may experience stress, anxiety, embarrassment, depression, or other negative emotions. These emotions, which can occur during or after participation in the research, are common in research involving sensitive topics such as sexual preferences or behavior. Social and economic harms are another type of risk. Participants in research that focuses on mental illness, illegal activities, and even certain diseases such as HIV may risk being labeled or stigmatized if precautions are not taken to provide adequate privacy and confidentially. A person's economic status may be affected if costs are incurred for participating (e.g., transportation expenses to and from the study site) or by loss of employment (present or future) if a breach of confidentiality occurs (e.g., an employer discovers an employee is being treated for substance abuse).

One common problem—about which ethics guidelines are typically silent—is how we should conceptualize study participants (McRae et al. 2011a). Consider, for example, that cluster randomized designs and cohort studies commonly compare a group receiving active intervention with a parallel group receiving no intervention. Does the term "participant" apply to those receiving no intervention? This question has far-reaching consequences. If people who do not receive intervention count as participants, researchers may have obligations to them that otherwise would not exist. Another way to think about this is to identify who might be at increased risk, rather than who is a participant. For example, the U.S. National Bioethics Advisory Commission (NBAC) recommends that whenever researchers anticipate that risks will extend beyond study participants, researchers should try to minimize risks to nonparticipants (NBAC 2001).

The benefits of health research are any favorable or positive outcome received as a direct result of the research. Put simply, without the research, the outcome would not exist. Sometimes the benefits of health research extend beyond study participants to society; other times, however, research participants do not benefit. And in other instances, only a few participants might benefit. Researchers should thoroughly consider what to do in all these scenarios and how benefits could be provided to those in need. Sometimes research involves reimbursement, incentives, or other tangible goods. Although such items may be provided when someone agrees to participate in research, these items should not be considered benefits arising from the research procedures. In some contexts, such as prisons, offering anything in return for participation in research may be viewed as pressure to participate and therefore should be carefully considered.

The risks of research must be reasonable when compared to the anticipated benefits. This can be difficult to assess because risks will vary depending on the study population. For example, research procedures considered safe for healthy adults may be risky for adults with compromised health or for vulnerable populations such as children, pregnant woman, or seniors. Even if the potential benefits are the same, if the risks differ, the risk/benefit balance is affected. Another consideration for evaluating risks and benefits is the expected result of the research. A higher level of risk may be acceptable if the research can reasonably be expected to benefit the participants. If there is no expectation that the research participants will benefit, the same level of risk may be unacceptable.

Foreseeing the benefits and harms in a study can be challenging. Striking a balance between the two can be difficult and, at times, controversial. A good example of this is the discussion generated by a series of studies conducted in Baltimore that assessed different methods for reducing the exposure of children to lead paint in older rented properties (Mastroianni and Kahn 2002). In this case, the fact was already known that exposure of children to lead is dangerous. However, due to the high cost of removing lead-based paint (the known, best solution), the researchers assessed the effectiveness of cheaper, partial methods of abatement for reducing or even removing the risk of exposure. If found to be effective, these alternative methods would allow treatment of more homes at the same cost, potentially benefiting more children. Monitoring during the study found that some children in the alternative abatement options had elevated blood lead levels. Some health officials believe that the research should not have gone ahead because of this likelihood. Others think that the research was justified because the children were not exposed to any greater level of lead, and in most cases, significantly less than if the research had not been conducted. In other words, no child was put at greater risk through participation, and all children benefited from blood monitoring. This study demonstrates the complexities of evaluating risks and benefits in public health research.

9.3.3 *Protection of Vulnerable Populations*

Although all segments of society should have the opportunity to participate in research, vulnerable populations may need additional protections to prevent coercion or exploitation. The definition of what it is to be vulnerable is contested (Chap. 7). However, NBAC (2001) defines vulnerability in the context of research as a condition, either intrinsic (e.g., mental illness) or situational (e.g., incarceration), that increases some participants' risk of being harmed. Regardless of how we define vulnerability, it is often interpreted to require special protections for the safety and well-being of populations such as children, prisoners, pregnant women, mentally disabled people, and economically or educationally disadvantaged people. The CIOMS (2002) international guidelines suggest that special justification is required for inviting vulnerable people to serve as research subjects and, if they are selected, the means of protecting their rights and welfare must be strictly applied. The history of research is replete with examples of unethical treatment of vulnerable populations (Chap. 2).

Despite such worries about protecting vulnerable populations, a strong equity-based argument can be made for ensuring that they are appropriately represented in health research, unless the rationale for not including them is clear and compelling (CDC 1996). To exclude vulnerable populations violates the spirit of the principle of justice, which requires fair distribution of risks and benefits of research. Inclusion of vulnerable populations may require accommodations to address the specific nature of the vulnerability; however, once these accommodations are in place, vulnerable people with the cognitive capacity to provide informed consent should exercise autonomous choice about their participation. For example, it seems arbitrary to exclude pregnant women from research as a matter of course rather than making a decision based on an assessment of risk levels, the ability to control risks, and the likelihood of direct benefit to the participant.

9.3.4 Returning Research Results

Public health research tends to focus on population-level research questions. In some cases, for example where data have been anonymized, even when an issue relevant to the clinical care of one or more individuals in the data set is discovered, there is nothing that can be done about it. However, in other cases, public health data sets or surveillance data might hold information that could be crucial to the care of individuals.

When and how should individual-level data, including incidental and secondary findings, be communicated to research participants? The primary argument for an ethical imperative to offer participants research findings, both summary and individual results, rests on the principle of respect for persons; however, the principles of beneficence and justice are also frequently cited (Presidential Commission for the Study of Bioethical Issues 2013; Miller et al. 2008; Fernandez et al. 2003). The word "offer" is important because giving people the right to decline results is also an expression of respect for persons. The ethical justification for a "duty to disclose research results," especially individual-level data, has been challenged due to the potential harms of disclosure (Miller et al. 2008). Miller and colleagues argue that the lack of consistent policy guidance for disclosures and the ambiguity about what to disclose undermines any generalized ethical duty to disclose. Clearly, before making a decision to return results, especially individual-level data, the potential benefits and harms from disclosure must be carefully assessed.

The research consent process should describe plans for returning results or provide an option for not receiving results. The consent process should explain the potential harms and benefits associated with receiving research results, the possible strengths and limitations of the results, and the options for follow-up and support if unanticipated consequences occur. If a decision is made to return results, careful considerations must be given to how the results will be returned (e.g., in person, over the telephone, through a letter), whether opt-in or opt-out procedures will be used, and when the results should be returned. Fernandez and colleagues (2003) argue that "research results should, in general, be delayed until the results are published or until they have undergone peer review and been accepted for publication." This recommendation is based on the need to ensure the integrity of the interpretation of the data and to prevent disclosure of inaccurate information.

To illustrate the diversity of opinion about sharing research data, some researchers have taken the obligation for disclosure further by advocating that research participants be granted access to their raw data via a data repository before these data are analyzed (Lunshof et al. 2014). Lunshof and colleagues suggest that access to raw personal data would increase transparency, personal choice, and reciprocity. Further, such access could equalize the relationship between those who donate data and those who use data for research. However, this rather utopian view raises issues with potential breaches of confidentiality, so more discussion is needed. More discussion is also needed about participants increasingly sharing information about research studies through social media, which can result in breaches of confidentiality and further challenge the integrity of research (Lipset 2014).

9.3.5 Conflicts of Interest

The potential for conflicts of interest occurs when an individual or group has multiple interests, one of which can compromise the integrity or impartiality of the other. Research involving human subjects often creates this potential when researchers are also involved with participants in the role of health care providers or through engagement with communities in the context of public health research. In resource-poor contexts, the economic impact of the research enterprise can be of such magnitude that it has sociopolitical ramifications or complexities with potential to spur conflicts of interest. Discussion about conflicts of interest raises issues about integrity in public health and even the very concept of public health as an activity (Coughlin et al. 2012).

Shrinking budgets for public health activities have led many health departments, even those in resource-rich countries, to explore alternative approaches to financing public health research, leading to questions about what constitutes an appropriate partnership and to concerns about real or perceived conflicts of interest. For example, should governments collaborate with vaccine manufacturers to research potential adverse effects of a vaccine? Should researchers collaborate with soda manufactures to study the association between sugar-sweetened beverages and obesity? The U.S. Institute of Medicine (IOM) Committee on Conflicts of Interest in Medical Research, Education, and Practice defines conflict of interest as "a relationship that may place primary interests (e.g., public well-being or research integrity) at risk of being improperly influenced by the secondary, personal interests of the relationship (e.g., financial, professional, or intellectual gains)" (IOM 2009). When Bes-Rastrollo and colleagues (2013) studied systematic reviews of the association between sugar-sweetened beverages and weight gain, they found instances where conflicts of interest influenced scientific findings. The systematic reviews that identified sponsorship or conflicts of interest with food or beverage companies were five times more likely to report "no positive association" between consumption of sugar-sweetened beverages and weight gain or obesity than the reviews that reported having no industry sponsorship or conflicts of interest. These findings point to the need for guidance on how to identify and avoid conflicts of interest with potential to influence outcomes of public health research, especially when the research shapes public policy (IOM 2014).

9.3.6 Conducting Research during Public Health Emergencies

Sometimes the traditional elements of research ethics are inappropriate frameworks for decision making. Let's consider, for example, a decision being contemplated to conduct research during a public health emergency. The research is deemed vitally important to analyze what happened during the emergency, to plan for future scenarios, and to prevent death and illness during disasters. However, such research raises concerns, including the appearance that health officials are more interested in expanding knowledge than in responding to the disaster and that researchers are insensitive to more urgent needs of affected individuals. Still, the case can be made for a strong, ethical imperative that obligates public health officials to conduct research that could yield data useful in preventing future death and illness during disasters (London 2016). The chief ethical task for conducting research during a disaster is to secure future benefits for people without sacrificing the rights or interests of research subjects (Jennings and Arras 2008; WHO 2015). So to justify research during a disaster, public health officials must first demonstrate a real need for the research, which includes its social and scientific value (anticipated results). Generally speaking, research that can be conducted in a nonemergency setting should not be conducted during an emergency response.

If the decision is made to conduct research during a public health emergency, some unique ethical concerns must be considered: the research should not detract resources and personnel from emergency response activities; research activities should be prioritized by highest social and scientific value; and, as people in an emergency are often affected physically and psychologically, and sometimes traumatized, they should be considered a vulnerable population (Jennings and Arras 2008; WHO 2015). At the very least during an emergency, keep in mind that some people may not be able to make reasoned, informed decisions to participate in the research. Consequently, adequate means of protection for participants must be in place. The procedures for an ethics committee review may need to be modified for disaster research projects (Lurie et al. 2013). Possible approaches for ensuring appropriate review include developing just-in-case protocols and establishing centralized or specialized ethics review committees that can approve disaster research protocols quickly (Médecins Sans Frontières 2013).

9.4 How Ethical Challenges Can Arise in Public Health Research: Lessons Learned from Cases

The cases presented in this chapter illustrate some of the ethical challenges raised by public health research. These challenges range from compliance with research ethics guidelines to the need to address the economic and political implications from the wider societal context in which public health research occurs. Social, economic, and political factors can directly lead to ethical challenges or may affect a researcher's ability to comply with ethical guidelines.

The case by Boulanger and Hunt illustrates how well-intentioned international efforts to improve access to health care in resource-poor countries can have unintended consequences that present ethical complications. The case raises various interconnected issues that have to do with researchers' responsibilities and obligations and with conflicts between individual and public goods. Within a collaborative international public health research project, such conflicts can easily arise when local investigators find themselves serving multiple roles that create potential conflicts of interest. Boulanger and Hunt provide an excellent summary of the responsibilities and obligations of researchers, including to

- Protect participants from harm and ensure they benefit from the research whenever possible;
- Support and protect research staff, especially students;
- Support and respect research collaborators, building local capacity when possible; and
- Support the research enterprise, which includes building public trust, maximizing the relevance and usefulness of the research, and disseminating findings.

Central to this case is a local researcher's uncovering of how informal fees for obstetric care are being diverted to senior hospital administrators. The local researcher has a dilemma. If he reveals this ethically dubious informal fee structure, he will not only jeopardize his standing at the hospital, but he could also undermine the availability of obstetric care to women in his community. The director of the research program must ethically weigh the research goal of improving access to health care services with supporting the interests of the research staff while also maintaining good relations with local health agencies. In many contexts, this case would be a clear-cut whistleblower issue demanding revelation. However, where informal fees are standard practice, part of the political culture, or the health infrastructure is already fragile or minimal, the issue becomes complicated, forcing one to prioritize competing values and moral considerations.

The case by Makhoul and colleagues involves research on mental health concerns among youth in a Palestinian refugee camp. The case highlights cultural and social factors that may influence the consent process, especially the power dynamics within communities. Beyond addressing central bioethical and medical principles of trust and respect for persons, the case points to the need for considering broad public health concepts such as respect for community values, empowerment, and advocacy. This case also illustrates how researchers are almost always drawn into a community's political dynamics by the economic influence of research in resource-poor settings. Efforts by community members to avoid alienating groups that contribute resources to the community may act as a subtle form of pressure to participate in the research.

The case by Kasule and colleagues illustrates the difficult practical choices that resource-poor countries face in processing the increasingly complex volume of research to be ethically reviewed. In these countries, public health officials struggle to complete basic administrative and regulatory aspects of research review and oversight, let alone provide conditions for careful, conscientious ethical analysis. This scenario questions the adequacy of training for members of ethics review committees. Failure to adequately train committee members and fund research oversight will result in lost opportunities and revenues, setting back a resource-poor country's research or health infrastructure for years. But funding an organization to develop research oversight may divert funds from other more urgent public health needs. Trading short-term public health solutions for long-term research funding presents a classic case of resource allocation and prioritization. Kasule and colleagues consider the pros and cons of reliance upon outside ethics review committees, which might save money at the expense of having less control of oversight.

The case by Kanekar describes the use of an Internet-delivered safe sex health promotion intervention for young black men who have sex with men. This case raises a number of practical and ethical considerations and questions that arise in public health research. How does one differentiate research from public health practice? What approaches are required to serve vulnerable populations? How can one use innovative techniques to target hard-to-reach populations? What are the best ways to protect the privacy of participants and ensure confidentiality of data? How can one reconcile or accommodate conflict among research partners who perceive their primary role or function in radically different ways (e.g., medical provider versus epidemiologist)?

9.5 Conclusions

Many ethical issues can arise in public health research. The social, economic, and political context within which the research enterprise functions further complicates the ethical landscape. Traditional approaches for considering research ethics issues emerged from biomedical research and initially emphasized ethical considerations at an individual level. However, research in public health demonstrates why this traditional approach to ethics should be expanded. A public health approach to research ethics is apt because it considers community values, the interdependence of citizens, social or population benefit, and social justice. However, as explained in Chap. 1, there is more to ensuring ethical conduct and scientific integrity in public health research than having an ethical review committee apply rule-based guidelines. Researchers need to be familiar with the ethical considerations unique to public health and have sufficient training and experience to exercise moral judgment in all phases of research.

References

Beauchamp, T.L., and J.F. Childress. 1979. *Principles of biomedical ethics*. New York: Oxford University Press.

Bes-Rastrollo, M., M.B. Schulze, M. Ruiz-Canela, and M.A. Martinez-Gonzalez. 2013. Financial conflicts of interest and reporting bias regarding the association between sugar-sweetened beverages and weight gain: A systematic review of systematic reviews. *PLoS Medicine* 10(12): e1001578. doi:10.1371/journal.pmed.1001578.

Centers for Disease Control and Prevention (CDC). 1996. *Inclusion of women and racial and ethnic minorities in research*. http://www.cdc.gov/maso/Policy/Inclusion%20of%20Women%20and%20Racial%20and%20Ethnic%20Minorities%20in%20Research10-18-2007.pdf. Accessed 24 Sept 2014.

Centers for Disease Control and Prevention. 1999. *Guidelines for defining public health research and public health non-research*. http://www.cdc.gov/od/science/integrity/docs/defining-public-health-research-non-research-1999.pdf. Accessed 24 Sept 2014.

Centers for Disease Control and Prevention. 2010. *Distinguishing public health research and public health nonresearch*. http://www.cdc.gov/od/science/integrity/docs/cdc-policy-distinguishing-public-health-research-nonresearch.pdf. Accessed 24 Sept 2014.

Coughlin, S.S., A. Barker, and A. Dawson. 2012. Ethics and scientific integrity in public health, epidemiological and clinical research. *Public Health Reviews* 34(1): 1–13. http://www.publichealthreviews.eu/upload/pdf_files/11/00_Coughlin.pdf. Accessed 24 Sept 2014.

Council for International Organizations of Medical Sciences (CIOMS). 2002. *International ethical guidelines for biomedical research involving human subjects*. Geneva: CIOMS. http://www.cioms.ch/publications/layout_guide2002.pdf. Accessed 24 Sept 2014.

Council for International Organizations of Medical Sciences. 2009. *International ethical guidelines for epidemiological studies*. Geneva: CIOMS. http://www.ufrgs.br/bioetica/cioms2008.pdf. Accessed 24 Sept 2014.

Dawson, A. 2009. The normative status of the requirement to gain an informed consent in clinical trials: Comprehension, obligations, and empirical evidence. In *The limits of consent: A socio-ethical approach to human subject research in medicine*, eds. O. Corrigan, J. McMillan, K. Liddell, M. Richards, and C. Weijer, 99–114. Oxford: Oxford University Press.

Dickert, N., and J. Sugarman. 2005. Ethical goals of community consultation in research. *American Journal of Public Health* 95(7): 1123–1127.

Fairchild, A.L., and R. Bayer. 2004. Ethics and the conduct of public health surveillance. *Science* 303(5658): 631–632.

Ferdandez, C.V., E. Kodish, and C. Weijer. 2003. Informing study participants of research results: An ethical imperative. *IRB: Ethics & Human Research* 25(3): 12–19.

Flicker, S., R. Travers, A. Guta, S. McDonald, and A. Meagher. 2007. Ethical dilemmas in community-based participatory research: Recommendations for institutional review boards. *Journal of Urban Health: Bulletin of the New York Academy of Medicine* 84(4): 478–493.

Garrard, E., and A. Dawson. 2005. What is the role of the research ethics committee? Paternalism, inducements, and harm in research ethics. *Journal of Medical Ethics* 31(17): 419–423.

Institute of Medicine (IOM). 2009. *Conflicts of interest in medical research, education, and practice*. http://www.iom.edu/Reports/2009/Conflict-of-Interest-in-Medical-Research-Education-and-Practice.aspx. Accessed 24 Sept 2014.

Institute of Medicine. 2014. *Conflict of interest and medical innovation: Ensuring integrity while facilitating innovation in medical research: Workshop summary*. Washington, DC: The National Academies Press.

Jennings, B., and J. Arras. 2008. *Ethical guidance for public health emergency preparedness and response: Highlighting ethics and values in a vital public health service*. http://www.cdc.gov/od/science/integrity/phethics/docs/White_Paper_Final_for_Website_2012_4_6_12_final_for_web_508_compliant.pdf. Accessed 24 Sept 2014.

Lipset, C.H. 2014. Engage with research participants about social media. *Nature Medicine* 20(3): 231. doi:10.1038/nm0314-231.

London, A.J. 2016. Research in a public health crisis: The integrative approach to managing the moral tensions. In *Emergency ethics: Public health preparedness and response*, eds. B. Jennings, J.D. Arras, D.H. Barrett, and B.A. Ellis, 220–261. New York: Oxford University Press.

Lunshof, J.E., G.M. Church, and B. Prainsack. 2014. Raw personal data: Providing access. *Science* 343(6169): 373–374. doi:10.1126/science.1249382.

Lurie, N., T. Manolio, A.P. Patterson, F. Collins, and T. Frieden. 2013. Research as a part of public health emergency response. *New England Journal of Medicine* 368(13): 1251–1255. doi:10.1056/NEJMsb1209510.

Marshall, P.A. 2007. Ethical challenges in study design and informed consent for health research in resource-poor settings. In *Special topics in social, economic and behavioral (SEB) research, Report number 5*. Geneva: World Health Organization.

Mastroianni, A.C., and J.P. Kahn. 2002. Risk and responsibility: Ethics, Grimes v Kennedy Krieger, and public health research involving children. *American Journal of Public Health* 92(7): 1073–1076.

McRae, A.D., C. Weijer, A. Binik, J.M. Grimshaw, et al. 2011a. When is informed consent required in cluster randomized trials in health research? *Trials* 12: 202. doi:10.1186/1745-6215-12-202.

McRae, A.D., C. Weijer, A. Binik, A. White, et al. 2011b. Who is the research subject in cluster randomized trials in health research? *Trials* 12: 183. doi:10.1186/1745-6215-12-183.

Médecins Sans Frontières. 2013. *Research ethics framework: Guidance document*. Brussels: Médecins Sans Frontières. http://fieldresearch.msf.org/msf/bitstream/10144/305288/5/MSF%20Research%20Ethics%20Framework_Guidance%20document%20(Dec2013).pdf. Accessed 24 Sept 2014.

Miller, F.G., and A. Wertheimer. 2007. Facing up to paternalism in research ethics. *Hastings Center Report* 37(3): 24–34.

Miller, F.A., R. Christensen, M. Giacomini, and J.S. Robert. 2008. Duty to disclose what? Querying the putative obligation to return research results to participants. *Journal of Medical Ethics* 34(3): 210–213. doi:10.1136/jme.2006.020289.

National Bioethics Advisory Commission (NBAC). 2001. *Ethical and policy issues in research involving human participants*. Bethesda: NBAC. https://bioethicsarchive.georgetown.edu/nbac/human/overvol1.pdf.

Nuremberg Code. 1947. Trials of war criminals before the Nuremberg Military Tribunals under Control Council Law No. 10, Vol. 2, pp. 181–182. Washington, DC: U.S. Government Printing Office, 1949. http://www.hhs.gov/ohrp/archive/nurcode.html. Accessed 24 Sept 2014.

Presidential Commission for the Study of Bioethical Issues. 2013. *Anticipate and communicate: Ethical management of incidental and secondary findings in the clinical, research, and direct-to-consumer contexts*. Washington, DC: Department of Health and Human Service.

Public Health Functions Steering Committee. 1994. *Essential public health services*. http://www.health.gov/phfunctions/public.htm. Accessed 24 Sept 2014.

Public Health Leadership Society. 2002. *Principles of the ethical practice of public health*. http://phls.org/CMSuploads/Principles-of-the-Ethical-Practice-of-PH-Version-2.2-68496.pdf. Accessed 1 Feb 2013.

Sim, J., and A. Dawson. 2012. Informed consent and cluster-randomized trials. *American Journal of Public Health* 102(3): 480–485. doi:10.2105/AJPH.2011.300389.

U.S. Department of Health and Human Services. 2009. *Code of Federal Regulations, Title 45, Part 46, Protection of Human Subjects*. http://www.hhs.gov/ohrp/humansubjects/guidance/45cfr46.html. Accessed 24 Sept 2014.

U.S. National Commission for the Protection of Human Subjects of Biomedical and Behavioral Research. 1979. *The Belmont report: Ethical principles and guidelines for the protection of human subjects of research*, Publication No. (OS) 78-0012. Washington, DC: U.S. Government Printing Office.

United Nations. 1948. *Universal declaration of human rights*. http://www.un.org/en/documents/udhr/. Accessed 24 Sept 2014.

Verweij, M., and A. Dawson. 2009. Public health research ethics: A research agenda. *Public Health Ethics* 2(1): 1–6. doi:10.1093/phe/php008.

Weijer, C., and E.J. Emanuel. 2000. Protecting communities in biomedical research. *Science* 289(5482): 1142–1144. doi:10.1126/science.289.5482.1142.

Willison, D., N. Ondrusek, A. Dawson, et al. 2014. What makes public health studies ethical? Dissolving the boundary between research and practice. *BMC Medical Ethics* 15: 61. doi:10.1186/1472-6939-15-61.

World Medical Association. 1964/2013. *Declaration of Helsinki—Ethical principles for medical research involving human subjects*. http://www.wma.net/en/30publications/10policies/b3/. Accessed 24 Sept 2014.

World Health Organization (WHO). 2015. Ethics in epidemics, emergencies and disasters: Research, surveillance and patient care. Training manual. Geneva: WHO.

9.6 Case 1: To Reveal or Not to Reveal Potentially Harmful Findings: A Dilemma for Public Health Research

Renaud F. Boulanger
Biomedical Ethics Unit
McGill University
Montréal, QC, Canada,

Matthew R. Hunt
School of Physical and Occupational Therapy
McGill University
Montréal, QC, Canada

Centre for Interdisciplinary Research on Rehabilitation
Montréal, QC, Canada
e-mail: matthew.hunt@mcgill.ca

This case is presented for instructional purposes only. The ideas and opinions expressed are the authors' own. The case is not meant to reflect the official position, views, or policies of the editors, the editors' host institutions, or the authors' host institutions.

9.6.1 Background

In 1987, African health ministers met in Mali to address access to quality primary health care, particularly in rural areas (Anonymous 1988). The resulting Bamako Initiative promoted universal accessibility, though it drew some early criticism for its support of user fees (McPake et al. 1993). For the next decade, user fees were implemented in many African countries to finance health care services. The World Bank supported the measure as part of its Structural Adjustments Programs, which also included austerity measures, trade liberalization, and privatization (McIntyre et al. 2006). However, user fees have since been shown to create access barriers that tend to affect the poor disproportionately (Macha et al. 2012), suggesting that many vulnerable individuals have been prevented from accessing needed health care services. Against this backdrop, mounting international pressure led to the reform of many user-fees programs, particularly in the last decade. One primary strategy for increasing health care access has been the introduction of selective exemptions of user fees for specific groups (Ben Ameur et al. 2012; Meessen et al. 2011; Ridde et al. 2012). Although this strategy was originally planned in the Bamako Initiative, it was not uniformly implemented. Given the scale of the changes that user fees removal implies for health care systems, there is ongoing research to evaluate their impact (Lagarde and Palmer 2011). Health system investigations such as these may raise ethical questions (Hyder et al. 2014), especially since they involve the study of a public health intervention, often focus on individuals in extreme poverty, and tend to be international and collaborative in nature.

Collaborative international public health research offers the opportunity to build local capacity (Mayhew et al. 2008). However, such research raises a number of issues about researchers' obligations and responsibilities. First is the responsibility to protect research participants from harm, an obligation recognized by all research ethics guidelines. This duty of protection is heightened when the research participants are from vulnerable populations (Hurst 2008), especially when they are recruited from extremely impoverished populations. Researchers' responsibilities toward research participants also include ensuring that they benefit from the results of the research whenever possible. For example, the *International Ethical Guidelines for Biomedical Research Involving Human Subjects* directs that "any intervention or product developed, or knowledge generated, will be made reasonably available for the benefit of that population or community" (Council for International Organizations of Medical Sciences 2002, guideline 10). A second researcher responsibility is to support students and staff hired as part of the research project and to protect them from harm (Wilson 1992). This responsibility can be thought of both as the duty of an employer and the fiduciary duty of an academic supervisor and must extend to situations of whistle-blowing. Third, researchers involved in collaborative research have a responsibility to colleagues and collaborators, especially given that research may play a crucial role in capacity building (Garcia and Curioso 2008). Although partnerships with local researchers have been touted as highly valuable (Costello and Zumla 2000), these ties may also result in unexpected ethical dilemmas for local researchers if conflicts arise between their research activities and their established local obligations and responsibilities (Richman et al. 2012). A fourth responsibility of researchers is dedication to the research enterprise. The conduct of public health research can have significant implications for the well-being of large segments of the population, but it requires the trust of the public and of relevant authorities. Endangering the relationship of trust in the context of one specific public health study may jeopardize or ruin other research initiatives (Corbie-Smith et al. 1999). Finally, a fifth responsibility of publicly funded researchers is their duty to the public in whose name they conduct research. Good stewardship requires that researchers strive to maximize the relevance and usefulness of their efforts and that they disseminate their findings (Arzberger et al. 2004). Researchers conducting collaborative international public health research may encounter ethically challenging conflicts among these five lines of responsibilities.

9.6.2 Case Description

Dr. Milena A. is the principal investigator of a large research program that is examining approaches for decreasing inequities in access to health care services in a low-resource setting. She works for an American university, and her research is funded by a U.S. agency. One member of her research team, Dr. Timothy N., is a local physician studying toward a public health degree at Milena's institution. He is back in his country after finishing his coursework and is ready to conduct fieldwork research. Timothy has taken leave from his position at a local hospital to pursue his studies and, although he wants to continue his clinical work at the hospital, he also wants to expand his focus to include population-level health issues and, eventually, work with his country's ministry of health. His studies are co-funded by Milena's research grant and by the ministry of health.

Timothy's research consists of an examination of the impact of his country's recent abolishment of health care user fees for children younger than 5 years. User fees had been implemented uniformly in the 1990s without special consideration for poorer families with young children. Initial indicators suggest that health care services continue to be underused in some districts, especially by poor children, despite the recent removal of user fees. Despite the limited uptake, the ministry of health touts the policy abolishing user fees for children younger than 5 years as an important success. Timothy is conducting his study at several urban health centers, including the hospital from which he is currently on leave. The research project has received ethics approval from Milena's institution and from the relevant local review boards.

Recently, Timothy requested a meeting with Milena saying that he needed advice. He reports that he has identified a system of informal fees that undermines the ministry of health's official policy by making health care once again too expensive for many families with young children. From what Timothy understands, the fees are levied primarily to fund better obstetric care locally, but some indicators point toward senior administrators keeping a small share for themselves. Timothy worries that making his findings public is too risky for him, especially since his involvement in this fieldwork is well-known. He does not think it possible to share his findings without identifying himself as the source of the information. His hospital is one of the sites where he has identified the system of informal payments. He also has good reasons to believe that some members of the ministry of health are already aware of the situation but have not taken action to address it. Disseminating his results will jeopardize his employment at the hospital, his relationships with government officials, and, potentially, the plans to improve obstetric care.

Milena is also conflicted. She recognizes that she has multiple roles, responsibilities, and interests, and that individual and communal goods are at stake. Identifying and seeking to address informal payment structures could improve accessibility of health care services for children, which is the primary goal of her research program. However, the team has responsibilities to Timothy as their student and colleague. Demanding that he upend his career, either for their benefit or for the improvement of health care accessibility, might fail to respect him as an individual. In addition, bringing the situation to light could embarrass the ministry of health. Because the research program depends on the ministry of health's authorization, tensions in relationships could lead to premature termination of the research. Such an event would have unpredictable outcomes on the careers of everyone on the research team and on the future of health care accessibility locally.

9.6.3 Discussion Questions

1. How should Milena and Timothy prioritize their responsibilities, and what should they ultimately do?
2. What preemptive actions could the research team have taken to limit the likelihood that the situation described above would happen?
3. How should the fact that, aside from Timothy, the research team members are not citizens in the country where they are conducting research be considered in the assessment of their obligations?
4. Is this a case where developing partnerships with local researchers might be counterproductive? Or, could a more robust partnership with local researchers have positioned the team to better address this issue?
5. How would the ethical analysis differ if, instead of identifying unequal access due to informal fees, Timothy had observed that those exempted from the fees were being offered a lower standard of care than patients whose fees were not waived?

References

Anonymous. 1988. The Bamako initiative. *Lancet* 2(8621): 1177–1178.

Arzberger, P., P. Schroeder, A. Beaulieu, et al. 2004. Promoting access to public research data for scientific, economic, and social development. *Data Science Journal* 3: 135–152.

Ben Ameur, A., V. Ridde, A.R. Bado, M.G. Ingabire, and L. Queuille. 2012. User fee exemptions and excessive household spending for normal delivery in Burkina Faso: The need for careful implementation. *BMC Health Services Research* 12: 412. doi:10.1186/1472-6963-12-412.

Corbie-Smith, G., S.B. Thomas, M.V. Williams, and S. Moody-Ayers. 1999. Attitudes and beliefs of African Americans toward participation in medical research. *Journal of General Internal Medicine* 14(9): 537–546.

Costello, A., and A. Zumla. 2000. Moving to research partnerships in developing countries. *British Medical Journal* 321(7264): 827–829.

Council for International Organizations of Medical Sciences. 2002. *International ethical guidelines for biomedical research involving human subjects*. http://www.cioms.ch/publications/layout_guide2002.pdf. Accessed 27 Dec 2012.

Garcia, P.J., and W.H. Curioso. 2008. Strategies for aspiring biomedical researchers in resource limited environments. *PLoS Neglected Tropical Diseases* 2(8): e274. doi:10.1371/journal.pntd.0000274.

Hurst, S.A. 2008. Vulnerability in research and health care: Describing the elephant in the room? *Bioethics* 22(4): 191–202. doi:10.1111/j.1467-8519.2008.00631.x.

Hyder, A.A., A. Rattani, C. Krubiner, A.M. Bachani, and N.T. Tran. 2014. Ethical review of health systems research in low- and middle-income countries: A conceptual exploration. *American Journal of Bioethics* 14(2): 28–37. doi:10.1080/15265161.2013.868950.

Lagarde, M., and N. Palmer. 2011. The impact of user fees on access to health services in low- and middle-income countries. *Cochrane Database of Systematic Reviews* 4: CD009094. doi:10.1002/14651858.CD009094.

Macha, J., B. Harris, B. Garshong, et al. 2012. Factors influencing the burden of health care financing and the distribution of health care benefits in Ghana, Tanzania and South Africa. *Health Policy and Planning* 27(suppl 1): i46–i54.

Mayhew, S.H., J. Doherty, and S. Pitayarangsarit. 2008. Developing health systems research capacities through north–south partnership: An evaluation of collaboration with South Africa and Thailand. *BMC Health Research Policy and Systems* 6: 8. doi:10.1186/1478-4505-6-8.

McIntyre, D., M. Thiede, G. Dahlgren, and M. Whitehead. 2006. What are the economic consequences for households of illness and of paying for health care in low- and middle-income country contexts? *Social Science & Medicine* 62(4): 858–865.

McPake, B., K. Hanson, and A. Mills. 1993. Community financing of health care in Africa: An evaluation of the Bamako initiative. *Social Science & Medicine* 36: 1383–1395.

Meessen, B., D. Hercot, M. Noirhomme, et al. 2011. Removing user fees in the health sector: A review of policy processes in six sub-Saharan African countries. *Health Policy and Planning* 26(suppl 2): ii16–ii29. doi:10.1093/heapol/czr062.

Richman, K.A., L.B. Alexander, and G. True. 2012. Proximity, ethical dilemmas, and community research workers. *American Journal of Bioethics Primary Research* 3(4): 19–29. doi:10.1080/21507716.2012.714837.

Ridde, V., E. Robert, and B. Meessen. 2012. A literature review of the disruptive effects of user fee exemption policies on health systems. *BMC Public Health* 12: 289. doi:10.1186/1471-2458-12–289.

Wilson, K. 1992. Thinking about the ethics of fieldwork. In *Fieldwork in developing countries*, ed. S. Devereux and J. Hoddinott, 179–199. New York: Harvester Wheatsheaf.

9.7 Case 2: Ethical Challenges in Impoverished Communities: Seeking Informed Consent in a Palestinian Refugee Camp in Lebanon

Jihad Makhoul, Rima Afifi, and Rima Nakkash
Department of Health Promotion and Community Health,
Faculty of Health Sciences
American University of Beirut
Beirut, Lebanon
e-mail: ra15@aub.edu.lb

This case is presented for instructional purposes only. The ideas and opinions expressed are the authors' own. The case is not meant to reflect the official position, views, or policies of the editors, the editors' host institutions, or the authors' host institutions.

9.7.1 Background

Beginning in 1948, the United Nations Relief and Works Agency (UNRWA) established camps in Lebanon to house refugees from Palestine. As of 2013, 12 camps remained (UNRWA 2013). The typical UNRWA camp houses three generations of refugees, most of whom are unemployed and face economic hardships from state-imposed legal and political restrictions (Chaaban et al. 2010). Camp housing is substandard, usually lacking adequate health care and educational infrastructures. A household survey of camp residents older than 15 years found that the mean length of school attendance is 6–7.5 years, the mean yearly household income is below $3,000, and more than half the respondents consider themselves poor (Makhoul 2003; Khawaja et al. 2006).

Family structures in the camp vary, ranging from matriarchal families, extended families, and traditional patriarchal families to even modern families where parents jointly make decisions. These family structures also include complex formations where, for example, a remarried father lives with his new wife and stepchildren. In such complex families, children often have several guardians or authority figures. Sociocultural conceptions shared by parents and social workers stress the reliance of children on parental decisions—parents know what is best for children, while children know they must obey parental decisions.

In resource-poor settings like the camps, many nongovernmental organizations (NGOs) supplement UNRWA services, thereby gaining influence. The perceived power that the local Palestinian NGOs hold in the community derives from years of providing supplemental economic and social services to residents. Not surprisingly, if an NGO is politicized, it also will hold political power. In this context, if an NGO agrees to participate in a project, residents may agree to participate without paying close attention to the details or the scope of work. They participate either because they trust the NGO to decide on their behalf or because they want to avoid being perceived as opposing an organization that provides them with needed services. Similarly, international NGOs hold perceived power by providing essential services and distributing needed supplies, especially during emergencies. Universities can acquire such power, even unintentionally, not only from the prestige and status that educational institutions generally enjoy, but also from the potential benefits that research projects bring to the camps. Intentional or not, exercising such power can raise unanticipated problems for the research enterprise.

To protect research participants, some national and international commissions have published guidance documents about equitable distribution of benefits and respect for autonomy, beneficence, and social justice. These documents include the *Nuremberg Code* (1947), the *Declaration of Helsinki* (World Medical Association 1964), The *Belmont Report* (National Commission for the Protection of Human Subjects of Biomedical and Behavioral Research 1979), and the *International Ethical Guidelines for Biomedical Research Involving Human Subjects* (Council for International Organizations of Medical Science 2002). Even though these international guidelines acknowledge the need to consider culture and community, they lack adequate guidance for community-based public health research (Racher 2007; Bledsoe and Hopson 2009). In addition, these guidelines are difficult to apply in nonbiomedical research contexts in community settings. This difficulty could be attributed to applying guidelines without first considering local contexts (Dawson and Kass 2005; Benatar 2002; Chilisa 2009). Many community-oriented practitioners find the principles too limiting to guide public health research ethics in community settings and recommend incorporating broader conceptions of respect, trust, inclusion, diversity, participation, empowerment, and advocacy (Racher 2007; Bledsoe and Hopson 2009).

Biomedical guidelines often clash with community interactions, especially in the nonindustrialized world (Bledsoe and Hopson 2009; Matsumoto and Jones 2009; Chilisa 2009). One such clash occurs between individual-oriented societies and more collectivist societies that view personhood and individual decision making through the lens of a person's relation to society (Marshall and Baten 2003). Another clash occurs between the artificially impersonal character of research environments and the centrality of relationships and partnerships in communities. Randomized clinical trials (RCTs), for example, require control of all possible confounders, a nearly impossible standard to achieve in close-knit and dense community settings (Makhoul et al. 2013). Implementing ethical guidelines in the context of power dynamics (Marshall and Baten 2004), like the pronounced power that males wield over females in patriarchal societies, can instigate numerous clashes. In communities like refugee camps that offer few economic or career opportunities, the perceived power that NGOs and, even more so, academic institutions wield is a force that must be taken into account. In such restricted settings, the power dynamics between researchers and research subjects can take on a subtle coercive character.

These same tensions, challenges, and dynamics will emerge in any efforts to obtain informed consent to participate in research. The emergence may stem from failure to appreciate the unique complexity of local familial, cultural, and political structures, or it may represent limitations in the principles being applied.

9.7.2 *Case Description*

A community coalition, initiated by researchers from a nearby university, has been meeting for more than a year to prioritize health concerns for youth in a Palestinian refugee camp near Beirut, Lebanon. The camp is a typical UNRWA camp and includes six elementary schools. The coalition comprises camp residents including youth (17–25 years), UNRWA representatives, camp NGO workers, and members of the university research team. The coalition has decided to focus on the mental health of younger adolescents (11–13 years) in this Palestinian refugee camp and to develop a research intervention on this issue. Cross-sectional studies and evaluation of interventions that link social and life skills to mental health outcomes strongly support the view that these skills enhance the mental health of youth; however, most of the evidence comes from industrialized settings.

The goal of the intervention is to enhance positive mental health by increasing the social and life skills of young adolescents, who will be recruited through the schools. The six elementary schools have comparable resources and student profiles. Each school has been randomly assigned either to the intervention or to the control arm of the study, and only fifth and sixth graders will participate. Participating students in the intervention group will receive 45 extracurricular sessions of 1½h each over 9 months and gain skills in solving problems, making decisions, building self-esteem, and enhancing relationships with peers, parents, and teachers. Parents of the students in the intervention group will receive 15 1-h group sessions, and teachers in the intervention schools will be offered six workshops addressing the same topics. Students randomized to the control group will receive 10 sessions over the course of 9 months, but their parents will not participate in the program. However, because teachers often work in more than one camp school, some teachers at the control schools may participate in the intervention workshops. All participants in either the intervention or control condition must complete pre- and post-assessment questionnaires that measure mental health and social and life skills before and after the intervention and at 6 months follow-up.

Recruitment into the research project will unfold in phases. Toward the end of the school year preceding the intervention, parents will be invited to an informational session about the project that will take place in one of the camp schools. After the informational session, meetings will take place with individual families in their homes to recruit students entering grades 5 and 6. Some youth (ages 17–23 years) who live in the camp will receive training to become part of the recruitment team. These youth will visit the homes of all potential intervention and control participants to explain the study and to obtain parental consent. If the parents consent, students will be invited to the school for further discussion (to ensure confidentiality and autonomy of decision making). Once the study has been explained to them, they'll be asked individually to give their assent.

You are a member of the university research team leading the effort to obtain informed consent. You would like to obtain consent and assent in accordance with standard international procedures, but you realize their application may need to be adjusted to the context of the camp. In particular, you have considered what role principles such as trust, inclusion, diversity, and broad community participation should play in the research project. That is why you chose to have older youth from the camp obtain both parental consent and student's assent, but you are concerned about potential problems that this approach may encounter. Also, given the power dynamics and conditions in the camp, you would like the research team to consider how this project can be used to spearhead a discussion with the community coalition about larger issues of empowerment and advocacy. With this in mind, you plan to address the following questions with your research team.

9.7.3 Discussion Questions

1. How could the history of Palestinian refugee camps potentially impact the informed consent process and the success of this intervention?
2. Who are the stakeholders in this case, and what stake, for or against, do they have in the research project? How would you deal with those who believe the project is not in their or the community's interests?
3. What are the advantages and potential disadvantages of using older youth to obtain parental consent and student's assent? What other steps could be taken to enhance the informed consent seeking process in such social contexts?
4. What incentives, if any, should be given for participation? To whom should these incentives be given? Given the limited opportunities for the inhabitants of the refugee camps and the perceived power of NGOs, at what point would incentives become compulsive to encourage participation?
5. How do relationships of power influence the application of informed consent procedures specifically, in this context? What steps can be taken to minimize the effects of power?
6. What bearing, positive or negative, does the background of the researchers have on the researcher-participant interaction, especially for researchers who have never lived in such camp settings and would be considered outsiders to the camp community?
7. Beyond the informed consent process, are the researchers simply teaching the adolescents how to adjust to an oppressive arrangement instead of exploring, providing and validating strategies to transform the situation? If so, what are some alternative intervention strategies that could foster the latter?
8. By almost any measure, the camp environment is abnormal for a developing adolescent. Given that social determinants severely challenge the health of all members of the camp community, how should the researchers take into account the unusual and extreme circumstances of the adolescents as they implement and evaluate interventions that aim to change individual-level circumstances and attributes?

References

Benatar, S.R. 2002. Reflections and recommendations on research ethics in developing countries. *Social Science & Medicine* 54(7): 1131–1141.

Bledsoe, K.L., and R.K. Hopson. 2009. Conducting ethical research and evaluation in underserved communities. In *The handbook of social research ethics*, ed. D.M. Mertens and P.E. Ginsberg, 391–406. Thousand Oaks: Sage Publications.

Chaaban, J., H., Ghattas, and R.R., Habib, et al. 2010. *Socio-economic survey of Palestinian refugees in Lebanon*. American University of Beirut (AUB) and the United Nations Relief and Works Agency for Palestine Refugees in the Near East (UNRWA). http://fafsweb.aub.edu.lb/aub-unrwa/files/AUB_UNRWA_report_final_draft.pdf. Accessed 3 Jan 2013.

Chilisa, B. 2009. Indigenous African-centered ethics: Contesting and complementing dominant models. In *The handbook of social research ethics*, ed. D.M. Mertens and P.E. Ginsberg, 407–425. Thousand Oaks: Sage Publications.

Council for International Organizations of Medical Sciences. 2002. *International ethical guidelines for biomedical research involving human subjects*. http://www.cioms.ch/publications/layout_guide2002.pdf. Accessed 18 Feb 2014.

Dawson, L., and N.E. Kass. 2005. Views of US researchers about informed consent in international collaborative research. *Social Science & Medicine* 61(6): 1211–1222.

Khawaja, M., S. Abdulrahim, R.A. Soweid, and D. Karam. 2006. Distrust, social fragmentation and adolescents' health in the outer city: Beirut and beyond. *Social Science & Medicine* 63(5): 1304–1315.

Makhoul, J. 2003. Physical and social contexts of the three urban communities of Nabaa, Borj el Barajneh Palestinian Camp and Hay el Sullum. Unpublished report. CRPH, American University of Beirut, Lebanon.

Makhoul, J., R. Nakkash, T. Harpham, and Y. Qutteina. 2013. Community based participatory research in complex settings: Clean mind–dirty hands. *Health Promotion International* 29(3): 510–517. doi:10.1093/heapro/dat049.

Marshall, A., and S. Batten. 2003. Ethical issues in cross-cultural research. In *CONNECTIONS'03*, ed. W.M. Roth, 139–151. http://www.google.com/url?sa=t&rct=j&q=&esrc=s&source=web&cd=1&cad=rja&uact=8&ved=0CCEQFjAAahUKEwjO7JWKuujIAhXK7CYKHdNyANc&url=http%3A%2F%2Fejournal.narotama.ac.id%2Ffiles%2FEthical%2520Issues%2520in%2520Cross-Cultural%2520Research.pdf&usg=AFQjCNG04xJ3QFK7bIjX_EQUvwrwZRacxg. Accessed 25 Feb 2016.

Marshall, A., and S. Batten. 2004. Researching across cultures: Issues of ethics and power. *Forum Qualitative Sozialforschung/Forum: Qualitative Social Research* 5(3): Article 39. http://nbnresolving.de/urn:nbn:de:0114-fqs0403396. Accessed 3 June 2015.

Matsumoto, D., and C.A.L. Jones. 2009. Ethical issues in cross-cultural psychology. In *The handbook of social research ethics*, ed. D.M. Mertens and P.E. Ginsberg, 323–336. Thousand Oaks: Sage Publications.

National Commission for the Protection of Human Subjects of Biomedical and Behavioral Research. 1979. *The Belmont report: Ethical principles and guidelines for the protection of human subjects of research*. http://www.hhs.gov/ohrp/humansubjects/guidance/belmont.html. Accessed 3 Jan 2013.

Nuremberg Code. 1947. Trials of war criminals before the Nuremberg Military Tribunals under Control Council Law No. 10, Vol. 2, pp. 181–182. Washington, DC: U.S. Government Printing Office, 1949. http://www.hhs.gov/ohrp/archive/nurcode.html. Accessed 23 Feb 2014.

Racher, F.E. 2007. The evolution of ethics for community practice. *Journal of Community Health Nursing* 24(1): 65–76.

United Nations Relief and Works Agency (UNRWA). 2013. *Lebanon*. http://www.unrwa.org/etemplate.php?id=65. Accessed 4 June 2013.

World Medical Association. 1964. *Declaration of Helsinki: Ethical principles for medical research involving human subjects*. http://www.wma.net/en/30publications/10policies/b3/. Accessed 23 Feb 2014.

9.8 Case 3: Improving Review Quality and Efficiency of Research Ethics Committees to Enhance Public Health Practice in Africa

Mary Kasule
Office of Research and Development
University of Botswana
Gaborone, Botswana
e-mail: mary.kasule@mopipi.ub.bw

Douglas Wassenaar
South African Research Ethics Training Initiative, School of Applied Human Sciences
University of KwaZulu-Natal
Pietermaritzburg, South Africa

Carel IJsselmuiden
Council on Health Research for Development
Geneva, Switzerland

School of Applied Human Sciences, South African Research Ethics Training Initiative, University of KwaZulu-Natal, Pietermaritzburg, South Africa

Boitumelo Mokgatla
Africa Office for Council on Health Research for Development
Gaborone, Botswana

Mapping African Research Ethics Review and Medicines Regulatory Capacity, Gaborone, Botswana
mokgatla@cohred.org

This case is presented for instructional purposes only. The ideas and opinions expressed are the authors' own. The case is not meant to reflect the official position, views, or policies of the editors, the editors' host institutions, or the authors' host institutions.

9.8.1 Background

Many low- to middle-income countries in Africa face a tremendous burden of infectious diseases. Tuberculosis (TB) causes particular concern, with incidence rising and the greatest prevalence in children. Compounding this concern is the lack of an easy-to-use and accurate diagnostic test (World Health Organization 2012). To address these challenges, the World Health Organization's (WHO) 2011 global plan to stop TB by 2050 urgently calls for more research to develop diagnostics, drugs, and vaccines. WHO's call reinforces the 2008 Global Ministerial Forum on Research for Health held in Mali, which recommended that each country allocate 2 % of health ministry funds to health care research (Yazdizadeh et al. 2010). All research involving human subjects will require review by institutional review boards (IRBs) or, as they are generally known in Africa, research ethics committees (RECs). But to expedite the process of high-quality ethical reviews necessary to keep pace with these new research initiatives, a corresponding investment in REC funding and training should be made.

In TB-endemic areas of Africa, the volume and complexity of research have increased without a corresponding strengthening in the capacity of local RECs (WHO 2011). At least 190 RECs operate throughout Africa, but the quality and capacity of each vary widely (IJssemuiden et al. 2012). Although some RECs still lack adequate research regulatory frameworks, the major challenge to strengthening capacity is lack of funding (Kass et al. 2007). This means, for example, that few, if any, African RECs have tools like electronic information management systems to coordinate submissions efficiently. It also means that few have trained REC administrators, a gap rightly identified as the missing link to improved quality and throughput of ethical review (IJsselmuiden et al. 2012). These factors can delay ethical reviews and create problems with quality and consistency (Milford et al. 2006; Kass et al. 2007). Whenever significant research funds are wasted on managing inefficient RECs, fewer funds are available to study ways to improve public health care services (Tully et al. 2000). This waste of resources on inefficient ethical review affects the timeliness of health services, which, in turn, affects subsequent health care policy and decision making. Ironically, such wastefulness poses an unethical barrier to potentially beneficial public health research activities. Worse, these inefficiencies can cost research institutions a chance to compete for grants that require prior ethical review of research proposals by the country's internal REC.

In Africa, external grants are often used to fund health research activities, whereas REC funding typically is either nonexistent or constrained by more pressing health care needs. Attempting to prioritize and allocate resources for activities with outcomes linked to funding puts policy makers in a dilemma. On the one hand, diverting funds from the immediate treatment of life-threatening diseases to a weak, inefficient REC can waste critical resources. On the other hand, not allocating funds to strengthen RECs can lead to the loss of external research funding, the very research that could reduce the burden of disease in the long run. Moreover, external funding, though filling a critical gap, often heightens the tensions at play in prioritizing between immediate needs for health care and long term needs for research and RECs.

9.8.2 Case Description

A multinational pharmaceutical company put out a call for proposals to research institutions in sub-Saharan Africa to apply for a research grant. The 3-year grant, which provides 500,000 U.S. dollars per year to develop an effective paediatric TB diagnostic tool, would involve conducting clinical trials in five African TB-endemic countries. Successful award of the grant is contingent upon timely review of the proposal by the applicant's national REC.

In one country eligible for the grant, the ministry of health (MoH) encouraged its National Tuberculosis Research Centre to apply. The grant funding would have boosted the country's long-term efforts to strengthen the capacity of its public health research by restructuring its TB treatment protocol. The Research Centre promptly submitted a proposal to the national REC, which levies 10 % of the grant as overhead to sustain the REC.

Despite the overhead funding, the country's national REC lacks an administrator formally trained in research ethics and a robust ethics review structure. Although the REC receives more than 100 applications annually, it only meets every 3 months, often missing deadlines, because it cannot afford essential tools to coordinate submissions efficiently. To have a proposal reviewed; applicants have to submit 20 hard copies of the research application form and 10 copies of all other study materials. The review procedure typically forces the principal investigator of a clinical trial to submit nearly 20 kg of paper copies, a considerable sum in supplies and manpower. Despite its high profile, the TB Research Centre's grant application does not prove to be an exception to the notoriously slow review process.

Professor Y, a highly capable public health specialist, directs the public health department in the local MoH. She also lectures at a local medical school, serves as Principal Investigator (PI) of an ongoing TB clinical trial in the country, and has extensive experience at all levels of REC activity and oversight. Unfortunately, Professor Y has never had formal training in research ethics, which is critical for anyone involved in managing REC activities. Because of her background, Professor Y became aware of the delays in reviewing the TB Research Centre's application. Recognizing its importance to the country, Professor Y offered to serve as the primary reviewer for the proposal. Professor Y called an ad hoc REC meeting. At this meeting, the other members, who had only received copies of the grant application form to prepare for their review, unanimously agreed to outsource review of the protocol because they lacked the expertise to evaluate the application. Amid these delays, institutions in other countries competing for the same grant, having already received ethical clearance from their RECs, were awarded the grant. Not only did the delays cost the country a funding opportunity to enhance its public health research capacity, but preparing the application also wasted precious time and scarce resources.

In response to this bungled opportunity, the MoH set up a task force to analyse the situation and offer recommendations. In its report, the task force recommended allocating more resources to RECs to strengthen capacity. Due to budget constraints, the MoH had to divert the money allocated to RECs from the antiretroviral program. Meanwhile, the MoH recommended temporarily outsourcing all REC services to a U.S. based clinical research organization.

9.8.3 Discussion Questions

1. What ethical tension or challenges could result from the insufficiencies in REC capacity that forced the MoH's decision to divert funds from the antiretroviral program to strengthen REC capacity?
2. How should a country prioritize between the need to foster research, which can have significant long-term impact and immediate health care needs?
3. Funding for the research grant and temporary outsourcing of ethical reviews will come from multinational or U.S. based partners. What are the advantages and disadvantages for developing countries to accept such funding? What impact does accepting such funding have on a country's ability to determine its own health priorities?
4. Professor Y has public health credentials, TB expertise, and extensive experience as an REC administrator. The case suggests that had she followed the procedures for the review process, the grant application might have been successful, even though she apparently lacks formal ethics training.
   (a) According to international research ethics regulations, what procedures should Professor Y have followed when distributing the proposal for review, allocating reviewers, and setting up the REC meeting?
   (b) How critical is formal ethics training to serving on an REC or to overseeing the development of REC capacity nationwide?
   (c) Is it a good use of time for someone like Professor Y to be serving administratively on an REC?
   (d) Would you recommend that the MoH create a permanent position for a trained research ethics administrator solely responsible for REC administration issues instead of allowing volunteers like Professor Y, who have multiple roles and responsibilities, to oversee the activity?
5. Given the cultural and economic differences between developed Western nations that sponsor research and African host countries, should formal ethics training to prepare for serving on an REC be modelled on Western training or on some other model?
6. Keeping the interests and values of all stakeholders in mind, consider the best ways to address the strengthening of REC capacity in African low- to middle-income countries at the local and global levels.

References

IJssemuiden, C., D. Marias, D. Wassenaar, et al. 2012. Mapping African ethical review committee activity onto capacity needs: The MARC initiative and HRWEB's interactive database of RECSs in Africa. *Developing World Bioethics* 12(2): 74–86.

Kass, N.E., A.A. Hyder, A. Ajuwon, et al. 2007. The structure and function of research ethics committees in Africa: A case study. *PLoS Medicine* 4(1): e3. doi:10.1371/journal.pmed.0040003.

Milford, C., D. Wassenaar, and C. Slack. 2006. Resources and needs of research ethics committees in Africa: Preparations for HIV vaccine trials. *IRB: Ethics & Human Research* 28(2): 1–9.

Tully, J., N. Ninis, R. Booy, and R. Viner. 2000. The new system of review by multi-centre research ethics committees: Prospective study. *British Medical Journal* 320(7243): 1179–1182.
World Health Organization (WHO). 2011. *An international road map for tuberculosis research: Towards a world free of tuberculosis*. Geneva: World Health Organization.
World Health Organization (WHO). 2012. *Global tuberculosis report 2012*. Geneva:World Health Organization. http://apps.who.int/iris/bitstream/10665/75938/1/9789241564502_eng.pdf. Accessed 3 June 2015.
Yazdizadeh, B., R. Majdzadeh, and H. Salmasian. 2010. Systematic review of methods for evaluating healthcare research economic impact. *Health Research Policy and Systems* 8: 6. doi:10.1186/1478-4505-8-6.

9.9 Case 4: Internet-Based HIV/AIDS Education and Prevention Programs in Vulnerable Populations: Black Men Who Have Sex with Men

Amar Kanekar
Department of Health, Human Performance and Sport Management
University of Arkansas at Little Rock
Little Rock, AR, USA
e-mail: axkanekar@ualr.edu

This case is presented for instructional purposes only. The ideas and opinions expressed are the author's own. The case is not meant to reflect the official position, views, or policies of the editors, the editors' host institutions, or the author's host institution.

9.9.1 Background

Since surfacing more than 30 years ago, the HIV/AIDS pandemic has devastated populations worldwide. Various factors have contributed to this epidemic, such as lack of awareness of HIV status, stigma, homophobia, negative perceptions about HIV testing, socioeconomic factors, behavioral risk factors, and high prevalence of sexually transmitted diseases (Centers for Disease Control and Prevention 2015). In the United States, one goal of the national HIV/AIDS strategy is to reduce HIV-related health disparities. Any reduction in the collective risk of acquiring HIV will require behavior change interventions in communities with the highest HIV prevalence. However, extending the reach of HIV/AIDS preventive interventions in remote areas with limited access to HIV testing and prevention services has proved difficult (Office of National AIDS Policy 2012).

The challenge of reaching some populations has led many practitioners to consider innovative intervention methods that rely on technologies such as the Internet and mobile telephones. Public health professionals are using these technologies to deliver health education to vulnerable populations in big cities, small towns, and hard-to-reach rural areas. In particular, the past decade has seen more health communication efforts using the Internet to prevent HIV and sexually transmitted diseases (Bull et al. 2007, 2009; Rietmeijer and McFarlane 2009). Studies of interventions that use Internet chat rooms, online modules, and health intervention websites show promising results that bode well for the future of these technologies (Chiasson et al. 2009; Moskowitz et al. 2009).

Studies conducted with marginalized and vulnerable populations such as black men who have sex with men (MSM) can pose difficulties. On the technology front, many difficulties reflect the Internet's relative novelty for conducting studies and the consequent lack of clarity in dealing with the rules, language, and norms of a virtual community culture compared with a traditional community culture (Loue and Pike 2010). On the allocation front, having limited resources usually implies that tailoring interventions to a specific group will mean forgoing benefits to another group. Still, in promoting the health of populations, public health professionals must strive to distribute resources fairly while responding to the specific needs of racial, ethnic, and cultural groups. These concurrent goals require maintaining a delicate balance between targeted and population interventions. On the ethics front, because some projects straddle the line between research and practice, public health professionals can become unsure about whether the ethical guidelines of research or of community work should govern their actions. They must bear in mind that trust, which is essential for conducting community-based participatory research, becomes more crucial when working with vulnerable populations, which tend to show a high degree of mistrust (Loue and Pike 2010). Those who study vulnerable populations need to negotiate community entry either by developing trust or by working closely with local practitioners and building upon established trust.

In the United States, the HIV/AIDS epidemic has hit the African-American population hardest, with black men accounting for 70 % of new HIV infections. Between 2006 and 2009, new HIV infections increased 48 % among black 13- to 24-year-old MSM (Centers for Disease Control and Prevention 2015); by 2009, 37 % of new HIV cases among black men were from black MSM. Given this high prevalence, before the end of 2015, the U.S. national HIV/AIDS strategy calls for a 20 % increase in the proportion of African Americans diagnosed with HIV who have an undetectable viral load (Office of National AIDS Policy 2012). Already, information about HIV issues affecting young MSM (Mustanski et al. 2011) is widely available on the Internet, including messages about how to reduce risk (Hightow-Weidman et al. 2011) and interventions to prevent HIV risk behaviors among MSM (Rhodes et al. 2010) and blacks who inject drugs (Washington and Thomas 2010). Studies show that online delivery of HIV counseling and behavioral interventions for MSM at high risk for HIV are successful, suggesting that the future holds great promise for Internet-delivered interventions for this vulnerable population (Chiasson et al. 2009; Moskowitz et al. 2009).

9.9.2 Case Description

Dr. Albert, a social scientist, and Dr. Baines, a community worker, are employed by a public health agency in a medium-size U.S. town. The agency has asked them to determine whether a skill-based, Internet-delivered intervention to promote safer sex among young Black MSM will increase HIV knowledge and increase the frequency of using safer-sex practices.

Project participants will be recruited via the Internet in gay chat rooms and be verified electronically by using Internet Protocol and Microsoft Access usernames and passwords (Bull 2011). Participants will be surveyed before they begin the training modules and again at 1- and 6-week intervals after completing the modules. Participants will be randomly assigned to control and experimental arms. Those in the control arm will receive 6 h of online training about health and well-being (e.g., nutrition, physical activity, stress reduction). The experimental arm will receive a 6-h online program including two 1-h modules on each of the following topics: (a) HIV/AIDS-related knowledge; (b) development and improvement of safe sex skills, such as partner communication and monogamous sexual relationships; and (c) self-efficacy in using condoms. The modules will include automated reminders for HIV testing. The study will measure improved knowledge on HIV/AIDS, partner communication about safer sex, and condom usage self-efficacy. Data will be analyzed using statistical software.

Dr. Albert thinks the results could be generalized not only to black MSM in the community but also to black MSM overall. He plans to write an article describing the results for publication in a scientific journal. Although Dr. Baines knows the impact of education on health, especially in underprivileged communities, she wants to educate only a subset of the community they will reach. Besides, since their work is for a public health agency, she believes the intervention ought to reach as many community members possible. She claims the project's goal is to provide a vulnerable and disadvantaged population with much needed education on health matters and health-promoting behavior and doubts their project constitutes research.

Dr. Albert worries that, because his colleague lacks academic rigor and underappreciates the role of evidence, she fails to appreciate the project's rationale and design and, as a result, is indifferent to the challenges the Internet poses (e.g., technology-induced bias, protection of confidentiality). Conversely, Dr. Baines believes Dr. Albert has missed the boat and is wasting resources, spuriously introducing statistical analysis of experimental and control arms into what the agency clearly had intended as an education intervention.

9.9.3 Discussion Questions

1. Is this a research project? Should approval from an ethics review committee be obtained? Or should the project be considered nonresearch because it will improve the health of the population? How should you decide?

2. Does the fact that the project is funded by a public health agency play a role in this discussion? Should public health agencies conduct studies to generate evidence about HIV education and prevention interventions? Should agencies focus on the delivery of interventions based on the existing evidence?
3. How is this black MSM population vulnerable, and how should this vulnerability be addressed in research and nonresearch interventions?
4. Do Dr. Albert and Dr. Baines have ethical obligations to other community populations? On what basis is the public health agency justified in advancing interventions that target only a subgroup of the community?
5. How should research studies on Internet-based interventions be conducted to ensure scientific validity, given the difficulties of knowing, for example, whether the participant meets the study's inclusion criteria? Which measures should be taken to protect the privacy and confidentiality of participants?
6. How should you decide what level and type of evidence you need to back a public health educational intervention? Should public health professionals always use science to validate educational interventions?

References

Bull, S. 2011. *Technology-based health promotion.* Thousand Oaks: Sage Publications.

Bull, S.S., S. Phibbs, S. Watson, and M. McFarlane. 2007. What do young adults expect when they go online? Lessons for development of an STD/HIV and pregnancy prevention website. *Journal of Medical Systems* 31(2): 149–158.

Bull, S., K. Pratte, N. Whitesell, C. Rietmeijer, and M. McFarlane. 2009. Effects of an Internet based intervention for HIV prevention: The Youthnet trials. *AIDS and Behavior* 13(3): 474–487. doi:10.1007/s10461-008-9487-9.

Centers for Disease Control and Prevention. 2015. *HIV Among African Americans.* http://www.cdc.gov/HIV/risk/racialethnic/aa/index.html. Accessed 2 June 2015.

Chiasson, M.A., F.S. Shaw, M. Humberstone, S. Hirshfield, and D. Hartel. 2009. Increased HIV disclosure three months after an online video intervention for men who have sex with men (MSM). *AIDS Care* 21(9): 1081–1089. doi:10.1080/09540120902730013.

Hightow-Weidman, L.B., B. Fowler, J. Kibe, et al. 2011. HealthMpowerment.org: Development of a theory-based HIV/STI website for young black MSM. *AIDS Education and Prevention* 23(1): 1–12. doi:10.1521/aeap.2011.23.1.1.

Loue, S., and E.C. Pike. 2010. *Case studies in ethics and HIV research.* New York: Springer.

Moskowitz, D.A., D. Melton, and J. Owczarzak. 2009. PowerON: The use of instant message counseling and the Internet to facilitate HIV/STD education and prevention. *Patient Education and Counseling* 77(1): 20–26. doi:10.1016/j.pec.2009.01.002.

Mustanski, B., T. Lyons, and S.C. Garcia. 2011. Internet use and sexual health of young men who have sex with men: A mixed-methods study. *Archives of Sexual Behavior* 40(2): 289–300. doi:10.1007/s10508-009-9596-1.

Office of National AIDS Policy. 2012. *National HIV/AIDS strategy: Update of 2011–2012 federal efforts to implement the national HIV/AIDS strategy*. http://www.aids.gov/federal-resources/national-hiv-aids-strategy/implementation-update-2012.pdf. Accessed 2 June 2015.

Rhodes, S.D., K.C. Hergenrather, J. Duncan, et al. 2010. A pilot intervention utilizing Internet chat rooms to prevent HIV risk behaviors among men who have sex with men. *Public Health Reports* 125(suppl 1): 29–37.

Rietmeijer, C.A., and M. McFarlane. 2009. Web 2.0 and beyond: Risks for sexually transmitted infections and opportunities for prevention. *Current Opinion in Infectious Diseases* 22(1): 67–71. doi:10.1097/QCO.0b013e328320a871.

Washington, T.A., and C. Thomas. 2010. Exploring the use of Web-based HIV prevention for injection-drug-using black men who have sex with both men and women: A feasibility study. *Journal of Gay & Lesbian Social Services* 22(4): 432–445. doi:10.1080/10538720.2010.491747.

Index

A
ACA. *See* Patient Protection and Affordable Care Act (ACA)
Acceptable risk, 180–183
Access to care, 95, 99–100
Accountability, 15, 245–247, 249, 265
Accountability for reasonableness, 28
A1C Registry, 39, 50–54
Adolescent mental health, 307
Adverse events, 41, 264, 265
Advertising, 53, 148, 154–156, 159
Advocacy, 185, 267, 269, 297, 306, 308
Africa, 121, 148, 182, 310–313
African-Americans, 45, 165, 221
Aggregate population health, 65. *See also* Population health
AIDS, 314
AIDS exceptionalism, 257
Alabama, 38, 44–50, 53, 54
Allocation, 62–70, 72, 73, 101, 227, 252, 260–262, 276, 315
AMR. *See* Antimicrobial resistance (AMR)
Anthrax attack, 126
Anthrax disease, 126. *See also* Inhalation anthrax
Anthrax vaccine, 101, 125–128
Anthrax vaccine adsorbed (AVA), 126
Antibiotic resistance, 130, 193
Antibiotics, 126, 127, 192, 193, 270
Antimicrobial resistance (AMR), 192
Antiretroviral therapy (ART), 109, 258, 260–262
Anti-vaccination movement, 104
Anxiety, 112, 291
Apathy, 232
Aristotle, 14, 15
ART. *See* Antiretroviral therapy (ART)
Assent, 22, 307
Asylum seekers, 209, 232, 233, 235–239
Autism, 104, 106
Autonomy, 13, 16, 17, 19–21, 23–26, 37–39, 53, 95–97, 100, 116, 150, 168, 169, 181, 183, 222, 237, 289, 306, 307
AVA. *See* Anthrax Vaccine Adsorbed (AVA)

B
Bacillus anthracis, 126
Bamako Initiative, 301
Behavioral health. *See* Behavioral health treatment
Behavioral health treatment, 75, 77, 78
Belmont report, 21, 22, 49, 247, 286, 306
Beneficence, 19, 22, 23, 49, 286, 289, 306
Bioethics, 4, 19–23, 28, 37, 47, 48, 81, 170, 203–205, 219, 247, 251, 286
Biomedical research, 20, 25, 180, 247, 252, 286–289, 297, 301, 306
Biotechnology (ethical challenges of), 21, 217
Bioterrorism, 101, 133
Bloodspot screening, 97, 111–114
Bloomberg, M., 53
Breast cancer, 142
Breast-feeding, 212
Breast screening, 143
Buck v. Bell, 43, 44
Built environment, 179
Bulgaria, 150, 172–175
Bulgarian Health Act, 173

D.H. Barrett et al. (eds.), *Public Health Ethics: Cases Spanning the Globe*, Public Health Ethics Analysis 3, DOI 10.1007/978-3-319-23847-0

C

Canadian Immigration and Refugee Protection Act (IRPA), 238
Case-control study, 212
Casuistry, 38, 39
Cataract, 66
CBPR. *See* Community-based participatory research (CBPR)
CDC. *See* Centers for Disease Control and Prevention (CDC)
CEA. *See* Cost-effectiveness analysis (CEA)
CEDAW. *See* Convention on the Elimination of All Forms of Discrimination against Women (CEDAW)
Centers for Disease Control and Prevention (CDC), 4, 31, 38, 39, 44, 45, 50, 109, 120, 121, 126, 137, 158, 164, 222, 245, 257, 260, 267, 288, 293, 314, 315
Central America, 218
CER. *See* Comparative effectiveness research (CER)
Childbirth, 100, 116, 117
Child health, 262, 276
Childhood obesity, 149, 158–161
Childhood vaccination, 97, 105
Children, 10, 29, 31, 40, 41, 43, 48, 73, 75–78, 96, 97, 101, 148, 149, 154–156, 158–161, 164, 168, 169, 174, 179, 196, 200, 210, 213, 218, 231, 232, 238, 275, 277, 280, 289, 292, 302, 305, 310
Chile, 129
Choice
  healthy, 160
  personal, 23, 25, 26, 111–114, 294
  voluntary, 140, 158
Cholera and outbreak, 244, 250, 270, 272
Cholera vaccines, 270
Chronic disease prevention, 137, 138, 140–151, 153–165, 167–170, 172–175
Chronic diseases, 38, 137–140. *See also* Noncommunicable diseases
Cigarette use, 173
CIOMS. *See* Council for International Organizations of Medical Sciences (CIOMS)
Climate change, 179, 184, 250
Clinical ethics, 4, 19–24, 37–39
Clinical guidelines, 72, 88
Clinical trials, 40, 247, 263, 264, 288, 312
Cluster randomized trials, 286, 290
Cold War, 231, 242, 243, 248–250
Coliform bacteria, 197
Collaboration(s), 7, 20, 23, 24, 32, 81, 82, 123, 197, 223, 241–243, 245–249, 263, 276, 281, 282, 286
Collective health, 32, 243–244
Colom, A., 49
Colombia, 66, 72, 73
Colonial rule, 242
Commercial sex work, 46, 47, 121, 123. *See also* Prostitution
Common morality, 13
Common rule, 20, 21
Commonwealth v. Henning Jacobson, 41
Communicable disease, 129
Communitarian values, 71
Community-based participatory research (CBPR), 290, 315
Community health, 4, 6, 10, 26, 39, 210, 227
Community participation, 71, 308
Comparative effectiveness research (CER), 63, 64
Compensation, 102, 133, 218, 264, 265, 273
Compliance, 15, 18, 19, 72, 100, 102, 133, 185, 236, 277, 287, 296. *See also* Noncompliance
Compulsory treatment program, 224
Conditional cash incentive scheme, 116–118
Conflict, 12, 13, 18, 21, 27, 31, 40, 66–68, 73, 85, 93, 96, 146, 168, 169, 174, 181, 182, 199, 242, 250, 259, 268, 277, 294. *See also* War and warfare
Conflicts of interests, 21, 142, 149, 294–296
Consent, 20, 22, 23, 25, 30, 31, 48, 169, 218, 219, 247, 258, 264, 280–283, 286, 289. *See also* Informed consent
Consumers, 71, 146–148, 168, 183
Convention on the Elimination of All Forms of Discrimination against Women (CEDAW), 122
Coordination, 133, 134, 244–245, 249
Corporate social responsibility, 148
Cost(s), 11, 15, 17, 29, 45, 61, 63, 65, 68, 71, 72, 75, 76, 78, 86, 137–139, 144, 151, 155, 158, 160, 161, 165, 168, 169, 174, 180, 236, 238, 247, 261, 263, 276, 277, 291, 292, 311, 312. *See also* Cost benefit; Cost effective; Cost saving
Cost benefit, 17, 182
Cost effective, 66, 67, 86, 88, 142, 144, 196, 261, 265
Cost effectiveness, 11, 15, 64, 66, 68, 72, 141, 150
Cost-effectiveness analysis (CEA), 63
Cost savings, 17
Council for International Organizations of Medical Sciences (CIOMS), 20, 205, 264, 280, 281, 293, 301, 306

Counseling and testing, 257, 258
Crib death, 212
Criminalization of infectious disease transmission, 98
Criminal laws, 120, 121
Culturally appropriate research, 280
Cutler, J.C., 47

D

DALY. *See* Disability-adjusted life year (DALY)
Decision-making process, 11, 67, 69–70, 72, 73, 149, 150, 169
Declaration of Helsinki, 20, 44, 246, 264, 286, 306
De-identified data, 281, 282
Denormalization, 163
Dental caries, 168–170
Deportation, 210, 232, 233
Detention policies, 231
Diabetes, 39, 50–54, 137, 141, 160, 277
Diarrheal diseases, 40, 196, 271
Dilemmas, 13, 72, 99, 100, 121, 156, 159, 182, 274–278, 296, 300–303, 311
Directly observed therapy, short-course (DOTS), 236
Disability-adjusted life years (DALYs), 64, 172, 196
Discrimination, 8, 9, 98, 100, 109, 158, 182, 183, 232, 233, 237, 244, 249, 250, 252, 257, 258, 280
Disease burdens, 8, 10, 68, 137, 150, 172, 196, 242, 252
Disease prevention and control, 5, 96–102, 104–107, 109–114, 116–118, 120–123, 125–135
Disease screening, 95, 97–98, 223
Disincentives, 98, 159
Disparities, black-white, 67
Disparities, health, 8, 67, 252, 314
Distributive and social justice, 163
Distributive justice, 29
Diversity, 14, 105, 106, 177, 180, 183, 294, 306, 308
Division of Venereal Disease, 45
DOTS. *See* Directly observed therapy, short-course (DOTS)
Drinking water quality, 196
Drug resistance, 97, 100, 267
Drug supply, 236, 267, 268
Drug trials, 20, 263–265

Duties, 15–18, 23, 53, 54, 97, 98, 102, 138, 203, 204, 206, 208, 238, 250, 287, 293, 301, 302

E

Economic analysis, 63
Economic development, 137, 157, 177, 182, 184, 189
Economic measures, 275, 277
Economic systems, 177, 184
Ecosystems, 177, 179, 180, 183–185
Effectiveness, 6, 10, 26, 29, 40, 45–47, 53, 63, 64, 67, 144, 163, 168, 222, 237, 252, 290, 292. *See also* Cost effectiveness
Efficiency, 6, 62–66, 68, 72, 169, 222, 310–313
Efficiency frontiers, 63
Emanuel, E., 247
Emergency model, 112
Emergency response, 95, 101–102, 227, 245, 295
Emergency Use Authorization (EUA), 126
Emigration, 230
Empowerment, 99, 252, 297, 306, 308
Enforcement, 18, 41, 70, 98, 133, 192, 244
Environmental hazards, 178
Environmental health, 38, 177–181, 184, 185
Environmental health risks, 177. *See also* Environmental hazards
Equity, 4, 8–9, 22, 23, 27–29, 53, 66, 67, 71, 73, 86, 91, 141, 182, 183, 188, 209, 237, 251
Essential public health services, 6, 44, 54, 285
Ethical conduct of research with human subjects, 286
Ethical reviews, 20, 48, 288, 298, 311
Ethical standards, 13, 15, 241, 253, 279–283
Ethics (difference from morality), 4, 10, 13, 14
Ethics frameworks, 4, 26, 38, 52, 53, 96, 246–253
Ethics review, 20
Ethics review committees, 20, 287, 296, 297
EUA. *See* Emergency Use Authorization (EUA)
European Region, 104, 172, 173
European Union (EU), 173, 230, 281
Evacuation, 102, 132–135, 200

F

Fair chances, 62–65
Fair distribution, 9, 293

Fairness, 28, 44, 47, 64, 65, 70, 91, 133, 181–183. *See also* Fair chances; Fair distribution; Fair outcomes
Fair outcomes, 71
Fluorides, 150, 168. *See also* Water fluoridation
Food and beverage marketing, 153–157. *See also* Food promotion
Food promotion, 154, 156
Food and beverage preferences, 154
Foreign assistance, 275
Framework convention on tobacco control, 148, 244–245
Free choice, 16, 17, 23, 25, 70
Freedom, 22, 30, 41, 42, 76, 101, 102, 107, 138, 139, 182, 248, 250, 263. *See also* Free choice; Free will
Free will, 16

G

Gates Foundation, 261
Gender inequality, 121
Generalizable knowledge, 287, 288
Global collaboration, 241, 247, 248
Global Fund, 243, 246, 261
Global health, 99, 184, 241–253, 257, 269
Globalization, 241–246, 249, 250, 281
Global public health, 32, 109, 151, 184, 192, 199–201, 241–253, 256–265, 267–273, 275–278, 280–283
Goodin, R.E., 204, 205, 207–210
Government(s), 7, 9, 10, 25, 32, 40, 43–47, 49, 50, 52, 53, 76, 78, 81, 140, 144–148, 150, 154, 155, 158–160, 169, 170, 174, 178, 184, 187–189, 199, 203, 214, 218, 219, 241–245, 247–250, 253, 263, 264, 267–269, 271, 273, 275, 294, 303
Greece, 150, 167–170
Guatemala STD studies, 38, 44–50
Guideline(s), 5, 13, 18, 20, 44, 48, 88, 142, 192, 193, 196, 197, 204, 205, 214, 215, 244, 247, 264, 268, 280, 282, 286, 289, 293, 296, 306, 315
Guiding Principles on Business and Human Rights, 250

H

Haiti, 270–273
Harm principle, 25, 26, 159
Harms, 39, 43, 47, 48, 53, 143–145, 148, 156, 159–161, 168, 177, 182, 183, 201, 204, 206, 207, 209, 210, 244, 247, 250, 275, 277, 280
Health-adjusted life-year measures, 64
Health-based targets, 196
Health care access, 122, 301, 303
Health care associated infections, 192
Health care costs, 138, 158, 160
Health care personnel, 131, 193
Health care staff, 193
Health care worker(s), 130, 193, 226, 227. *See also* Health care personnel; Health care staff
Health communication, 315
Health disparities, 8, 67, 252, 314
Health equity, 4, 8–9, 22, 23, 29, 53, 164, 165, 180, 184, 186–190, 227, 251
Health impact assessment, 189
Health inequities, 8, 9, 22, 251
Health interventions, 7, 10, 17, 23, 24, 27, 39, 43, 50, 53, 63, 66, 163–165, 170, 227, 252, 301, 315
Health maximization, 65, 67, 68
Health outcomes, 9, 63, 64, 66, 72, 116, 150, 154, 163, 181, 196, 227, 251, 252, 282, 307
Health priorities and resource allocation, 61, 63–73, 75–78, 80–82, 84, 85, 87–92
Health promotion, 9, 66, 71, 73, 137, 138, 140–151, 153–165, 167–170, 172–175, 177, 214, 297
Health promotion incentives, 95, 100–101
Health reform, 71
Health risk assessments, 141
Health status indicators, 276
Helmet rules, 200
Hepatitis, 221, 223
HIV/AIDS, 20, 64, 121, 196, 243, 244, 249, 252, 257, 258, 260–262, 271, 315, 316
  among African-American men, 315
  education, 314–317
Hobbes, T., 248
Human dignity, 248
Human immunodeficiency virus (HIV), 31, 49, 98, 99, 109, 120–122, 188, 221, 223, 236, 237, 244–246, 252, 256–261, 291, 314–316
  criminalization, 98, 120–124
  infections, 109, 121, 122, 221, 260, 261, 315
  prevention, 109, 122, 256–258, 314
  surveillance, 122
  testing, 97, 98, 109, 121–123, 257–259, 314, 316
  testing policy, 256–259
  transmission, 98, 99, 108–110, 121, 223
Human research regulations, 280

Human-rights, 9, 29, 99, 101, 121, 122, 181, 231–233, 246, 248–251, 257, 258, 268, 275. *See also* Human rights frameworks; Human rights theory
Human rights abuses, 232
Human rights frameworks, 246, 249, 250
Human rights theory, 248
Hurst, S.A., 204, 208, 301

I

ICER. *See* Incremental cost-effectiveness ratio (ICER)
Immigration, 30, 97, 209, 231, 233, 237
Incarceration, 220–224, 292
Incidental and secondary findings, 293
Inclusion, 68, 262, 269, 293, 306, 308
Incremental cost-effectiveness ratio (ICER), 64
India, 100, 116–118, 244, 250, 263, 264, 280
Indian Council of Medical Research, 264
Individual behavior, 138, 140, 164, 180
Individualism, 22, 24, 42, 43, 49, 54
Individual liberty, 27, 31, 42, 43, 50, 96, 181
Individual rights, 26, 37, 43, 101, 180–183
Inequalities, 67, 116, 163, 164, 169, 183
Infant mortality, 67, 252, 264, 271, 276
Infants, 109, 112, 212–214, 280
Infection (active and latent), 236, 237
Infectious diseases, 30, 38, 39, 41, 45, 50, 96, 98, 99, 177, 179, 180, 188, 196, 199, 222, 223, 236, 241, 257, 273, 282, 310
Influenza, 226, 228
Information, 4, 29, 31, 32, 37, 53, 102, 105, 112–114, 127, 138, 139, 141, 142, 148, 156, 159, 185, 196, 245, 259, 281, 282, 286, 288–290, 293, 294, 303, 311
Informed choices, 112, 160
Informed consent, 20–23, 46–49, 95, 97, 98, 101, 120, 126, 127, 219, 247, 251, 252, 257, 264, 265, 279–283, 289, 290, 293, 305–308. *See also* Consent
Informed consent (in STD experiments), 47, 49
Inhalation anthrax, 126
Injection drug use, 220–224
Injustice, 8, 210, 214, 231
Inmates, 209, 221
Institutional review board (establishment of), 48
Institutional review boards (IRBs), 20, 49, 244, 281, 282, 311
Interdependence, 7, 24, 25, 27, 206, 298
International aid workers, 199, 244
International Bioethics Committee of UNESCO [IBC], 205
International collaboration, 8, 241–253, 257–265, 267–273, 275–278, 280–283. *See also* Global collaboration
International Conference on Harmonisation of Good Clinical Practice (ICH-GCP), 264
International Covenant on Civil and Political Rights (ICCPR), 248, 250
International Covenant on Economic, Social and Cultural Rights (ICESCR), 145, 248, 249
International Declaration on Human Genetic Data, 251
International Ethical Guidelines for Biomedical Research Involving Human Subjects (CIOMS), 20, 286, 288, 301
International Ethical Guidelines for Epidemiological Studies, 286
International Monetary Fund (IMF), 242
Internet-delivered interventions, 315, 316
Intersectoral, 7, 24, 155, 251
Intervention ladder, 146, 147
Investigational new drug (IND), 126
In-vitro fertilization (IVF), 218
IOM. *See* U.S. Institute of Medicine (IOM)
Iraq, 250, 276
IRPA. *See* Canadian Immigration and Refugee Protection Act (IRPA)
IVF. *See* In-vitro fertilization (IVF)

J

Jacobson, H., 38, 41–44, 50, 53, 54
Jacobson v Massachusetts, 38–44
Janani Suraksha Yojana (JSY), 116–118
Jenner, E., 40
Jew Ho *v*. Williamson, 43
Justice, 7, 8, 13, 20, 22, 23, 29, 44, 47, 49, 53, 86, 164, 165, 169, 181, 215, 222, 248, 286, 293. *See also* Injustice

K

Kant, I., 15, 16
Knowles, John H., 138, 139

L

Lang and Rayner models for public health
- biomedical model, 178
- ecological model, 178
- sanitary-environmental model, 178
- social-behavioral model, 178
- techno-economic model, 178

Latin America, 71, 116, 168, 195

Law, 4, 6, 10, 12, 16–18, 23, 28, 31, 38, 41–43, 76, 77, 87, 88, 146, 148, 150, 174, 180, 217, 218, 231, 237, 242, 249, 250
Least infringement, 26, 29, 53
Lebanon, 305–308
Lewis, David, 113, 206
Liberty, 17, 22, 25, 26, 28, 41, 43, 54, 96, 101, 133, 145, 182
Lifestyles, 50, 73, 138–140, 159, 163–165, 179
LMICs. *See* Low- and middle-income countries (LMICs)
Locke, J., 248
Low- and middle-income countries (LMICs), 137, 150, 168, 199, 242–245, 247, 249, 250, 252, 253, 256, 310

M
Maastricht Treaty, 231
Managed competition, 71
Mandatory notification, 129
Mandatory treatment, 95–97, 100
Mandatory vaccination, 40, 43, 95–97, 102–107. *See also* Childhood vaccination
Māori, bed-sharing, 213, 214
Māori population, 212
Marginalized populations, 133, 204–215, 217–219, 221–224, 226–233, 236–239, 287
Market(s) (and regulations), 146
Massachusetts, Board of Health, 41
Mass evacuation, 102, 132–135. *See also* Evacuation
Maternal-child health, 67
Maternal mortality, 116, 217, 276
Maximizing strategy, 65. *See also* Health maximization
MDGs. *See* Millennium Development Goals (MDGs)
Measles, 96, 102–107, 236
Media campaigns, 149, 158–161
Medicaid, 51, 68, 160
Medical tourism, 216–219
Medication(s), 30, 100, 130, 140, 244, 252, 253, 261, 262, 265–269. *See also* Medicines
Medicines, 21, 22, 25, 37, 61, 127, 236, 265, 271, 277
Mental health, 68, 131, 158, 231, 249, 252, 297, 307. *See also* Mental illness
Mental illness, 68, 73, 75, 76, 178, 224, 230, 291, 292
Men who have sex with men (MSM), 262, 297, 314–317
Methicillin-resistant *Staphylococcus aureus* (MRSA), 181, 182, 191–194
Middle East and North Africa (MENA) region, 275. *See also* Middle East
Migration, 185, 230–232
Migration management (MM), 231
Millennium development goals (MDGs), 184, 195, 243, 249, 252
Mill, J.S., 15, 25
Minimal/least infringement principle, 26, 53
Minimal risk, 290
Mining, 177, 180, 184, 186–190
Mining health and social impacts, 139
Modifiable risk factors, 212, 213
Mongolia, 184–190
Morality, 10, 13, 14. *See also* Common morality
Moral marker of vulnerability, 209
Mother-to-child HIV transmission (MTCT), 108–110
Motorcycles, 181, 182, 199, 200
Motor vehicles, 199. *See also* Motorcycles
MRSA. *See* Methicillin-resistant *Staphylococcus aureus* (MRSA)
MSM. *See* Men who have sex with men (MSM)
Multidrug-resistant TB (MDR-TB), 29, 130, 236, 268
Multinational, 157, 247, 264, 265, 281, 312
Multinational research, 279–283
Multiple sclerosis (MS), 66, 228

N
Nanny state, 53, 144
National Bioethics Advisory Commission (NBAC), 247, 291
National Commission for the Protection of Human Subjects of Biomedical and Behavioral Research (National Commission), 21, 48, 49, 286, 306
National Institute of Clinical and Health Excellence (NICE), 65
NBAC. *See* National Bioethics Advisory Commission (NBAC)
Needle sharing, 223
Negative right of populations, 277
Neoliberal concerns, 73. *See also* Neoliberal values

Neoliberal values, 71
Net benefits, 17, 22, 182
Netherlands, 113, 192, 212
Newborn bloodspot screening (NBS), 97, 111–114. *See also* Bloodspots screening; Residual bloodspots
Newborns, 30, 31, 219
New York City Department of Health and Mental Hygiene (NYC DOHMH), 51
New Zealand, 213
New Zealand Cot Death Study (NZCDS), 211–215
NICE. *See* National Institute of Clinical and Health Excellence (NICE)
Nonbiomedical research, 306
Noncommunicable diseases, 39, 50, 52, 54, 68, 137, 154, 172
Noncompliance, 18, 100, 131, 133
Nongovernmental organizations (NGOs), 32, 181, 197, 199, 245, 267, 269, 271, 305, 306
Nonmaleficence, 19, 22, 23
Nonmodifiable risk factors, 212
Non-paternity, 112
Nonprofit organizations, 199, 200
Norms, 19, 25–29, 31, 32, 38, 148, 160, 210, 250, 251, 262, 282, 315
Nuffield Council on Bioethics, 146, 159, 168, 169, 280, 281
Nuremberg Code, 20, 44, 286, 305

O

Obesity, 26, 68, 82, 140, 143, 149, 150, 154, 158–165. *See also* Childhood obesity; Obesity costs; Obesity prevention
Obesity costs, 159
Obesity prevention, 149, 157, 159–161
Obligations, 8, 11, 15–18, 21, 22, 26, 32, 38, 52, 62, 63, 98, 123, 133, 138, 148, 170, 208, 217, 244, 246, 247, 250, 251, 259, 291, 294, 296, 301, 302
Occupational health and safety, 177, 180, 181
OECD. *See* Organisation for Economic Co-operation and Development (OECD)
Office the United Nations High Commissioner for Human Rights (OHCHR), 249
Opt out/opt in, 30, 52, 53, 112, 113, 294
Oral diseases, 150, 168, 169
Oral health care, 169
Oral health policies, 168
Organisation for Economic Cooperation and Development (OECD), 158, 159, 231
Overweight, 137, 140, 158, 161

P

PAHO. *See* Pan American Health Organization (PAHO)
Palestine, 305
Palestinian, 307
Palestinian refugee camp, 297, 305–308
Panama, 217, 218
Pan American Health Organization (PAHO), 104, 129, 130, 241
Pandemic(s), 20, 27, 28, 67, 68, 226, 227, 314
Pandemic influenza, 62, 101, 245
Pandemic planning, 226–229
Parental consent, 30, 31, 114, 307, 308
Parents, 4, 10, 15, 30, 31, 76, 77, 140, 149, 156, 157, 159–161, 210, 212–214, 232, 289, 305, 307
Parity between mental and physical health coverage, 76
Parran, T., 47
Participant, 293
Participation, 5, 7, 29, 44, 46, 49, 62, 71, 121, 170, 184, 185, 237, 245, 247, 264, 268, 281, 290–293, 306
Paternalism, 21, 25, 95, 96, 150, 159, 168, 169, 183, 208
Paternalistic, 21, 26, 100, 146, 182, 183, 289
Paternity, 112. *See also* Non-paternity
Patient Protection and Affordable Care Act (ACA), 63, 68, 76, 77
Patriarchal societies, 306
PAWS. *See* Pervasive arousal withdrawal syndrome (PAWS)
PCSBI. *See* Presidential Commission for the Study of Bioethical Issues (PCSBI)
Peace Corps, 181, 199, 200
Penalties, 72, 98, 122, 140, 141, 275
PEPFAR (The United States President's Emergency Plan for AIDS Relief), 261
Personal autonomy, 21, 22, 25–26, 47, 174
Personal responsibility, 138, 139, 141, 145, 150, 163–165. *See also* Individual behavior
Personal safety, 182, 199–201
Pervasive arousal withdrawal syndrome (PAWS), 232
Pharmaceutical companies, 211, 217, 250, 263–265, 312
PHS, 6, 21, 38, 44–50, 53, 54, 65, 112, 275, 280, 285

Points of dispensing (PODs), 127
Policy, 10, 12, 13, 15, 21, 30, 39, 43, 48, 49, 51, 53, 54, 62–64, 66–68, 78, 84, 85, 90, 91, 138–141, 144, 146, 148, 149, 151, 154–157, 159, 162, 167–170, 172, 177, 180, 182–184, 188, 191–194, 200, 242–246, 249–252, 257–260, 263, 267, 270, 273, 275, 281, 293, 302, 311
Policy interventions, 139, 155
Political, 8, 10, 11, 18, 19, 22, 24–27, 29, 31, 32, 37–39, 42, 44, 54, 68, 76, 78, 81, 138, 143, 146, 148, 150, 160, 169, 170, 178, 180, 181, 185, 188, 230, 236, 242, 246, 248, 250, 252, 267, 268, 271, 275, 277, 278, 286, 287, 296, 297, 305, 307
Population, 4–10, 23, 26, 31, 37–39, 44, 47, 49–54, 62, 65–69, 73, 80, 82, 85, 89, 141, 143, 144, 150, 156, 163, 164, 168, 173, 178, 180–183, 187, 188, 195, 241–243, 245, 247, 249–252, 260, 261, 263, 264, 271–273, 277, 278, 282, 286–288, 292
  benefits, 23, 180–183, 298
  health, 6, 27, 50, 61, 62, 66–69, 96, 137, 138, 148, 156, 243, 244, 249, 251
  health interventions, 38
Population health, 6, 27, 50, 61, 62, 66–69, 96, 137, 138, 148, 156, 243, 244, 249, 251
Poverty-reduction, 116
Power, 25, 26, 41, 43–45, 54, 148, 178, 180, 181, 183, 275, 276
  perceived power, 306, 308
  political power, 305
  power dynamics, 297, 306, 307
Perilous path to peace, 274–278
Practical ethics, 3, 19
Precedents, 9, 29, 50, 54, 259
Pre-exposure prophylaxis programs (PrEP), 260
Pregnancy, 19, 109, 116, 212, 213, 216–219
PrEP, 260–262
Presidential Commission for the Study of Bioethical Issues (PCSBI), 45–47, 126, 293
Presumptive norm, 25, 26, 28, 29, 31
Presumptive values, 25–27, 31
Prevention, 5, 7, 38, 39, 45, 50, 71, 73, 78, 80, 81, 84, 87, 138, 142, 144, 145, 147, 149, 154, 158–161, 165, 168–170, 192, 200, 212, 213, 215, 222, 237, 251, 272, 314–317
Prevention *vs*. treatment, 257
Primary prevention, 38, 141, 143
Principles, 4, 7, 10, 11, 13–24, 26, 27, 32, 37, 38, 42, 43, 49, 53, 54, 65, 68, 78, 80, 81, 86, 138, 141, 151, 168, 242–244, 246–248, 251, 258, 259, 285, 286, 288, 293, 306, 308
Principles of Biomedical Ethics, 286
Principles of the Ethical Practice of Public Health, 285
Principlism, 20–23
Prioritizes, 4, 7, 12, 18, 21, 37, 73, 169, 296, 307, 311
Priority setting, 62–73, 227, 228
Priority setting in health care, 87–89. *See also* Health priorities and resource allocation
Prisoners, 46, 47, 221–223
Privacy, 29, 30, 39, 52–54, 97–99, 113, 114, 291, 297
Procedural justice, 29, 169
PROCET. *See* Program for Control a nd Eradication of Tuberculosis (PROCET)
Profession(al), 13, 15, 19, 21, 22, 24, 27, 32, 38, 47, 50, 54, 72, 81, 141, 143, 144, 149, 157, 169, 180, 182, 185, 189, 192, 194, 209, 219, 228, 249, 269, 282, 288, 289, 314, 315
Program for Control and Eradication of Tuberculosis (PROCET), 129
Proportionality, 29, 96
Prostitution, 98, 120, 121, 123
Public health (definition of), 5, 37
Public health emergencies, 106, 245, 287, 295, 296
Public Health leadership Society, 7, 15, 285
Public health policies, 23, 53, 69, 95, 97, 98, 100, 101, 113, 178, 250
Public health research, 38, 44–46, 48, 49, 177, 178, 286–297, 301–303, 305–308, 310–316
Public health research *vs* public health practice, 38
Public health service model, 112
Public health services, 23, 65, 275
Public health surveillance, 39, 40, 51, 183, 288
Public hospitals, 71–73
Public-private partnership(s), 68

Q

QALY. *See* Quality-adjusted life year (QALY)
Quality-adjusted life year (QALY), 17, 64–66
Quality assurance, 112

R
Racism, 46, 49
Randomized controlled trials, 141, 142, 286
Refugees, 209, 231, 237, 305–307
Regulations, 6, 18, 20, 21, 23, 28, 38, 40, 42, 43, 49, 66, 70, 113, 121, 129, 146, 148, 155, 173, 179, 183, 185, 188, 217, 218, 236, 238, 244, 252, 263–265, 280, 281, 286, 287, 289
Reproductive technology, 217
Research, 5, 7, 12, 18, 20–22, 25, 38–40, 44, 45, 47–49, 51, 53, 54, 72, 88, 141, 142, 150, 154, 205, 222, 223, 241, 244, 246, 247, 250–252, 262–265, 268, 269, 279–283, 288, 289, 292–295, 311, 315. *See also* Research funding
Researchers' obligations and responsibilities, 301
Research ethics, 4, 18–23, 37–39, 47, 264, 281
Research ethics committees (RECs), 289, 310–313
Research funding, 312
Research oversight, 287, 297
Residual bloodspots, 114
Resource allocation, 227, 276, 297
Resource allocation decisions, 61–63, 70
Resource allocation (in public health versus medicine), 61, 63–68, 70–73, 75–78, 80–82, 84, 85, 87–92
Resource shortages, 227
Respect, 7, 9, 12, 13, 16, 19, 22–25, 29, 30, 48, 181, 250, 259, 262, 282
Respect for persons, 19, 22–24, 48, 49, 286, 293, 297
Returning research results, 293, 294
Revisability condition, 69
Right to health, 4, 8, 16, 99, 100, 122, 138, 145, 249, 250
Risk(s), 8, 11, 12, 17, 20, 22, 28, 30, 31, 47–52, 54, 61, 67, 72, 78, 137, 138, 140–143, 146, 148, 150, 155, 158, 160, 163, 165, 169, 170, 172, 173, 178, 181, 252, 253, 260–262, 264, 265, 267, 269, 273, 280, 292, 293, 315
  benefit analysis, 291, 292
  management, 180, 183, 196
  reduction, 180
Road safety, 199
Rockefeller Foundation, 241
Roma people, 232
Rousseau, J.-J., 248
Rule-based guidelines, 298
Ryan White Care Act, 120

S
Safe deliveries, 116
Safe drinking water, 181, 195
Safety, 5, 6, 11, 12, 21, 41–43, 221
Safe water, 182, 195–198. *See also* Safe drinking water; Drinking water quality
Sanctions, 133, 244, 250, 274–278
Sanitation, 5, 39, 45, 50, 144, 195, 196, 200, 236, 270–273, 275
Scandinavia, 192
Schools, 37, 43, 82, 146, 155, 159, 160, 168, 174, 218, 232, 233, 262, 277
Screening, 29–31, 76, 141, 142, 164, 257
Secondary prevention, 39, 50, 141–143
Secondhand smoke, 161, 173
Self-determination, 29, 52, 242
Self-regulation models, 149
Self-regulatory approaches, 155
Self-regulatory codes, 155. *See also* Self-regulatory approaches
Sequential Organ Failure Assessment (SOFA) scores, 91
Serodiscordant couples, 260–262
Sexually transmitted infections (STI), 121, 122
SIDS. *See* Sudden Infant Death Syndrome (SIDS)
Siracusa principles, 237
Smoke free legislation, 173
Smoking, 138–141, 148, 150, 151, 160, 161, 163, 172–175, 210, 212, 213, 245
  bans, 160, 174
  in public places, 150, 172–175
Smoking-related causes of death, 172
Social-compact theory, 42
Social conditions, 9, 164, 248, 252
Social consensus, 11, 23, 27
Social contract theory, 24, 248. *See also* Social-compact theory
Social determinants, 8, 158–159, 165, 252
Social determinants of health (SDH), 8–9, 123, 179, 227, 246, 251–253
Social equity, 185
Social gradient, 163
Social justice, 4, 8–9, 21–23, 53, 180, 184, 227, 237, 251, 257, 298, 306
Social norms, 19, 27, 149, 160
Social welfare, 117
Socioeconomic conditions, 163
Socioeconomic disparities, 133
Solidarity, 7, 8, 24, 26–29, 31, 71, 169, 170, 206, 237, 267
Spain, 68, 96, 102, 105, 106, 168
Sponsorship, 156, 295

Stakeholder(s), 4, 10–13, 19, 26, 28–32, 37, 62, 67, 69, 73, 78, 82, 149, 150, 155, 169, 170, 175, 233, 244–246, 249, 265, 308, 313
Standards, 4, 6, 9–13, 15, 18, 27, 30, 42, 43, 51, 65, 66, 68, 76, 86, 88, 139, 148, 154, 159, 172, 241, 242, 246, 248, 250, 253, 257, 258, 279–283
Standards of care, 98
STD Prevention, 120–124
Stigma, 68, 75. *See also* Stigmatization and obesity stigma
Stigmatization and obesity stigma, 98, 99, 162–165, 257
Stock-outs, 244, 253, 266–269
Storage, 111–114, 196, 217, 267
Structural intervention, 120
Structural reform, 72
Students, 105, 182, 193, 296, 301, 303, 307
Sub-Saharan Africa, 110, 121, 185, 195, 197, 200, 236, 260–262, 312
Substance abuse, 123, 138, 221–223, 291
Sudden infant death syndrome (SIDS), 209, 211–215
Surrogacy and egg donor, 219
Surrogate pregnancy, 218. *See also* Surrogacy and egg donor
Surveillance, 5, 7, 95, 97–98, 106, 121, 227, 237, 245, 293
Sweden, 41, 230–233
Syphilis, 21, 31, 44–49, 237, 280
Syria, 250, 276–277

T

TB incidence and prevalence, 29, 97, 129, 130, 310
TB medication, 244, 253, 267–269
TB treatment, 96, 130, 131, 237, 268, 311
Terrorism, 101, 126, 275. *See also* Bioterrorism
Title 45, Part 46, of the Code of Federal Regulations, 286
Tobacco, 137, 139, 140, 146–148, 160, 172, 173
Trades, 65, 139, 146, 169, 187, 243, 275, 301
Transparency, 15, 28, 29, 62, 90, 168, 170, 237, 294
Transparent, 91. *See also* Transparency
Transportation safety, 182, 200, 201
Trauma, 178, 200, 233, 290
Treatment, 23, 29, 30, 45–49, 63, 64, 66, 68, 75–77, 81, 87, 88, 90, 92, 137, 141, 142, 168, 169, 244, 256–258, 265, 267–270
Triage, 67, 68, 278
Trust, 7, 21, 32, 40, 47, 49, 98, 175, 183, 296, 297, 302, 306, 308, 315
Truvada, 260–262
Tuberculosis (TB), 29, 40, 51, 81, 96, 129–131, 221, 310. *See also* TB incidence and prevalence; TB medication; TB treatment
  screening, 29, 235–239
  testing, 235–239
  treatment, 235–239
Tuskegee syphilis study, 46, 49. *See also* U.S. Public Health Service Syphilis Study at Tuskegee

U

U.K. Food Standards Agency, 154
U.N. Human Development Index, 271
U.N. Human Rights Council (HRC), 249, 250
Unintentional injury, 199
United Kingdom, 65, 147, 168
United Nations (U.N.), 81, 145, 230, 231, 242, 261, 271, 276–278
United Nations Educational, Scientific and Cultural Organization (UNESCO), 247
United Nations Relief and Works Agency (UNRWA), 305
United States, 20, 22, 30, 39–41, 44, 45, 47–51, 54, 61, 63, 67, 75, 84, 85, 137, 147, 148, 150, 158, 160, 163, 164, 168, 218, 221, 222, 242, 245, 261, 267, 275, 280, 315
Universal access, 23, 122, 301
Universal Declaration on Bioethics and Human Rights, 251
Universal Declaration on the Human Genome and Human Rights, 251
Unprotected water sources, 195
UNRWA. *See* United Nations Relief and Works Agency (UNRWA)
U.N. Universal Declaration of Human Rights (UDHR), 99, 230, 248, 286
U.N. Vienna Declaration and Programme of Action, 249
U.S. Advisory Committee on Immunization Practices, 126
U.S. Department of Health and Human Services, 18, 20, 21, 48, 49, 140, 281, 286, 288, 290

U.S. Department of Homeland Security (DHS), 126
Use of incentives for research, 263
User fees, 301, 302
U.S. Food and Drug Administration (FDA), 126, 260
U.S. Institute of Medicine (IOM), 6, 154, 294
U.S. Public Health Service, 21, 38, 44–50, 280
U.S. Public Health Service Syphilis Study at Tuskegee, 21, 281
Utilitarianism, 15, 17, 91, 181. *See also* Utility
Utility, 17, 26, 27, 29, 93, 123, 141, 143, 181, 247, 282

V
Vaccination, 6, 40–42, 73, 92, 277
Vaccine(s), 20, 39–41, 80, 270, 275, 277
Vaccine coverage, 104–106, 127
Values, 4, 7–13, 18, 19, 25–27, 31, 32, 37, 38, 43, 53, 54, 63, 64, 71, 73, 78, 82, 88, 91, 93, 141, 144, 150, 168, 170, 175, 246, 265, 278
Vertical transmission, 109
Vibrio cholera, 269, 272 (*see also* Cholera and outbreak)
Victim blaming, 140
Voluntary, 18, 30, 40, 140, 142, 148, 155, 159, 252, 257, 258, 281
Voluntary counseling and testing and HIV, 122
Voluntary *vs*. mandatory evacuation, 102
Vulnerability (definition of), 204, 209
Vulnerability, 252
Vulnerable, 180, 181, 187, 188, 199. *See also* Vulnerability
  groups, 48
  and marginalized groups, 162–165
  and marginalized populations, 133
  populations, 44, 47, 49, 134, 149, 180, 228, 278, 292, 293, 295, 297, 301, 314–317

W
Waivers of informed consent, 290
War and warfare, 126, 277
Water contamination, 196
Water fluoridation, 150, 167–170
Waterhouse, B., 40
Water quality testing, 197
Water Safety Plan (WSP), 196
Well construction, 181, 182, 195–198
Western, 3, 22, 222, 231, 243, 257, 258, 271, 276
WHO, 173
WIP. *See* Working Party on Infection Prevention (WIP)
Working Party on Infection Prevention (WIP), 192–194
Workplace hazards, 178
World Bank, 137, 172, 187, 188, 242, 261, 301
World Health Organization (WHO), 5, 49, 75, 80, 84, 90, 91, 137, 154, 158, 168, 173, 196, 199, 242, 263, 267, 269, 271, 275, 276, 280, 281, 286
World Health Organization Framework Convention on Tobacco Control, 173
WSP. *See* Water Safety Plan (WSP)

Y
Youth, 149, 153–157, 297, 307, 308

Z
Zucht v. King, 43

CPSIA information can be obtained
at www.ICGtesting.com
Printed in the USA
LVHW022221070222
710528LV00009B/397

9 783319 795386